W9-CFB-757

"I'm a psychoanalyst and clinical psychologist with no medical training, and I found *Handbook of Clinical Psychopharmacology for Therapists* to be a compelling and stimulating read, as well as a welcome addition to my reference shelf. This text is coherent and user-friendly, and reading it is a surprisingly pleasurable way to expand your knowledge in an area of clinical treatment usually not made this accessible to nonmedical professionals."

—Susan Flynn, PhD

"I recommend the *Handbook of Clinical Psychopharmacology for Therapists* to psychotherapists from various clinical trainings and diverse clinical orientations, as well as to nonpsychiatric physicians and their prescribing assistants. One of the most valuable elements of this text is the authors' reminder to consider when and how medication can be appropriate to treatment, and how the clinician is an essential part of the psycho-medical treatment team.

"If you have only one reference book on your shelf addressing the interface between clinical treatment and psychopharmacology, this should be it."

—Marvin B. Berman, PhD

"*Handbook of Clinical Psychopharmacology for Therapists* is a modern masterpiece written by a multidisciplinary team of distinguished practitioners. It is one of the most clearly written and reader-friendly yet comprehensive books on the subject of psychiatric diagnosis and psychotropic drug therapy. The *Handbook* is packed full of useful tables, figures, and illustrations that amplify the main text or can be used independently for a rapid introduction to the field or for reviewing the fundamentals. Covering both the spectrums of pathophysiology and the neurobiology of drug action, this slim, state-of-the-art-and-science text is truly a handbook worthy of the name and should be an essential resource for mental health professionals and students alike."

—Clifford N. Lazarus, PhD, licensed psychologist and director
of Comprehensive Psychological Services of Princeton,
author of *Don't Believe It for a Minute* and *The 60-Second Shrink*

"*Handbook of Clinical Psychopharmacology for Therapists* is a wonderfully useful and comprehensive book. It should be essential reading for all mental health professionals and for others like myself who have family members suffering from mental illness. Its great virtues are its clarity and its humane and informed sense of the diagnosis, treatment, and care of extraordinarily complicated conditions."

    —Jay Neugeboren, author of *Imagining Robert*

"This book belongs on the desk of every psychiatrist, clinical psychologist, social worker, or anyone who works with clients who are taking psychoactive drugs. Also, anyone teaching or interested in abnormal psychology will find it indispensible. The authors manage, with judicious use of well-designed tables and clear, concise writing, to fill a gap in the current literature. No other book with which I am familiar covers the history of psychiatric medicine as well as both the neurochemistry and clinical use of psychotropics. The authors make excellent use of case histories, which are always to the point. I cannot think of anything that could be added to this text, or any part of it I would want to change."

    —Harry Avis, PhD, professor of psychology at Sierra College and
      author of *Drugs and Life*

HANDBOOK
OF CLINICAL
PSYCHOPHARMACOLOGY
FOR THERAPISTS

SEVENTH EDITION

JOHN D. PRESTON, PSYD, ABPP
JOHN H. O'NEAL, MD
MARY C. TALAGA, RPH, PHD

NEW HARBINGER PUBLICATIONS, INC.

Publisher's Note

Care has been taken to confirm the accuracy of the information presented and to describe generally accepted practices. However, the authors, editors, and publisher are not responsible for errors or omissions or for any consequences from application of the information in this book and make no warranty, express or implied, with respect to the contents of the publication.

The authors, editors, and publisher have exerted every effort to ensure that any drug selection and dosage set forth in this text are in accordance with current recommendations and practice at the time of publication. However, in view of ongoing research, changes in government regulations, and the constant flow of information relating to drug therapy and drug reactions, the reader is urged to check the package insert for each drug for any change in indications and dosage and for added warnings and precautions. This is particularly important when the recommended agent is a new or infrequently employed drug.

Some drugs and medical devices presented in this publication may have Food and Drug Administration (FDA) clearance for limited use in restricted research settings. It is the responsibility of the health care provider to ascertain the FDA status of each drug or device planned for use in their clinical practice.

To the best of our knowledge, recommended doses of medications listed in this book are accurate. However, they are not meant to serve as a guide for prescribing of medications. Physicians, please check the manufacturer's product information sheet and the *Physicians' Desk Reference* for any changes in dosage schedule or contraindications.

Figures 6-A, 6-B, 6-E, 8-D, 8-E, 9-B, and 15-F have been previously published in *Clinical Psychopharmacology Made Ridiculously Simple*, 1994, MedMaster Inc., Miami, and are reproduced here with the permission of the copyright holder.

Handbook of Clinical Psychopharmacology for Therapists, Seventh Edition
Copyright © 2013 by John D. Preston, Psy.D., ABPP, John H. O'Neal, MD, and Mary C. Talaga, R.Ph., Ph.D.
New Harbinger Publications, Inc.
5674 Shattuck Avenue
Oakland, CA 94609
www.newharbinger.com

Cover design by Amy Shoup
Acquired by Melissa Kirk
Text design by Tracy Marie Carlson
Indexed by James Minkin

All rights reserved. Printed in the United States of America.

First edition printed from June 1994 to December 1996; Second edition printed from September 1997 to March 2001; Third edition printed from September 2001 to June 2004; Fourth edition printed from July 2004 to July 2007; Fifth edition printed from January 2008 to July 2009.

Library of Congress Cataloging-in-Publication Data

Preston, John, 1950-
  Handbook of clinical psychopharmacology for therapists / John Preston, PsyD, ABPP, John D. O'Neill, MD, and Mary C. Talaga, RPh, PhD. -- 7th edition.
    pages cm
  Summary: "This seventh edition of The Handbook of Clinical Psychopharmacology for Therapists includes the latest updates on medications for mental health disorders and their side effects along with a new chapter on the effects of withdrawing from medication. This essential guide to psychopharmacology has been adopted as a textbook at universities nationwide and is a must-have resource for every therapist's library"-- Provided by publisher.
  Includes bibliographical references and index.
  ISBN 978-1-60882-664-3 (hardback) -- ISBN 978-1-60882-665-0 (PBK e-book) (print) -- ISBN 978-1-60882-666-7 (ePub) (print) 1. Psychopharmacology--Handbooks, manuals, etc. I. O'Neill, John. II. Talaga, Mary C. III. Title.
  RC483.P737 2013
  616.89'18--dc23
                            2012034630

Seventh Edition

18 17 16

15 14 13 12 11 10 9 8 7

To my sweet granddaughters, River and Aurora.
—J. P.

To my patients, for they have been my best teachers.
—J. O.

To Layla, for the joy you bring into my life.
—M. T.

What is paraded as scientific fact is simply the current belief of some scientists. We are accustomed to regard science as truth with a capital "T." What scientific knowledge is, in fact, is the best available approximation of truth in the judgment of the majority of scientists who work in the particular specialty involved. Truth is not something that we possess; it is a goal toward which we hopefully strive ... the current opinion of the scientific establishment is only the latest and never the last word.

—M. Scott Peck, MD,
author of *The Road Less Traveled*

Contents

Part Three
Medications

Acknowledgments

Many thanks to our publisher, Dr. Matthew McKay, and our editors, Leslie Tilley, Melissa Kirk, and Kayla Sussell, for helping our ideas to take form.

To our families and friends, with deep appreciation, for their patience and encouragement throughout this project.

Finally, heartfelt thanks to our students and our patients. May this book reach many and hopefully contribute to our ongoing struggle to reduce emotional suffering.

Part One

Understanding Psychopharmacology: The Basics

Part one of this book briefly covers the development of psychopharmacology from a historical and sociological perspective and then goes on to provide an overview of neurobiology and pharmacology. The purpose of these chapters is not to provide a comprehensive discussion of the fields of pharmacology or neurophysiology, but is simply to familiarize you with the basic terminology and models of pharmacokinetics.

1

Introduction

This book is intended primarily for mental health professionals and those in graduate training in psychology, social work, psychiatric nursing, and counseling. The professional goal of most readers will be to provide services that aim to reduce emotional pain, to promote psychological growth and healing, and to foster the development of personal autonomy. To these ends, we in the field are trained in various theoretical approaches that attempt to explain the development of maladaptive lifestyles and subjectively painful psychiatric symptoms. These theories serve to give meaning and coherence to what we do in clinical practice and, most importantly, lay a foundation of understanding so that interventions make sense and further the goal of reducing suffering in ways that are effective.

Many schools of thought exist regarding the origins of mental health problems. As has been well documented in the history of psychiatry, as schools of thought evolve, controversy, dogma, and empassioned belief systems emerge. It may be inherent to the development and maturation of science that these emotionally toned belief systems and the resulting debates occur.

From the mid-1960s through the 1970s, polarization occurred within psychiatry between those advocating psychological theories (primarily psychodynamic and behavioral models) and those on the other side of the fence using biological and medical models. The disagreements that emerged were more than differences of opinion or dry debate. Each school attracted followers who had strong emotional investments in their perspective.

For many years this division resulted in the development of barriers between groups of mental health clinicians—and at times in fragmentation in care. Fortunately, during the past decade something has changed. We are beginning to witness a shift in thinking, as increasing numbers of practitioners and training institutes move away from egocentric and dogmatic positions and begin to embrace a more integrated approach with regard to both theories of etiology and methods of treatment.

New discoveries in the neurosciences, refined technical advances in psychotherapy, and a large number of outcome studies in both pharmacotherapy and psychotherapy have made it abundantly clear: People are complex. Mental health problems spring from many sources; and reductionist, unidimensional models are simply inadequate to explain the wide array of mental and emotional problems people experience. Likewise, no single approach to treatment works for all problems. Certain disorders clearly respond better to certain interventions, whereas others require alternative approaches.

In writing this book, although our primary focus is on psychopharmacology, we share a strong respect for what will be termed *integrative approaches* to treatment: recognition of the importance of varied treatments and collaboration among professionals from different disciplines.

We hope that you will find this book helpful as you engage in this most important profession and work toward the goal of reducing emotional pain.

History of Biological Psychiatry

In understanding psychopharmacology, it may be helpful if you are able to place it in a historical context. Let's take a brief look at this history as it unfolded.

In the late eighteen hundreds, psychiatry was clearly rooted in the medical model and the neurology of the day. Psychiatrists believed, almost exclusively, that mental illness could be attributed to some sort of biologic disturbance. The earliest attempts to approach the understanding of mental illness in this era involved two main areas of investigation.

On one front was the development of the first systematic nosologic system by Emil Kraepelin. This pioneering work laid the foundation for all later diagnostic schema (such as the *Diagnostic and Statistical Manual of Mental Disorders*, or *DSM*). And many of Kraepelin's original notions about the classification of major mental illness have stood the test of time. He was a brilliant investigator and the one most responsible for ushering in descriptive clinical psychiatry. However, his endeavors must have been accompanied by a good deal of frustration and impotence, since, despite the development of a systematic approach to diagnosis, Kraepelin and other psychiatrists of his time had few, if any, methods of treatment.

At the same time, the hunt was on for evidence of brain pathology, which was presumed to underlie mental illness. Research was conducted in neuroanatomy labs but yielded few concrete results. For example, the famous French neurologist Jean-Martin Charcot believed that hysterical conversation symptoms were undoubtedly due to some type of central nervous system lesion. He explained the fact that no demonstrable pathology could be isolated on autopsy by saying it simply suggested that somehow the lesion mysteriously disappeared at the time of death. We must bear in mind, however, that in all likelihood, these researchers and clinicians were desperate to find causes and cures and went at it by the means best known to them (biology) and using the scant technology available at the time.

Biological psychiatry got a shot in the arm in the late eighteen hundreds, as two discoveries were made. At the time, probably one half of those housed in asylums suffered from a type of psychotic-organic brain syndrome that ultimately was found to be caused by the *Treponema pallidum* bacteria (a central nervous system infection seen in the late stages of syphilis). It was also eventually discovered that some organic mental syndromes were due to pellagra (a disease associated with niacin and protein deficiency). These were important discoveries, and they fueled enthusiasm in biological psychiatry. It was just a matter of time, it was felt, before other biologic causes would be isolated and medical treatments developed. However, such discoveries did not occur until the middle of the twentieth century. For practical purposes, biological psychiatry came to a halt as it entered the nineteen hundreds.

The disappointments stemming from medical research on mental illness and the failure to develop any effective treatment probably increased the receptivity of psychiatry to divergent approaches. At this same time Sigmund Freud was assembling the basic notions of psychoanalysis. Freud's initial theory was strongly influenced by his own medical and neurological training (for example, his "Project for a Scientific Psychology," 1895), and many of his prevailing ideas continued to have their roots in biology, including drive theory, instincts, and psychosexual development. However, his newly emerging theory and techniques of treatment sparked interest in the use of novel, nonmedical approaches to treatment.

By the 1920s psychological (rather than biological) explanations for the development and treatment of psychopathology had found their place in clinical psychiatry, and by the 1940s psychodynamic thinking had permeated American psychiatry and become the dominant theoretical model. Yet these newly developed approaches proved to be inadequate in the treatment of the more serious forms of mental illness, such as schizophrenia and manic-depressive psychosis. In one of his last manuscripts, Freud himself admitted his disappointment in psychoanalytic methods for treating schizophrenia. He hypothesized that eventually it would be discovered that these grave mental disorders were due to some form of biologic abnormality, and that perhaps drugs would eventually be found to treat these illnesses.

Somatic Therapies

In the days of Kraepelin, pharmaceuticals were used to treat mentally ill patients. Generally, the drugs were prescribed to sedate wildly agitated psychotic patients. For example, Kraepelin listed in one of his textbooks the following group of recommended medications (Spiegel and Aebi 1989):

For Agitation	To Produce Sleep
Opium	Chloral Hydrate
Morphine	Ether
Scopolamine	Alcohol
Hashish	Chloroform
	Bromides

Kraepelin noted, however, that none of these preparations cured mental illness, that they were for short-term use, and that a number of them could lead to problems with addiction. All of these drugs achieved behavioral control by sedating patients; none really affected psychotic symptoms per se, nor did they have any impact on activating patients who were stuporous or clinically depressed.

Other somatic therapies were developed in the first half of the twentieth century, with variable results. Malaria therapy was conceived in 1917, insulin shock in 1927, psychosurgery in 1936, and electroconvulsive treatment (ECT) in 1938. All of these methods, as originally conceived, carried serious risks, and most demonstrated marginal effectiveness. Psychosurgeries were carried out by the thousands in the 1940s, resulting in rather effective behavioral control over agitated psychotic patients but at great human cost. Many, if not most, lobotomized patients were reduced to anergic, passive, and emotionally dead human beings.

Electroconvulsive treatment, conversely, was quite effective in certain groups of patients, such as those with psychotic depressive disorders. However, early methods of administration were fraught with dangerous complications and side effects, and ECT was used on a widespread basis, indiscriminately. Many patients were treated with it inappropriately and did not respond. (As shall be discussed later, in recent years significant advances have been made in ECT, and it now affords a highly effective, safe treatment for selected types of patients.)

Most severely ill patients in the late nineteenth and early twentieth centuries continued to be housed in overcrowded state mental hospitals and were "treated" using tried and true methods of the day: seclusion, restraint, and wet-sheet packs. Although seemingly inhumane procedures were employed, it may be important to consider that the psychiatrists of that era were relatively helpless in the face of very severe mental illnesses and that these approaches (although certainly misused at times) reflected their attempt to reduce the horrendous human suffering seen in thousands of severely ill people.

New Discoveries

In the 1950s, three new discoveries heralded the beginnings of a new interest in biological psychiatry. Interestingly, these three areas of investigation were conducted by separate groups of researchers, each with little knowledge of the work being done by their colleagues (Kety 1975).

Thorazine and other early psychotropic drugs

Immediately after World War II, medical researchers and chemists working for pharmaceutical companies were trying to develop a drug that would reduce the complications associated with shock following major surgery. In early 1951, a compound initially labeled #4560 RP was developed and testing with surgical patients was begun (Spiegel and Aebi 1989). The initial results were encouraging. Given preoperatively, it relaxed patients, somewhat reduced postoperative shock, and proved to be a good antiemetic (preventing postsurgical nausea). The finding that it produced noticeable sedation came as a surprise. In the aftermath of field trials with surgical patients, the pharmaceutical company Laborit decided to try this medication with restless, agitated psychiatric patients to help improve sleep, totally unaware that the drug would prove to have more widespread effects on the psychiatric patients who were tested.

Initial clinical trials first reported in 1952 resulted in marked behavioral changes when given to manic and schizophrenic patients. Not only did it produce a calming effect, but after a period of time it actually appeared to reduce psychotic symptoms, such as delusions and hallucinations. Additional studies were carried out the following year, and by 1954 the drug was approved for use. The new medication was given the generic name chlorpromazine; in the United States it was marketed under the brand name Thorazine. It received immediate acceptance, and by the end of 1954, for the first time ever, there was a marked decrease in the number of patients incarcerated in state mental hospitals: the first major breakthrough in psychopharmacology.

Other psychotropic medications were discovered during the 1950s. The first antidepressant was developed in 1952 (iproniazid, an MAO inhibitor), although clinical studies in humans did not take place until 1956. The first tricyclic antidepressant, imipramine (Tofranil), was developed in 1954 and entered the market in 1957. The first minor tranquilizer, meprobamate, was released in 1955, followed shortly by the safer benzodiazepine, chlordiazepoxide (Librium), in 1958. Finally, lithium carbonate, originally used as a sedative by J. Cade in 1948, began to be used to treat bipolar disorder (formerly called manic-depressive illness) in the early 1960s.

It is interesting to note that most of these psychopharmacological discoveries were accidental; that is, the drug companies were developing medications to treat other medical illnesses and just happened to find that the drugs could affect psychiatric symptoms. Also, these discoveries were made empirically; they were not developed as an outgrowth of a particular theory of neurochemical dysfunction, nor was the mechanism of action at all known. What was evident was that the medications worked and were far superior to any previous treatments for severe mental illness.

The synapse and neurochemical transmission

Although C. S. Sherrington inferred the existence of the synapse (the small space separating individual nerve cells) as early as 1906, the specific details of synaptic transmission were not fully understood for many decades thereafter. Sherrington's ideas involved a sort of telephone switchboard model of the nervous system, and neuronal messages were assumed to be transmitted via electrical stimulation. It was not until the 1950s that neuroscientists realized that communication between nerve cells, although partially electrochemical in nature, is largely due to the release of chemical substances. These chemicals, which transmit messages from one nerve cell to another, are referred to as neurotransmitters; other chemicals that play an indirect role in neurotransmission are called neuromodulators.

With this discovery, it became possible to imagine that certain neurologic dysfunctions might be caused by chemical irregularities, and that therefore it might be possible to develop drugs that could influence or alter neurotransmitter function.

Genetic studies

The third line of investigation involved both genetics and studies of familial patterns of mental illness. The earliest research in this direction was ultimately criticized for numerous methodological flaws. Yet some of the basic findings proved to be fundamentally correct. There is a strong genetic loading for certain mental illnesses, in particular for schizophrenia and bipolar disorder. (In recent times evidence has been obtained revealing genetic loadings for a number of mental disorders, although clearly the strongest evidence exists for bipolar disorder, attention-deficit/hyperactivity disorder, and some types of schizophrenia.)

Controversy

By the early 1960s then, it had been discovered that synaptic activation is chemical in nature; certain illnesses seem to be genetically passed on from generation to generation (and genetic factors are expressed biochemically); and newer drugs could significantly reduce psychiatric symptoms. The triangulation of this data provided rather strong support for a renewed interest in biological psychiatry. There was new hope for the millions of patients suffering from serious mental illness, and psychiatry had begun to step back into "real medicine" again.

However, despite the advances, these new treatments were plagued by a host of side effects—some unpleasant, some actually dangerous. These potent drugs were also often overused or were misused in certain treatment settings. Consequently,

Medications and the Media

Research studies and clinical experience certainly influence prescribing practices. However, in recent years the media has had a profound effect on public opinion and ultimately on clinical practice.

In the late 1980s, negative attention was focused on the drug Ritalin (methylphenidate), a widely prescribed stimulant used in the treatment of attention-deficit/hyperactivity disorder (ADHD). Andrew Brotman, summarizing the work of Safer and Krager (1992), states, "The media attack was led by major national television talk show hosts and in the opinion of the authors, allowed anecdotal and unsubstantiated allegations concerning Ritalin to be aired. There were also over twenty lawsuits initiated throughout the country, most by a lawyer linked to the Church of Scientology" (Brotman 1992, audiotape).

In a study of the effects of this negative media and litigation blitz, conducted in Baltimore County, Maryland, Safer and Krager (1992) found that the use of Ritalin had dropped significantly. From 1981 through 1987, the use of Ritalin had increased fivefold. However, in the two-year period during and just following the negative media attention, there was a 40 percent decrease in prescriptions for Ritalin. And this decrease occurred at a time when research on ADHD and stimulant treatment continued to strongly support the safety and efficacy of such medications. The authors go on to state that 36 percent of children who discontinued Ritalin experienced major academic maladjustment (such as failing grades or being suspended), and an additional 47 percent who

continued

controversy began to arise, both among professionals, and in the lay public and mass media.

Professional dissent

Within professional ranks, debate issued from two fairly discrete theoretical camps: those who were promedication and those who were pro-psychotherapy. Each group amassed impassioned arguments not only in favor of its own point of view, but also against the other school of thought, as set out below.

Promedication (antipsychotherapy)—arguments in favor of medication treatment as the treatment of choice:

- Because of its quantifiable nature—that is, the ability to monitor dosage—medication treatment can be studied much more systematically than psychotherapy.

- Medications act quickly to reduce painful and debilitating symptoms.

- The quicker response seen with medications can help to restore hope and reduce demoralization.

- Treatment with medications can be conducted in a much more systematic and standardized fashion, whereas psychotherapy relies heavily on the individual skill of the psychotherapist.

- Rapid and effective symptom relief can potentially reduce suffering to such an extent that the patient is better able to engage productively in psychotherapy. Likewise, the reductions of drive strength afforded by some psychotropic medications may operate to free up more psychic energy, which could then be channeled into adaptive ego functions.

- Medications can provide help to patients who have limited intellectual capacity, poor ego strength, or both; that is, drugs may be effective with people for whom psychotherapy is inappropriate.

- Psychotherapy is often prolonged and expensive, may be unavailable to many people, and is of unproven effectiveness (this was the case especially in light of the very limited psychotherapy outcome studies available in the 1950s and 1960s). Thus medications are much more cost-effective and more readily available to the general public.

Finally, those strongly wedded to a biochemical model of psychopathology contended that social, behavioral, and psychological approaches simply could not correct the underlying biologic abnormality responsible for major mental illnesses. Recent studies, however, have cast doubt on this hypothesis.

Pro-psychotherapy (antimedication)— arguments in favor of psychotherapy as the treatment of choice:

- Only psychotherapy, not medications, can address the complexity of human psychological functioning. Medications only treat symptoms, whereas psychotherapy focuses on the whole person or psyche.

- Psychotherapy aims toward personal growth and autonomy, whereas drugs are likely to foster dependency, either on the doctor or on the drug itself.

- Drugs can interfere with autonomy and expressions of free will, whereas psychotherapy honors these processes. The prescription of medications may, at least at an unconscious level, communicate the message that the drug will do the work, you don't have to. (Numerous documented instances of overuse of tranquilizing medications to achieve behavioral control provided fodder for this argument.)

- Medications may reduce anxiety and other forms of suffering to such an extent that people will be less motivated to engage in psychotherapy.

- Many drugs have undesirable or dangerous side effects, and some can lead to dependence and abuse.

- Medications ultimately do not solve problems, teach adaptive coping skills, mend broken hearts, or fill empty lives (Menninger 1963).

discontinued encountered mild to moderate academic problems. Concurrently, as Ritalin use (especially new prescriptions) decreased, there was a significant (fourfold) increase in the prescription of tricyclic antidepressants among ADHD children. It is important to note that tricyclics, although often used to treat ADHD, tend to have more troublesome side effects than Ritalin, and have been implicated in six reports of cardiac fatalities. Brotman (1992) concludes, "When there are reports in the media that lead to stigmatization of a certain drug ... there tends to be a move to other medications which have less notoriety, even if they may, in fact, be more problematic."

More recently, following wide acclaim as a new "breakthrough drug for depression" (Cowley et al. 1990), Prozac (fluoxetine) came under attack by consumer groups and, again, the Church of Scientology. The negative attention was sparked by a single article (Teicher, Glod, and Cole 1990) documenting the emergence or reemergence of suicidal ideas in six patients treated with Prozac. The six patients had been diagnosed as suffering from severe depressive disorders, and in no case were there actual suicide attempts following the onset of treatment with Prozac. But suddenly Prozac was thrust into a very unfavorable light and was the next drug in line to find itself the topic of television talk shows.

Subsequent studies have failed to find any evidence that Prozac is more likely to be associated with suicidal feelings than any other antidepressant (Fava and Rosenbaum 1991; Beasley and Dornseif 1991). In fact, in one study the incidence of suicidal

continued

ideations was greater in patients treated by placebo or imipramine (a tricyclic antidepressant) than by Prozac (Beasley and Dornseif 1991).

The Church of Scientology attempted to convince the Federal Drug Administration (FDA) to pull Prozac from the market. However, the FDA ruled against taking such action because there was no scientific evidence to support the claims made by the Church of Scientology (Burton 1991).

All medications produce some side effects. Reports of adverse effects, even if very infrequent, must be taken seriously and investigated systematically. There is a place for skepticism and scrutiny. However, one must consider the negative effect of unsubstantiated reports in the lay press. For example, the risk of Prozac-induced suicide appears to be *extremely* low, and the suicide rate in untreated major depression is reported to be 9 percent. Clearly, failure to treat carries the graver risk.

It is very likely that many seriously depressed people and parents of ADHD children have been understandably, and unnecessarily, frightened by negative, sensationalistic reports in the media. To quote Brotman (1992) again, "Pharmacotherapy does not exist in a social and political vacuum."

Although this debate continued throughout the 1960s and 1970s, clearly there were also a number of what G. L. Klerman (Beitman and Klerman 1991) calls "pragmatic practitioners"—those mental health professionals who used whatever approaches seemed to work. Certainly it was, and is, reasonable to consider that some disorders are best treated by psychotropic medications, others by psychotherapy, and it often makes sense to use a combination of both modalities.

Public opinion

A parallel to the professional debate began to occur within the general public. In institutes of higher education, the humanistic movement began to permeate not only departments of psychology but the global academic community as well. The post-McCarthy social climate was ripe for new attitudes that challenged political and social control and applauded the expression of free will, self-expression, and self-actualization. Reports began to surface regarding the abuse of psychiatric medication by the medical profession. Opponents to drug treatment accused the psychiatrists of using medications to achieve control. The term "chemical straitjacket" became popularized.

The 1970s saw the proliferation of new tranquilizers, and pharmaceutical companies reaped fortunes from the sale of well-known pills such as Valium and Librium. The vast majority of prescriptions written for minor tranquilizers (more than 90 percent) were written by family practice doctors, not psychiatric specialists. The "drugged state" was the fastest growing state in the union (Bly 1990). The inappropriate use and abuse of tranquilizers gained increasing public attention and even found its way into popular songs (the Rolling Stones' "Mother's Little Helper") and movies (*I'm Dancing as Fast as I Can*).

In the 1960s, the Church of Scientology was successfully sued by the American Psychiatric Association. In retaliation, it began a long, embittered assault on American psychiatry. Initially the Church of Scientology launched a negative campaign against the use of Ritalin, a psychotropic medication used to treat attention-deficit disorder. More recently it has orchestrated a move to shed negative light on the antidepressant Prozac (see sidebar on page 8).

Biological psychiatry was under attack. Although clearly there was a good deal of abuse and misuse of psychoactive drugs, there also continued to be decreasing numbers of people living in mental hospitals, and drug companies were at work developing newer and "cleaner" psychotropic medications, medications with fewer side effects.

Rapprochement: Biological and Psychological Perspectives

During the 1980s, a shift began in which increasing numbers of mental health practitioners and researchers widened their previously narrow views on etiology and treatment of mental illness. Increasingly, it became recognized that unidimensional models, whether psychological or biological, fell short of explaining the tremendous complexities of human psychological functioning and psychopathology. This transition to more complementary and integrated views of cause and cure can be attributed to several new developments:

- The side effects of medications historically resulted in very poor compliance rates among psychiatric patients, and the most effective medication available is useless if the patient doesn't take the drug as prescribed. Compounds introduced in the 1980s and early 1990s have yielded effective medications with much more user-friendly side-effect profiles.

- Discoveries have been made in which new medications and newer uses for existing medications provide very good results in treating certain types of mental illnesses, such as panic disorder and obsessive-compulsive disorder. This greatly increases the psychiatrist's arsenal of effective medications.

- A growing body of well-controlled research studies (double-blind, randomized, placebo-controlled) lend convincing support to the efficacy of psychotropic drugs.

- Neuroimaging techniques, such as PET and SPECT scans, allow researchers to view metabolic activity in the living brain. These technologies have been able to isolate localized brain abnormalities in certain mental disorders, including major depression, schizophrenia, ADHD, and obsessive-compulsive disorder. They can provide data on particular sites of drug action or binding, and can illustrate

Psychopharmacology and the "Managed Care" Dilemma

Since the advent of newer-generation psychotropic medication, many millions of people are receiving more effective treatment for a host of psychiatric conditions. For this we are grateful. However, it also has become abundantly clear that the effects of psychiatric drugs are limited. Under the best of all circumstances such treatments do not have an impact on all aspects of psychological suffering.

In our view, successful psychiatric treatment should always include psychotherapy. Only in the context of a healing relationship may many aspects of psychological dysfunction be adequately addressed. Numerous interpersonal, intrapsychic, spiritual, and existential dimensions of human functioning simply are not amenable to pharmacologic treatment.

In this book we acknowledge the many benefits of drug treatment; however, we must also share a concern: In these days of cost containment and managed care, individual human lives and quality-of-life issues are often ignored. It is a real concern that an automatic, knee-jerk reaction will be just to prescribe pills, when so much more is needed. We are treating people, not just nerve cells.

However, given the rising cost of pharmaceuticals, the most recent cost-containment strategies are as likely to focus on the use of psychiatric medication as well as on psychotherapeutic interventions. Paradoxically, perhaps as psychotropic drugs begin to account for an ever-increasing percentage of total health care expenditures, we will see best-practice guidelines influenced

continued

in a way that will support psychotherapy.

We hope that critical questions will be raised. Are medication treatment failures completely an effect of the drugs not working? Or could the relative lack of psychotherapeutic modalities be a contributing factor? Similarly, as the prescribing of psychotropics has become the first step in treatment, has that first step been taken before an accurate diagnosis was made? Are we medicating out of habit, when it is not really indicated? If the patient would benefit more from psychotherapy, are we doing more harm than good?

We remain hopeful that the pendulum will swing back to support what most practicing clinicians know to be true: the best outcomes result from appropriately balanced treatment that includes therapy and medications.

Human beings and their life problems are enormously complex. And it is the highly trained clinician who must ultimately decide which combinations of treatments are best suited for each individual client (*not* insurance companies, treatment manuals, or untrained technicians)!

changes between the pre- and post-treatment status of particular brain structures. Imaging techniques have added considerable "hard data" to various theories of biochemical etiology in selected mental illnesses.

■ Neuroimaging techniques have been accompanied by a host of new laboratory procedures that allow neuroscientists to assay the neurochemical by-products found in spinal fluid. Although early psychopharmacology was implemented without any real knowledge of the underlying pathophysiology, in the past decade, biochemical theories have gained tremendous scientific support.

These new developments in psychiatry and the neurosciences have been hard to ignore. Many formerly hard-line psychotherapists have been won over by the flood of research findings and their personal experiences in treating people with psychoactive drugs.

During this same period, important advances were made in the theory and practice of psychotherapy. During the late 1970s and 1980s the first truly well-controlled psychotherapy studies emerged (including the now popular meta-analyses). The results of these studies cast doubt on the findings of early research that had suggested that psychotherapy was ineffective (Eysenck 1965, for example). Of the many forms of psychotherapy that have been developed, the meta-analyses suggest that no single school of therapy is clearly superior and that psychotherapies across the board are often much more effective than no treatment.

Also during this time we witnessed the development of novel treatment approaches, such as cognitive behavioral psychotherapy (Beck 1976) and interpersonal psychotherapy (Klerman et al. 1984) as a treatment for particular disorders, such as depression and panic disorder. These approaches have appeal, in that they can be somewhat systematically applied (some even provide "canned" formats or "cookbooks"). Also, the methodology is a bit less reliant on the personal characteristics of the therapist. These approaches then lend themselves to a short-term format and can often be conducted in groups. And, finally, these psychotherapies can be more easily studied. Both cognitive behavioral and interpersonal psychotherapies have a solid track record of effectiveness (as is discussed further in the next chapter).

Finally, both clinical-anecdotal and research studies have emerged that support the combined use of pharmacotherapy and psychotherapy in the treatment of particular disorders. At times, the combined treatments have been shown to be superior to either single treatment alone.

For many in the mental health community, the writing on the wall has become far more legible: A single model for understanding and treating mental disorders is too narrow and is simply inadequate. As we shall be discussing in subsequent chapters, current evidence suggests that particular disorders do respond best to certain medical treatments, and for these, medications are the treatment of choice. Other disorders have little to do with biochemical dysfunction, and medications play little or no role in their treatment. And still other disorders require the skillful integration of biological and psychotherapies.

As the saying goes, when you only have a hammer, every problem looks like a nail. Fortunately, at the present time, mental health professionals have access to a "toolbox" of approaches that can, if employed appropriately, dramatically increase our effectiveness in reducing emotional suffering and promoting mental health.

Why Learn About Psychopharmacology?

In the United States, the majority of mental health services are provided by nonmedical therapists. Likewise, the majority of prescriptions for psychotropic medications are written by family practice and primary care physicians (see figure 1-A). Thus, even though psychiatrists represent the branch of medicine that specializes in psychopharmacology, they are directly responsible for providing only a fraction of professional services to the mentally ill. Consequently, it is becoming increasingly important for all mental health clinicians to have a basic familiarity with psychiatric medication treatment.

Many nonmedical psychotherapists are or will become strongly and rather directly involved in medication treatment. In some settings psychologists and social workers assume a major role in monitoring client responses to psychotropic medications. As primary therapist, these practitioners are in most frequent contact with clients and are in the best position to observe symptomatic improvement, side-effect problems, and issues involving medication compliance. When consulting with primary care physicians, or as a staff member in some HMO settings, nonmedical therapists who are well-versed in the use of psychiatric medications can play an active (albeit collaborative) role in recommending particular medications and dosage adjustments. In addition, the Department of Defense, in response to an inadequate number of psychiatrists available in the military, implemented a program to train a small number of psycholo-

Who Writes Prescriptions for Psychotropic Medications		
Class of Medications	**Psychiatrists (%)**	**Nonpsychiatric MDs (%)**
Antipsychotics	40	60
Antidepressants	15	85
Antianxiety	10	90
Hypnotics	11	89
Lithium	62	38
Source: Pomerantz et al. (2004)		

Figure 1-A

gists so that they are able to prescribe a limited formulary of psychiatric medications. Currently, properly trained psychologists can become licensed to prescribe psychiatric medications in the states of New Mexico and Louisiana. These various activities reflect quite direct involvement in medication treatment by nonmedical therapists.

In contrast, many nonmedical therapists have little to do with drug treatment. In some cases this may be due to the nature of their position in a particular treatment setting; in others it may have more to do with their own preferences and biases, such as opposition to medication treatment. However, we believe that, regardless of the degree of involvement and interest in medication treatment, it is increasingly important that all mental health therapists become acquainted with some basic notions regarding psychopharmacology.

Convincing evidence now exists that certain mental disorders are either caused or accompanied by neurochemical abnormalities. The failure to appropriately diagnose and medically treat such conditions can result in the use of ineffective or only partially effective treatments and hence in prolonged suffering. Aside from the obvious cost in human terms, prolonged inappropriate treatment results in excessive financial burdens for clients, their families, and the health care system.

In addition, to date there have been successful malpractice suits brought against therapists who failed to treat or refer for treatment patients suffering from particular disorders known to be generally responsive to medication.

All mental health professionals must be able to, at the very least, diagnose mental disorders that require psychotropic medication treatment so that appropriate referrals can be made. Differential diagnosis will be discussed in detail in this book.

In many cases, clients may not choose to see a psychiatrist, even when told by their therapists that medication treatment is indicated. This may be due to financial concerns or to the negative stigma some people believe is attached to psychiatric treatment. A viable alternative, in some cases, is referral to the family practice doctor. Many people suffering from emotional distress see their family physician first. This doctor may begin treatment with psychotropic medications and may also refer the patient for psychotherapy. In such cases, the nonmedical therapist may be in a key position to supply information regarding diagnosis and treatment response. Increasingly, family practice physicians and nonmedical therapists become partners collaborating on the treatment of many clients—especially those suffering from fairly uncomplicated depressive and anxiety disorders.

Effective consultation with family practice doctors and psychiatrists alike is enhanced by the nonmedical therapist's ability to accurately communicate and discuss diagnosis, target symptoms, presumed etiology, and possible treatments. We hope this book will provide a solid grounding in basic issues to help improve communication and cooperation between professionals.

Mental health treatment has moved increasingly toward greater acceptance of multidisciplinary and integrated treatment modalities. As sophistication in the diagnosis and medical treatment of mental disorders continues to develop, it will be important that mental health professionals not take a step backward. The polarization of models and professional "turf battles" of the 1960s and 1970s may have sparked useful and lively debate, but they also often resulted in a fragmentation of care. Ongoing knowledge of and respect for diverse models and collaborative involvement hold promise for increasingly effective efforts in treating mental illness.

2

Integrated Models

The decision about whether to use psychotropic medications in the treatment of psychiatric disorders is influenced by a number of factors. Unfortunately, often the decision is based largely on the clinician's a priori view toward treatment, deriving from his or her theoretical perspective. As we shall argue, the critical variable in this decision is more appropriately based on the diagnosis, and in particular on the presence or absence of key target symptoms that suggest the patient is experiencing some form of neurochemical disorder.

In broad and extremely heterogeneous groups of disorders, such as mood disorders, *some* may be largely or exclusively caused by biological factors. Other disorders in such groups share *some* symptoms with biologic-based mental illness, yet their etiology stems largely or exclusively from nonbiologic sources, for example, emotional, psychosocial, or cognitive sources. Thus a very important question to address when making a diagnosis and subsequent decisions about treatment is, "Is there any evidence to suggest that this person's problems are due to some form of biologic disturbance?" However, all too often this question is framed overly simplistically: "Is the disorder biological or is it psychological?"

The distinction between what is psyche and what is soma is ambiguous at best. Invariably, there is a complex interaction between psychological and biological factors in all cases of emotional disorder. This complexity will be the focus of this chapter.

Psychology and Biology: A Two-Way Street

A comprehensive discussion of the classic philosophical issue, mind-brain dualism, is beyond the scope of this book. (The reader is referred to Goodman 1991; Young 1987.) However, we would like to highlight a small number of cases and research studies that illustrate the interactive effects of biologic and psychologic factors.

Biological Factors' Impact on Psychological Functioning

Men ought to know that from the brain, and from the brain only, arise our pleasures, joys, laughter, and jests, as well as our sorrows, pains, griefs, and fears.... It is the same thing which makes us mad or delirious, inspires us with dread and fear, whether by night or by day, brings sleeplessness, inopportune mistakes, aimless anxieties, absentmindedness, and acts that are contrary to habit.

—Hippocrates

For the past two thousand plus years, there has been at least rudimentary recognition of the brain as the site of reasoning and emotions.

Early physicians were keen to note that brain injuries could result in profound changes in personality, cognition, and emotional control. And, as noted in chapter 1, in the earliest days of modern psychiatry the field was grounded in biological sciences and the medical model.

Two fairly common clinical examples serve as illustrations of how disordered brain functioning can lead to marked psychiatric symptomatology.

Case 1

Robert B. is a forty-two-year-old stockbroker. He has always been an ambitious, bright, energetic man. Despite normal stresses of daily life, he had never experienced major psychiatric problems until a month ago. For no apparent reason he began gradually to slip into a state of lethargy, fatigue, and low motivation. His normal zest for life diminished, his usual sharpness of wit became dull, and his sense of enthusiasm gave way to increasing blandness and emptiness. He was totally perplexed as he searched his recent life experiences to find the cause for his malady. None was to be found.

In the ensuing weeks he lost weight, frequently woke at 3:00 A.M. and was unable to go back to sleep, and lost all sexual desire for his wife.

Upon close investigation by his family physician, it was eventually discovered that the depressive symptoms began several weeks after he had started taking an antihypertensive drug to treat his high blood pressure. The medication was suspect and was eventually changed. Within a couple of weeks, the depression vanished.

This case illustrates how a medication can, at times, dramatically alter a person's brain chemistry, resulting in major psychiatric symptoms. In Robert's case, there was no evidence of long-standing psychological problems and no clear psychological stressors.

The brain can be seen, in a sense, as a tremendously complex biological ecosystem. As in other ecosystems, global functioning and survival depend on a large number of interrelated variables. At times, small changes in one aspect of the system influence a number of other variables—in essence, sending a ripple effect throughout the entire system. In the brain, often certain delicately balanced neurochemical systems can be altered (the term often used is *dysregulated*), resulting in a cascade of alterations affecting many other neurochemicals and the functioning of a host of brain structures. A drug, as in the example above, is but one of many variables that can result in neurochemical dysregulation and resulting psychiatric symptoms. (More will be said about other causes later in the chapter.)

Case 2

Elizabeth M. is a sixty-eight-year-old retired accountant whose passion is gardening. However, during the past three months she became unable to tend her garden for more than a few minutes at a time. She was almost constantly seized by tremendous restlessness and agitation, fretting, wringing her hands, and pacing about her house. "I feel like I am going to crawl out of my skin," she said.

Elizabeth lost twenty-five pounds over this three-month period and suffered fitful sleep. She also began to contemplate suicide. Her hopes for a well-deserved, peaceful retirement seemed to have been erased, as if she were plagued by some kind of curse. She could pinpoint absolutely no painful life events that might give meaning to her condition.

Fortunately, ultimately it was discovered that she was suffering from hyperthyroidism. Following successful treatment, she has been able to return to her garden and her life.

In this case, a metabolic disorder was the culprit. In the cases of both Robert and Elizabeth, neurochemical and hormonal factors grossly interfered with brain functioning. In both cases, the people were radically changed. Their perceptions were altered (pessimism, hopelessness), their sense of self was shaken, their emotions were out of control, and their physiological functioning had been derailed. Certainly they had strong emotional reactions to these changes (a phenomenon sometimes referred to as secondary emotional symptoms); however, in both cases the primary etiology was biological.

All mental health clinicians will encounter clients who present for treatment with presumed psychological problems but who, in fact, are suffering from biologically based disorders. Such disorders fall into three categories:

- Due to medical illnesses (such as hyperthyroidism)

- Due to drugs (prescribed, over-the-counter, or recreational)

- Endogenous mental illnesses[1]

Psychological Factors' Impact on Biological Functioning

For a very long time there has been some vague notion that emotional stress can affect physiology. For example, for hundreds of years it has been noted that severe stress can lead to disease. Family physicians have long noted that in the wake of tragic losses, the bereaved easily fall prey to illness. Yet not until this century did the psychology-biology interaction begin to be explored. Psychosomatic medicine was ushered in by the pioneering work of Franz Alexander in the 1940s. And an explosion of interest and research has been seen in the 1980s and 1990s in the emerging field of

---

1. The term *endogenous* means "arises from within." Certain psychiatric disorders have been found to be largely endogenous; that is, they arise spontaneously in the absence of provoking psychosocial stressors. The disorders can be attributed to a biological abnormality or a predisposition or vulnerability to dysfunction. Many of the so-called endogenous disorders appear to carry a genetic loading: they are passed from generation to generation and presumably can be linked to certain genetic factors. More will be said about endogenous psychiatric disorders in subsequent chapters.

psycho-neuro-immunology—the study of the effects of emotional factors on disease susceptibility and disease resistance.

It would require several textbooks to even begin to review the literature in psycho-somatics and psycho-neuro-immunology. We would, however, like to briefly discuss a few studies that shed some light on the issue of the interaction of psychology and biology and its relationship to mental illnesses. The first two of these studies involved experimentation with animals.

- E. Kandel and colleagues have studied the effects of environmental experiences and learning on the nervous system in the *Aplysia* (a marine mollusk). This animal is well suited for such a study because its nerve cells are quite large and easy to visualize. Also, it does respond well to learning experiments such as habituation, sensitization, and classical conditioning (Pinsker et al. 1970).

  The researchers were able to trace neural pathways from touch receptors in the mollusk's gill and siphon, through its primitive nervous system, and out into corresponding motor neurons. Using repeated exposures to mild aversive stimuli, the investigators were able to document specific biochemical changes at the synapse, as well as structural changes in specific nerve cells. Conclusion: environmental events and learning are actually accompanied by measurable changes in nerve cells; the animal's biology is altered.

- Neurologic changes have similarly been demonstrated in studies of learned helplessness in rats. In these classic studies, animals are exposed to extremely aversive conditions, from which they have no escape. After a period of exposure, the animals begin to exhibit marked behavioral changes: They become passive and immobile. And they fail to mount coping responses (escape) from later aversive situations from which escape *is* possible. In many respects, the animals have learned that they are helpless to respond, and then they come to take on characteristics that resemble major depression in humans. Interestingly, not only do these helpless rats behave in a depressed manner, but their biochemical functioning is altered. Measures of brain chemistry reveal neurochemical alterations that are identical to those seen in humans suffering from severe grief reactions or clinical depression. Again, environmental experiences have modified brain functioning (Weiss, Glazer, and Pohorecky 1976).

- In very similar ways, in numerous studies the biochemistry of people with reactive depressions has been shown to be markedly altered. For example, emotionally healthy individuals without a personal or family history of depression who encounter major psychosocial stressors (especially losses) can become depressed. Presumably such people are not especially at risk (biologically or psychologically) for depression, but nonetheless they become depressed in response to significant stressful events. Further, in the course of their reaction, *some* patients develop not only emotional symptoms (sadness, pessimism, low self-esteem) but also a host of biologic symptoms, such as sleep disturbances and marked biochemical abnormalities. The chemical dysfunctions include dysregulation of both neurotransmitters in the brain and hormones (for instance, adrenal hormones such as cortisol). Metabolic by-products of neurotransmitters have been measured in assays of spinal fluid and by way of brain-imaging techniques such as PET and SPECT scanning.

- Baxter et al. (1992) have convincingly demonstrated that psychotherapy can affect brain functioning. PET scans allow researchers to directly image living brain tissue and thus provide data on metabolic activity of specific areas of the brain. Studies using PET scans in severe obsessive-compulsive disorder reveal a localized brain abnormality: a metabolic disturbance in the head of the caudate nucleus, a brain structure that is part of the basal ganglia. In obsessive-compulsive disorder, when individuals are symptomatic, this abnormality is visible on PET scans. Yet following successful *behavioral* treatment (exposure and response-prevention treatments) the functioning of this brain area normalizes.

- Evidence also exists supporting the theory that the earliest episodes of affective illnesses in bipolar patients are often "reactive" in nature; that is, the initial episode is not an endogenous, biologic event but rather is evoked by psychological stressors. As a consequence of the initial episode, neurons in key areas of the limbic system may undergo a process of modification (neurochemically and even structurally), whereby the brain is changed more or less permanently. The result of this is that, following the first one or two episodes, the altered brain functioning leaves the nervous system at much greater risk for subsequent episodes and sets in motion an endogenous process whereby affective episodes can then occur spontaneously, even in the absence of psychological stress. From that point on, if the disorder is not controlled, each episode further affects the nervous system; the threshold for recurring episodes becomes progressively lower. This process is known as *kindling*. It begins as a response to external stressors and evolves into a largely biological illness.

These are but a few of many studies and clinical findings that collectively provide strong support for the idea that environmental and psychological factors can significantly affect biologic and neurologic functioning.

Biological-Psychological Interactions

It is very likely that complex, interactive effects exist between biological and psychological factors. It's never a question of all or none. In the case of Robert B., he was suffering from an endogenous depression and experiencing marked lethargy, poor concentration, and low motivation. This eventually led to performance problems at work and a number of critical remarks from his boss. These events began to fuel the flame of low self-esteem. Low self-esteem is generally not felt to be a primary symptom of biologically based depressive disorders, but it is almost universally seen to emerge as patients live with ongoing clinical depression.

Biologic effects may secondarily affect psychological functioning in a number of ways, among them:

- Altered perception. Biologic effects can contribute to the pessimistic thinking seen in depressive disorders and the tendency to anticipate fearful outcomes often seen in anxiety disorders.

- Increased emotional sensitivity and reduced emotional controls. Increased emotional arousal or pain may motivate a person to become more socially withdrawn and can often lead to a host of negative conclusions regarding personal competency, as in, "What's wrong with me? I'm crying like a baby."

- Decreased energy and arousal, poor concentration, and lowered motivation, which often leads to impaired performance in school and work.

- Sexual dysfunction, which can translate into interpersonal problems in intimate relationships.

- Bizarre behavior enacted during a manic or a psychotic episode. Such behavior can continue to be a source of tremendous personal embarrassment and shame long after the psychotic episode is resolved.

These consequences of a primarily biologically based mental disorder have an impact on the individual's sense of self-worth and competency in the world. Conversely, this increased level of despair can, in itself, operate to intensify the underlying biological abnormality.

Practical Implications

As previously mentioned, the question "Is this disorder psychological or is it biological?" is too simplistic. The more appropriate question is "To what extent is there evidence that biochemical factors may be contributing to a patient's current symptomatology?" This is much more than an academic question. To the extent that we can determine biologic etiology (or at least a degree of biologic dysfunction as a part of the more global disorder), pharmacologic treatments may be indicated. (How a biologic etiology and the need for medication are determined is addressed in detail in later chapters.)

Stimulus-Response Specificity

Stimulus-response specificity is a concept describing conditions where a very specific response can be predicted with tremendous regularity when a stimulus is applied. One example would be that an electrical shock to muscle tissue evokes a contraction. This model is appropriate for some types of medical interventions. For example, for acute cardiac and respiratory arrest, the techniques of cardiopulmonary resuscitation (CPR) can be used with most victims, regardless of their age, socioeconomic status, sex, or religious beliefs. When there is an obstructed airway, performing an emergency tracheotomy is appropriate for victims regardless of their emotional status, personality style, or level of psychosocial maturity. Likewise, some medications have fairly universal effects on all people; for instance, sodium pentothal produces unconsciousness (Deckert 1985).

Medical treatments in psychiatry generally *do not* follow the rule of stimulus-response specificity. Although the particular mechanism of drug action may be identified, the same medication given to two depressed patients, for example, may affect them very differently. Some of these differences may be traced to variations in metabolism from individual to individual (see chapter 4). Or the underlying biochemical abnormality in one depressed patient may be different than the abnormality in another depressed patient, and thus the medications affect different underlying disorders.

Beyond these physiological differences, however, the patients' responses may be influenced to a significant degree by a host of social, cognitive, and personality factors that have little or nothing to do with biology. In the realm of psychiatric medication treatment, sociocultural experiences and beliefs, personality style, and a vast number of personal psychodynamic factors can, and do, dramatically influence patient response. Psychological functioning cannot be understood using the simple, reductionist notions implied in stimulus-response specificity.

The good clinician *always* treats the person, not just the disorder. We may choose to influence nerve cells with psychotropic drugs, but the response will always be woven into the complex fabric of highly idiosyncratic personality factors. Therefore, successful pharmacologic treatment *always* requires a thorough knowledge of not only the diagnosis and pathology and the medications used, but the unique meaning of the treatment to the individual patient. Assembly-line psychotropic treatment often fails, not because medications are ineffective, but because clinicians do not take the time to understand their patients.

Unfortunately, in many overcrowded mental health clinics, some clinicians act as if stimulus-response specificity is appropriate. The result is that often these attempts at treatment efficiency and cost containment backfire. Many patients don't respond well and either must demand further outpatient services or continue to decompensate until they require hospitalization. And, of course, there is the human cost associated with prolonged suffering.

In the remainder of the chapter, we explore a number of ideas regarding psychological factors that have direct bearing on the outcome of medication treatment.

The Psychodynamics of Pharmacologic Treatment

When a prescription is written and a pill is taken, the effects of the medication are almost always influenced by a number of psychological factors. Some of these factors have to do with the commonly held beliefs regarding "drugs" and "illness" that are etched into the experience of most people in our culture. Other factors spring from highly personal, idiosyncratic sources, either in conscious awareness or buried deeply in the unconscious mind.

The astute clinician should continually ask the questions, "If medications are suggested or prescribed, how will this be perceived by my patient?" and "What personal meaning might be attached to this form of intervention?" Prescribing and recommending medication always occurs in an interpersonal context. It is not like a landscaper recommending and applying a particular fertilizer to your lawn. Rather, it can be a highly personalized communication between therapist and client, a communication ripe for all sorts of transference distortions and a type of interaction that *may* alter the nature of the therapeutic relationship.

In addressing these issues, we will first speak about rather common, generic themes and then go on to describe more unique, personal concerns. Let's consider some of the possible consequences.

Generic Meanings

In our culture, certain themes are evident in our clichés and language that link the taking of medicine with badness and punishment. The saying "Give him a taste of his own medicine" is but one example. One of the classic scenes from the *Our Gang* movie shorts has the wicked stepmother punishing Spanky and Alfalfa by making them swallow castor oil. Hearing bad news or carrying out unpleasant tasks is sometimes referred to as having to "swallow a bitter pill." Even in mature adults, these connections between "taking your medicine" and punishment may echo at unconscious levels.

Probably more common are notions regarding medication and "being sick." Many psychiatric patients may be able to view their difficulties honorably, as "problems in living," and yet feel shamed and humiliated by a suggestion that they take psychotropic medications. The unspoken meaning they perceive may be, "You need medications, thus you are sick." And being sick, in psychological terms, often carries its own assortment of negative connotations: weak, inadequate, crazy, deranged, and so on.

A common underlying concern sparked by the recommendation for psychotropics is, "The therapist must think I can't handle things on my own—thinks I need a crutch." This cannot only be wounding to the client's self-image, but may undermine the client's belief that the therapist is hopeful regarding his or her capacity for growth and healing.

Morality pervades many beliefs about the taking of drugs for emotional problems. Some people erroneously assume that all psychiatric drugs are alike. They conclude that all psychotropics are "tranquilizers," that all can lead to drug addiction, and that such dependence on drugs is little different than alcoholism. Thus, if you take drugs, you are bad or, at the very least, weak willed. This view of drugs as evil, or at least as dangerously addictive, is adopted by some 12-step chemical dependency programs. The lay leaders of some 12-step groups are understandably skeptical and afraid of drugs that can lead to abuse but may be ignorant of the fact that most psychotropic medications are not addictive at all. It is all too common for someone who has received a dual diagnosis of, for example, alcohol abuse and major depression to encounter tremendous pressure in his or her 12-step recovery program to discontinue anti-depressant medication. Fortunately, many recovery programs are learning about the appropriate use of some psychiatric medications and understand their role in treating dual-diagnosis clients.

Finally, psychiatric drugs are seen by some as an assault on free will and autonomy. Certainly this idea has been brought to our attention by media reports of instances in which psychotropic drugs have been used solely to achieve behavioral control. "Chemical straitjackets" and other forms of biological restraint, such as lobotomies, have been the subject of popular film and television productions (for example, *One Flew over the Cuckoo's Nest*, *Girl Interrupted*, and *A Beautiful Mind*). And clearly these abuses have and do occur. However, appropriately used medical interventions oftentimes work to free people and promote autonomy.

Case 3

Sara M. is a thirty-four-year-old stay-at-home mother. Over the past two years she has been plagued by devastating panic attacks and is unable to leave her home or to be alone. Her husband must have relatives stay with Sara or hire a "babysitter" to be with her when he goes to work. Sara is frightened, and she feels humiliated.

Sara initially balked at the suggestion that she take psychiatric medications. She saw the recommendation as an attack on her sense of adequacy and worth. However, after a period of psychotherapy, she did agree to take the medications. After eight weeks of treatment with paroxetine and clonazepam, she was free from panic attacks and began to venture out of her home for the first time in two years. Six months later she was reentering the mainstream of life and had just attended a performance of the local symphony. One of her greatest personal losses had been her inability to attend the symphony.

For Sara, the medication played a key role in reducing panic symptoms. But it was her own courage that enabled her to resume normal living, as she gradually chose to go outside her home or to spend time alone. In Sara's case, medications played a part in restoring her autonomy and bringing her back to life.

Case 4

One of the authors treated a young woman, Ellen G., who came for her first appointment at the mental health clinic with this opening line: "I'm starting to fall apart again. I guessed it was time to come in and start taking my Thorazine again." She had been treated with this antipsychotic drug off and on for the past three years and was now consulting with a new therapist. The therapist commented, "Well, maybe you're right about needing the medication again. But let's take some time to talk and see if we can understand what's going on for you."

As her story unfolded, it became clear that she was experiencing symptoms of a serious, delayed-onset post-traumatic stress disorder. In prior treatments, her therapists had never explored her circumstances beyond observing her feelings of panic, depersonalization, and confusion. They were quick to medicate her and seal over her distress.

In the current treatment, medications were not used. Months later this woman remarked, "That first day when you didn't just give me meds, but said 'Let's talk' ... [i]t was the first time I started to feel hopeful about therapy."

When medications are given, especially if they are offered or recommended early on in treatment, many clients' perception is, "They just want to drug me. They don't want to talk.... They don't want to hear my pain." Patients may feel they are being treated as a "case" (as in stimulus-response specificity), and the result can be a serious warp in the developing therapeutic alliance or even premature termination of therapy.

At times when therapists feel stuck with a client's progress, their own sense of futility or impotence may lead to the decision to try medications. This feeling of pessimism may be picked up on by the client. As Jerome Frank (1991) and others have argued, one of the most important roles therapists can play is to help maintain realistic hopefulness, especially during times when clients are feeling especially demoralized. Certainly, psychotropic medications may be indicated and can be crucial interventions with *some* "stuck" psychotherapy clients. However, the choice to medicate should be based on thorough consideration of diagnostic issues and not be simply a response to the therapist's own pessimism.

Personal Meanings

Just like any other type of intervention or communication in therapy, the therapist's behaviors and interactions can certainly be perceived in particular, unique ways by the client—ways that make sense when the client's psychodynamics are understood. Although such personal dynamics vary tremendously from person to person, we would like to address several fairly common examples that can be seen in clinical practice.

Dependent and borderline personality disordered patients

The request for medications (explicit or implicit) by dependent patients often conveys a need to be fed. Aside from direct medication effects, the gratification experienced by the patient when given drugs may account for symptomatic improvement. It is also important to note that once the therapist prescribes medications (however appropriate this may be), in some way he or she has strayed from a position of neutrality, and this may have consequences for the therapeutic relationship. Conversely, the choice not to prescribe or recommend medications may be seen as "withholding."

Obsessive-compulsive patients

People with obsessive-compulsive personality styles value control and precise intellectual scrutiny. Thus, when medications are prescribed, the therapist will often be confronted with (1) a request for detailed information about the medication and its side effects, (2) frequent discussions regarding medication response and side effects (even very minor side-effect problems), and (3) worries centering around loss-of-control experiences that may result from even very minimal side effects, such as a slight degree of sedation or dizziness.

Case 5

Albert K. is a fifty-four-year-old engineer receiving treatment for a major depression. This rigid, obsessional man came for his appointment a week after being started on antidepressants. During the past week he had written a computer program to track medication side effects on a daily basis, and he brought a data sheet with him to the session. The program addressed fifteen different side effects (which he had gleaned from the *Physicians' Desk Reference*); each one was rated daily on a scale of 1 to 10, and results were displayed in terms of daily scores and weekly averages and on bar graphs. This was Albert's style, his way of approaching medication treatment. The therapist thought it was a classic for obsessional patients and was impressed with Albert's program and charts.

Anxious patients

Individuals who suffer from severe anxiety disorders and, in particular, phobias and panic disorder already experience a significant amount of fearfulness in their daily life. Oftentimes when medications are prescribed, the medication itself becomes a new source of fear for these patients. This is frequently seen when such individuals are started on antidepressant medications. These medications may present some side effects, such as a rapid heart rate, and these are quickly interpreted by the anxious patient as a sign of increased anxiety and loss of control. This may lead to patients quickly discontinuing the medication or even therapy itself.

Paranoid patients

The issues encountered with paranoid patients often surround struggles over control and autonomy. These people are especially frightened by others assuming a position of control over them, and being "medicated" often touches on this theme. In more psychotic paranoid patients, this issue not uncommonly takes the form of delusions in which the patient feels the therapist is trying to poison him or her.

Depressed patients

Frequently, seriously depressed patients, when encountering very minor side-effect problems, complain bitterly about these difficulties or abruptly discontinue antidepressant medication treatment. It may be difficult to understand why a profoundly depressed person would abandon treatment when all he or she has encountered is a slightly dry mouth or minor degree of sedation. Yet it bears keeping in mind that such people are already exquisitely sensitive to discomfort, overwhelmed by psychological pain, and prone to tremendous pessimism. Although the therapist hopes for significant benefit from the antidepressant, the patient's experience is often focused on a here-and-now awareness of added discomfort and probably a persistently bleak view of the future.

Narcissistic patients

The never-ending search for the perfect relationship, the perfect job, and the perfect life that narcissistic patients pursue may extend to the demand for the perfect medication—which pharmaceutical companies have not as yet developed.

Medication as a tool for resistance

Across diagnostic groups, a common experience is for the patient to bring up medication and medication problems as a form of resistance. It is, of course, important to track medication responses and encourage patient-therapist dialogue regarding effects. However, when this topic comes to dominate too much of the therapy hour, it may be an indication that the subject is being used in the service of resistance. That is, the focus is shifted away from inner thoughts and feelings to symptoms and side effects. In addition, arguments or complaints regarding medication issues may also become an arena for struggles over control.

Countertransference issues

Medications are sometimes given to patients in a sort of "rescue response," when the therapist either fears the therapy is ineffective or is worried about the patient experiencing excessive emotional pain. Although certainly this may be appropriate at times, it can also be a countertransference problem that interferes with treatment.

A therapist will sometimes give medications to a patient to soften the blow of termination or to assuage the therapist's guilt over stopping treatment—a problem seen more commonly these days in short-term therapy clinics. Some clinics offer only limited psychotherapy but will allow patients to continue some form of contact with therapists—if they are on medications. So prescribing medications can be a way to "legitimize" continued contact and avoid the losses associated with termination.

It is not our goal to recommend specific solutions to these various client dynamics or countertransference problems but rather to highlight them as particular concerns. The well-trained therapist never views medication treatment in a vacuum or as a stimulus-response specific intervention. Alertness to these issues and a willingness to inquire about personal interpretation of the recommendation for medication are our best hedge against problems that can potentially derail treatment or contribute to poor medication compliance.

The Cultural Context of Psychopharmacology

It is beginning to be understood that the ways psychotropic medications are metabolized may vary (sometimes considerably) among ethnic groups. When metabolism rates are reduced, the result can be significantly higher blood levels of medications with consequent increases in side effects and possible toxicity. Accelerated metabolism of drugs can result in inadequate blood levels and ineffective treatment outcomes. Differences in *pharmacokinetics* (how the body affects drugs) do exist among ethnic groups. These factors can make the difference between success or failure in pharmacological treatment. The impact of ethnic variables regarding drug metabolism are discussed in detail in appendix B.

The impact of one's ethnic affiliation and culture on beliefs about medical treatment is a significant factor that is often overlooked in psychopharmacology. Beyond the physiological differences in medication responses, there are numerous factors that reflect cultural beliefs regarding views of mental illnesses and medical treatment in general. In many parts of the world, as is true in a multitude of subcultures in the United States, views about the causes of psychiatric symptoms and generally held beliefs about treatment may vary considerably.

In a now classic study (Lee, Wing, and Kong 1992) evaluated Chinese patients' responses to treatment with lithium. These subjects exhibited typical side effects from lithium; however, their overall responses to these side effects often were quite different from those usually seen in most patients treated in a Western culture. For example, although Caucasians treated in the United States complain of side effects (such as *polydipsia*: the need to drink a lot of water, and *polyuria*: frequent urination), their Asian counterparts often felt positive about these effects, because they were seen as a sign that the medication was cleaning out their bodies by removing toxins. Their view of potentially adverse effects was significantly influenced by their cultural context.

This example highlights the importance of learning about particular beliefs and concerns prior to treating those from different cultural backgrounds. Henderson (1995), for instance, has noted that Latinos and Asians often anticipate that medication responses will occur quickly. This is especially important to know, given the fact that most psychiatric medications require weeks before noticeable symptomatic improvement can be seen. For these reasons, it's essential to spend time acquainting oneself with preconceived notions about medicines and medication responses. Moreover, since there are many different ethnic and cultural groups in the United States, the clinician must always be sensitive to these differences and strive to learn as much as possible regarding the beliefs and attitudes of various groups.

Other factors related to cultural differences also must be evaluated, such as the frequency of alcohol use and smoking (which can have an impact on drug metabolism) in particular cultural groups; low-income groups often suffer from more general medical problems and thus may be taking more prescription drugs (setting the stage for potential drug-drug interactions). Many impoverished individuals also suffer from malnutrition. Unfortunately, access to medical and psychological treatment may also be influenced by one's socioeconomic status. This can be further complicated by lack of access to transportation or the high cost of transportation, financial limitations that have an impact on the ability to purchase medications, and a tendency to not seek out regular preventive medical services. Finally, not infrequently, people of color and those with very limited financial resources are seen for briefer and less frequent medical appointments

In numerous settings, indigenous healing traditions may represent dominant views about health. Many patients are reluctant to talk openly about such treatments to those who do not belong to their cultural group due to understandable concerns that their practices may not be understood or may be dismissed. Additionally, some healing practices may include the use of herbs, some of which may pose problems regarding drug-drug interactions. Cultural beliefs about treatment may also influence the issue of medication adherence.

If the clinician is insensitive to alternative beliefs regarding healing and psychological symptoms, not only may the current treatment be less than successful, but this may alienate patients to such a degree that they will be unlikely to seek out standard psychiatric treatment in the future. Thus it is important to clearly communicate to patients that you are very interested in knowing as much as possible about their unique cultural beliefs and to express a willingness to understand.

In addition, it may be helpful to know about particular cultural experiences and metaphors that can be used to help explain medication effects. For example, in agrarian cultures, the idea that it is necessary to prepare the soil and plant seeds well ahead of the harvest can be used as a familiar metaphor to illustrate how many psychiatric medications must be used for several weeks before symptom relief is experienced.

In the chapters that follow, we will discuss in detail the multitude of issues related to treatment planning and specific pharmacologic strategies. Needless to say, no medication can be effective if people do not take the drug, and issues of personal beliefs, personality dynamics, and culturally influenced attitudes are critical to evaluate and understand patients' responses to medication. The art of psychopharmacology treatment requires a sound understanding of psychiatric diagnosis and the evaluation of treatment options, but ultimately, it also requires cultural sensitivity and sound clinical judgment to address concerns that can either make or break it in terms of successful outcomes.

3

Neurobiology

The Nervous System on a Cellular Level

This chapter provides an overview of neurobiology in order to create a foundation for subsequent chapters that address biologic etiologies and pharmacology. For the interested reader, sidebars contain more technical and detailed discussions.

The Nerve Cell

The human brain contains approximately 100 billion nerve cells (also referred to as *neurons*). Although there are numerous types of nerve cells, most function in a similar fashion. The proper functioning of the nervous system depends on communication between the neurons. Structurally, all neurons are composed of a cell body, dendrites, axon, and terminal boutons (see figure 3-A). *Dendrites* are short, branched structures projecting out from the cell body. They receive and conduct information to the cell body; there may be one or many dendrites on each cell. Extremely fine projections on the dendrites are called *dendritic spines*. Spines are common locations for synapses. The *axon* is a long fiber that ends in enlarged structures called *terminal boutons*. The axon serves to conduct impulses away from the cell body.

Within the cell body lie a number of tiny structures responsible for moment-to-moment operation and survival of the cell. Each neuron receives oxygen, glucose, and a host of other molecules from capillaries that lie adjacent to the cell. Some of the more important molecules delivered to the nerve cells via the bloodstream are amino acids, which serve as the building blocks for proteins.

Each cell must manufacture a multitude of proteins, which are then used for many different purposes, including the production of receptors, enzymes that regulate intracellular biochemical processes, growth factors, and structural elements of the cell. Each cell also produces its own messenger molecules (*neurotransmitters*), which are secreted

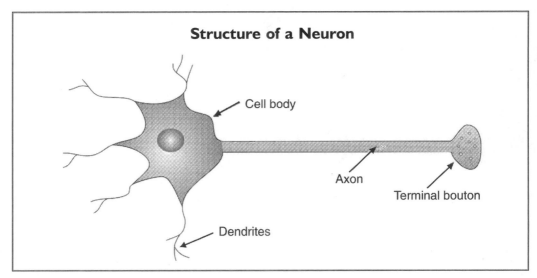

Structure of a Neuron

Cell body

Axon

Terminal bouton

Dendrites

Figure 3-A

by the cell and which then may influence the functioning of adjacent neurons. Because of this influence on adjacent neurons, neurotransmitters are sometimes referred to as *first messenger* molecules.

Intercellular Communication

When nerve cells are activated and produce a nerve impulse, the resulting surge of electrochemical energy begins in the cell body and is rapidly passed along the axon (i.e., away from the cell body) ending in the terminal bouton. Here, the impulse causes the release of neurotransmitter molecules into the tiny space between nerve cells referred to as the *synapse*. The human brain's 100 billion nerve cells are richly interconnected, making approximately 100 trillion synapses. Yet in almost all instances, the nerve cells do not actually touch one another; they are separated by this tiny space. Communication between nerve cells requires the action of neurotransmitting molecules that deliver stimulation (and thus information) across the synapse. Let's see how this works and also how it can malfunction.

Conduction and Transmission

The process of nerve activity begins with stimulation of the cell. A variety of molecules, called *ligands*, may be able to bind to and activate receptors. Such molecules include neurotransmitters, hormones, and certain drugs. The activation of excitatory receptors on the dendrites or the cell body results in a brief change in electrical potential from the cell's resting state. This change is called an *action potential*. The action potential is converted into a nerve impulse as it spreads throughout the dendrites, cell body, and ultimately down the axon. At the nerve ending, the nerve impulse performs the critical function of causing the release of neurotransmitting chemicals into the synapse. The neuron that releases the neurotransmitters is called the *presynaptic* neuron; the neuron that receives the neurotransmitters is called the *postsynaptic* neuron. The process of impulse movement along the axon is referred to as *conduction*; *transmission* refers to the passage of the impulse across the synaptic space.

Neurotransmitter molecules are manufactured in the cell body and are then transported down the axon for storage in tiny containers (*vesicles*). While enclosed in vesicles, the neurotransmitters are protected from destruction by enzymes that reside in the fluid within the presynaptic terminal bouton. Upon receiving stimulation from the action potential, the vesicles migrate toward the cell membrane, fuse with it, and for a microsecond create a pore (a tiny gateway in the cell membrane), discharging their contents into the synapse. Receptors are on the adjacent, postsynaptic membrane (see figure 3-B).

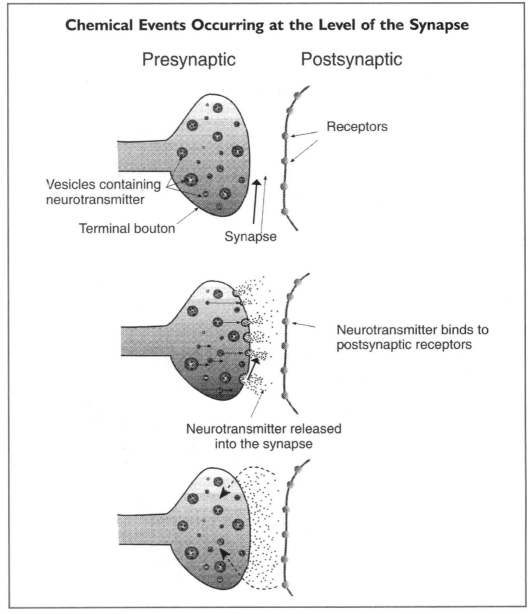

Chemical Events Occurring at the Level of the Synapse

Presynaptic   Postsynaptic

Receptors

Vesicles containing neurotransmitter

Terminal bouton

Synapse

Neurotransmitter binds to postsynaptic receptors

Neurotransmitter released into the synapse

Figure 3-B

Messenger Molecules

In detailed discussions of neurotransmission, distinctions are
often made in describing specific
types of neurotransmitters, also
referred to as *neuromodulators*.
Categorization models are based
on properties such as the size or
type of molecule, or the location of
synthesis within the neuron.

These models undergo nearly
continuous revision as new information is discovered. Regardless
of classification criteria, there are
two very important and basic
properties common to most
neurotransmitters. The first is that
these chemicals are found within
neurons and released as a result
of the nerve impulse. The second
is the ability of all neurotransmitters to produce a physiological
effect on a neuron. A neurotransmitter classification system that
includes the biogenic amines, the
neuropeptides, and the amino
acids is useful for understanding psychopharmacology. Within
each category there are numerous
specific chemicals.

When narrowly defined, the
biogenic amines comprise only
epinephrine, norepinephrine, and
dopamine. However, in a broader
and more practical sense, serotonin, histamine, and acetylcholine are often also included.

Endorphins and *enkephalins* are
examples of neuropeptides. They
are sometimes called naturally
occurring opioid peptides because
of their ability to bind to the same
receptors as morphine. Other
important peptides that will be
discussed in this book are corticotropin releasing factor (CRF)
and substance P.

In this family of neuropeptides,
there are numerous substances
with purported effects on such
diverse physiological systems
as pain response, memory and

continued

The Effects of Receptor Binding

Neurotransmitter molecules, when released
into the synapse, are capable of binding to specific
receptors (for example, dopamine molecules bind
only to dopamine receptors and have no direct
impact on other receptors). *The binding of neurotransmitters to receptors is the primary means by which one
nerve cell can influence the functioning of other neurons.*

The effects of receptor binding vary tremendously depending on which type of receptor is
involved. Functionally, some neurotransmitters
are excitatory, since they activate adjacent neurons,
and others are inhibitory (i.e., acting like a brake
when turned on; they have the impact of reducing nerve cell excitability). One notable exception
is seen with the serotonin system in the brain. The
molecule serotonin is not itself inherently excitatory or inhibitory. It all depends on which type of
serotonin receptor is activated. Currently fourteen
subtypes of serotonin receptors have been discovered. Most are inhibitory, although some are excitatory. Thus, if serotonin levels are increased in the
entire brain, it will have multiple effects (Barnes
and Sharp 1999).

When neurotransmitters are released into the
synapse, some molecules bind to receptors, some
are chemically destroyed by enzymes found in
the extracellular fluid, and many are rapidly reabsorbed into the presynaptic neurons. The reabsorp-
tion is accomplished by way of a *reuptake transporter
pump* (see figure 3-B). This is a protein structure in
the cell membrane. Neurotransmitter molecules
reenter the nerve cell and are repackaged in the
vesicles. This is a sort of molecular recycling that
allows neurotransmitters to be used again and
again.

Many of the currently available antidepressants operate via reuptake inhibition, where the
drug molecule enters the reuptake pore and blocks
it. The result is that the neurotransmitters released
into the synapse stay there longer and thus may
have a greater effect on the postsynaptic neuron.
Ultimately, neurotransmitters die off and disappear due to enzymatic degradation, thus making it
essential for nerve cells to continuously manufacture new neurotransmitters to replenish those that
have been lost.

Across the Synapse: Receptors and Intracellular Actions

Receptors are protein molecules that have been produced in the neuron and are embedded in the cell membrane. A portion of the molecule is exposed on the surface of the neuron membrane, and the other end penetrates into the cell. The exposed portion has certain binding sites where messenger molecules are able to attach themselves, and thus activate the receptor.

Most nerve cells have between 2,000 and 3,000 receptors on the surface of the cell body and dendrites. Any given cell may have dozens of receptor subtypes on its surface (e.g., a dopamine cell may have dopamine receptors, but it may also have serotonin receptors, opiate receptors, and so forth, allowing it to be influenced by a host of neurotransmitters and hormonal molecules). Most receptors are on the surface of the cell, although some reside within the cell body.

The absolute number of receptors and the ratio of inhibitory-to-excitatory receptors (brakes and accelerators), which ultimately help determine sensitivity/excitability levels of the cell, are partially determined by genetics, the inherent nature and makeup of the cell. However, it is important to note that populations of receptors are significantly influenced by external factors (such as the impact of stressors or drugs). (See the sidebar entitled "Impact of Stress on Receptors.")

The life span of receptors is between twelve and twenty-four hours. After this period of time, they wear out or are reabsorbed into the cell. Thus, throughout an individual's life span, nerve cells must be capable of continuously monitoring receptor populations and replacing lost receptors. Also, the cell must be able to adjust receptor populations in accord with environmental demands (see sidebar entitled "Impact of Stress on Receptors"). Thus, nerve cells are by no means static. In order to handle stressors, they are ever-changing, and it is remarkable how the nervous system is able to do this so effectively (at least, most of the time).

One way to categorize receptors is from a *functional* standpoint based on the end result of neurotransmitter-receptor coupling. The most basic distinction is inhibitory versus excitatory. That is, when activated by a messenger molecule, will the impact on the cell be in the direction of increased or decreased neuronal excitation?

learning, appetite, and temperature regulation.

Amino acid neurotransmission is pervasive throughout the brain. Quantitatively, amino acids constitute the majority of all transmitters in the brain. There are several amino acid neurotransmitters with relevance in neuropsychiatry. Glutamate, which is highly concentrated in the brain, and aspartate, which is localized in the spinal cord, are excitatory. Gamma aminobutyric acid (GABA), heavily distributed in the brain, and glycine, primarily found in the spinal cord, are inhibitory. The neurotransmission of amino acids is a major focus of neuropsychiatric disease-state research and drug development.

Advances in neurotransmitter research have challenged the classic criteria for neurotransmitter typology (Snyder and Ferris 2000). The gases nitric oxide and carbon dioxide are identified as atypical neurotransmitters. They are distinct from typical neurotransmitters in that they are not stored in presynaptic vesicles and do not interact via a postsynaptic receptor complex. Mirror-image amino acids, known as *enantiomers,* are also being studied to determine if they possess the requisite properties to be considered neurotransmitters. One such molecule, D-serine, may prove to have a role in the etiology and treatment of schizophrenia.

It has been proposed that D-serine and glutamate combine to activate NMDA receptors. The atypical feature of D-serine is that it resides in the glia (the supporting cells surrounding neurons), rather than in neurons. Another proposed novel neurotransmitter is adenosine, which has neuroactive properties, yet is neither a biogenic amine nor an amino acid.

Impact of Stress on Receptors

Many biological systems are said to be "regulated systems." This means that organisms, organ systems, tissues, or individual cells, to assure survival, may alter their functioning (chemical functioning and even structure/morphology) to accommodate to changing environmental circumstances. However, there is also an inherent tendency to return to baseline or "homeostasis" after an environmental disturbance has ended. Should such disturbance last a long time (as is the case with chronic stress or drug abuse), cells can react in a number of ways (e.g., by developing tolerance, adjusting excitability levels, and so on).

Neuronal adaptations take place via the mechanisms of up-regulation or down-regulation. Chronic exposure to high levels of stress causes a bombardment by certain excitatory neurotransmitters. This often leads to a down-regulation (reduction in the number and density) of excitatory receptors. Conversely, abnormally low levels of certain neurotransmitters or hormones may spur the up-regulation of excitatory receptors as an attempt of the cells to normalize the activity/firing rates of neurons. This is but one form of biological flexibility and adaptation seen in response to changes in the external environment (Post, Weiss, and Leverich 1994; Post and Weiss 1997).

Assessing the status of receptor density in certain brain regions is one way to identify particular types of pathology (e.g., depression) and/or psychotropic medication effects.

Typically, the terms *up-regulation* and *down-regulation* refer to changes in the number of receptors. However, the terms are used sometimes to refer to changes in overall neurotransmitter systems (e.g., *up-regulating brain serotonin* may refer to an increase in global central nervous system (CNS) serotonin activity).

Another way to consider receptors is from a *mechanistic* standpoint. In other words, how does the ligand-receptor activity occur? The majority of receptor activities can be categorized into five basic types, which are often referred to as *signaling mechanisms*. Signaling mechanism research has become increasingly important for understanding biological functioning (and malfunctioning) and provides an expanding platform for new drug development. In neuropsychiatry, two of the most relevant types of signaling mechanisms are the *ion-channel mediated process* and the *G-protein mediated second messenger system* described in the sidebar called "Into the Neuron: Second Messenger Systems and Gene Expression." These two mechanisms are also known as *ionic* or *metabotropic*, respectively.

Ionic actions take place when receptors are associated with ion channels. Ion channels are tiny pores on the surface of nerve cell membranes. When neurotransmitters, drugs, or other ligands bind to these receptors, it causes the ion channel to open transiently, thus allowing certain ions (electrically charged molecules, e.g., chloride or sodium) to pass throughout the membrane. (During the momentary opening of channels, the membrane is said to be *permeable* to certain molecules.) Ionic actions are responsible for rapid and transient changes in nerve cell activity, e.g., as occurs with neuronal firing underlying sensory perception or voluntary muscle action.

Most psychiatric medications do not operate via ionic receptors. One exception are the minor tranquilizer/benzodiazepine drugs that facilitate the opening of chloride-ion channels. Once these drugs enter the central nervous system (CNS), they are able to produce a rapid onset of actions (i.e., tranquilization).

Metabotropic actions, in contrast, are not rapidly occurring; rather, they involve gradual changes in neuronal functioning that take place over hours, days, weeks, or even months. When ligands bind to these receptors, they operate by activating what are referred to as *second messenger systems* within the cytoplasm of the cell. This process is said to involve a cascade of chemical actions that ignite a number of intracellular biochemical events. These alterations in the cell's inner chemical microenvironment operate to change or regulate cellular activity, partly by influencing gene expression. For details see the sidebar called "Into the Neuron: Second Messenger Systems and Gene Expression."

Most psychiatric medications operate by acting on metabolic receptors, and this explains, in part, why most of these drugs require several weeks of administration before the onset of noticeable symptomatic improvement.

Neuronal Malfunction

A number of things can go amiss at the cellular level in the brain, with consequent psychiatric symptoms. Most of the time, these pathologic cellular changes take place after a period of time during which particular neurons are bombarded by extreme amounts of excitation spurred by psychological stresses or drug abuse. Gradually the internal chemistry and even the structure of key nerve cells develop abnormalities leading to neuronal malfunctions. Let's take a look at several common dysfunctions that are believed to underlie major mental illness (these abnormalities will be explored in greater detail in later chapters).

- The initial synthesis (production) of neurotransmitters may be inhibited, thus little neurotransmitter is available for release.

- Neurotransmitters may be subject to excessive degradation by enzymes (such as MAO, monoamine oxidase).

- Certain biologically based disorders or drugs may either facilitate or inhibit the release of neurotransmitters by the presynaptic bouton.

- The process of reuptake absorption may be altered. For example, cocaine abuse leads to a blocking of dopamine reuptake pores. In clinical major depression, reuptake of serotonin, norepinephrine, and/or dopamine may become accelerated.

- Receptors may be either abnormally up-regulated or down-regulated (see sidebar "Impact of Stress on Receptors"), causing neurons to malfunction.

- Pathological alterations can occur in gene expression due to marked changes

Into the Neuron: Second Messenger Systems and Gene Expression

Through metabolic receptor action (also referred to as *G-protein-linked receptors*), drug molecules and other ligands are able to activate G-proteins (tiny protein molecules that lie adjacent to the interior surface of the cell membrane). The activation of G-proteins is the starting point for a diverse array of biochemical changes that can then take place within the cell. G-proteins act like molecular switches activating enzymes in the cytoplasm. G-protein activation also can have an impact on ion channels (not opening them per se, but rather, altering their intrinsic excitability). But their more common role is the activation of a number of enzymes, collectively referred to as *second messengers*. Second messengers are usually small, water-soluble molecules found in the cytoplasm.

The primary means of second messenger activation is by way of a biochemical reaction referred to as protein phosphorylation. Second messengers regulate enzymes referred to as protein kinases, which transfer phosphate groups from adenosine triphosphate (ATP) onto specific protein substrates, while protein phosphatases basically do the opposite (i.e., they remove phosphates). Altered proteins then are "activated" and capable of bringing about several different changes in cellular functioning including:

1. Inactivation of ion channels or, conversely, activation of other ion channels

2. Turning on the production of neurotransmitters

3. Effects on gene expression (i.e., turning on genes) (Hyman and Nestler 1996; Post, Weiss, and Leverich 1994; Post and Weiss 1997)

Gene Expression: Within the nucleus of all human cells are twenty-three pairs of chromosomes. Each chromosome is comprised of long, double-stranded DNA molecules. Embedded in the DNA are

continued

genes (sequences of nucleotides). Each cell contains all the genes for the entire human body (i.e., the human genome), although each cell accesses and expresses only those gene sequences responsible for the functioning of that particular cell. Gene sequences are the molecular blueprints for the production of proteins (which are subsequently manufactured in the cell and yield a host of molecules that have numerous important functions, e.g., receptors, growth factors, enzymes, and so on).

For genes to have an effect on cellular functioning, they first must be accessed and activated (i.e., gene expression). Specific gene expression may be an endogenous process but may also be influenced by environmental stimulation (e.g., activated by stressors and by certain drugs, which can turn genes on or off, and can thus influence the rate of protein synthesis). Gene expression involves several steps. Transcription factors activated by second messengers attach to specific areas of the DNA molecule (promoter sites) and, in turn, activate genes (expose them and initiate the process of gene transcription onto messenger RNA molecules). Messenger RNA molecules (mRNA; also proteins) align alongside the DNA and make a copy of the gene sequence (much as a CD is used to copy data from a computer hard drive). Then the mRNA exits the nucleus and travels to a part of the cell known as the *endoplasmic reticulum*. Here it attaches to ribosomes, where proteins are constructed.

Next, transfer RNA (tRNA) collects amino acids from the cytoplasm and helps to arrange them in the particular sequence encoded on the mRNA. The result is a chain of amino acids that, when complete, forms a protein. The final molecules are referred to as a *gene product*. Second messengers either may facilitate or interfere with gene expression. And, ultimately, stimulation by neurotransmitters influenced by stressors or drugs will thus have an impact on second messengers. Additionally, stress hormones such as glucocorticoids, thyroid, and sex hormones also can influence the rate of gene expression.

in second messengers (see sidebar entitled "Into the Neuron: Second Messenger Systems and Gene Expression") and may result in numerous abnormal cellular responses, including cell growth, altered receptor sensitivity, dendrite retraction, loss of dendrite spines, and/or cell death (*apoptosis*).

The Impact of Neuronal Malfunction

Nerve cells in the three critical neurotransmitter systems (dopamine, serotonin, and norepinephrine) in total represent less than 1 percent of total brain neurons. Yet malfunctions in any of these systems can result in marked dysregulation of the brain and, at times, in catastrophic psychiatric symptoms. Sometimes the changes in the nervous system are relatively transient; for example, as with those that occur with certain adjustment disorders. At other times, the impact is greater and more long-lasting, but it is also subject to eventual spontaneous remission, as is the case in some types of major depression. However, in many psychiatric disorders, the underlying biological changes can, without treatment, be more or less permanent and often progressive (e.g., bipolar disorder).

Neuroanatomy

Advances in the neurosciences, especially newer neuroimaging techniques (such as functional MRI, PET, and SPECT scanning), have allowed researchers to identify more precisely which brain structures are implicated in the cognitive, perceptual, and emotional aspects of brain functioning. Likewise, such techniques have made possible the delineation of the brain structures and neurotransmitter systems that appear to malfunction in cases of primary brain pathology and in neurochemically medicated psychopathologies.

Although volumes have been written about neuroanatomy and brain functioning, in this discussion we will touch only on those brain structures believed to be relevant to the study of psychiatric disorders. What follows represents a very brief overview of functional neuroanatomy, which will lay the groundwork for specific material presented in the chapters that follow.

Brain Structures

For practical purposes, the brain can be divided into three basic units: the brain stem (a) and adjacent structures, the central core of the brain (b) (including the limbic system, diencephalon, and basal ganglia), and the cerebral cortex (c) (see figure 3-C). Clearly, the highest area of the brain, the cerebral cortex, is responsible for much of what is termed human: perception; complex cognitive processes; reality testing; and initiation of behavior, judgment, and so forth. Interestingly, however, the major biological dysfunctions seen in psychiatric disorders are thought to take place primarily outside of the cortex proper.

Major mental illnesses appear to involve neurochemical dysfunctions occurring in various subcortical areas: the limbic system, basal ganglia, reticular system, and brain stem. These brain structures are complexly interconnected and play critical roles in mediating primary affective states and a host of biological rhythms and drives (such as sleep, sex, and hunger).

Figure 3-D outlines the basic structures found in these important areas of the CNS, with reference to their various normal functions and the hypothesized psychopathology associated with each brain structure. However, it is important to note that few, if any, psychiatric disorders have been associated with pathology or dysfunction of any single brain structure, although specific neuroanatomical areas have been clearly implicated in playing a special role in certain mental disorders.

Every region of the brain is activated and controlled by specific nerve cells. Billions of interconnecting nerve cells orchestrate the complex interactions necessary to carry out a host of functions ranging from basic instincts, reflexes, and life support, such as regulation of blood pressure, to highly developed abilities, such as abstract thought. When all is working as it should, people are able to respond to physiological and psychological demands in a normal and adaptive fashion.

However, brain functioning can be derailed by damage to brain tissue, via trauma, toxins, or disease, or by malfunction occurring in nerve cells. At times, such dysfunctions may affect only a tiny percentage of brain neurons. Yet the results can be devastating. The specific nature and location of brain dysfunctions will be revisited in later chapters as the physiological bases of major mental disorders are explored. Here, an overview of functional neuroanatomy is presented (see figure 3-E). It focuses only on those brain structures and systems currently believed to underlie psychiatric disorders.

The Hypothalamus

This primitive brain center is about the size of a pea and lies at the base of the brain. It is a complex structure and is responsible for regulating a host of biologic functions, including the following: the circadian rhythm, sleep cycles, appetite, sex drive, and regulation of both the autonomic nervous system and almost all of the endocrine glands. The now-familiar neurotransmitters, serotonin, norepinephrine, and dopamine, are thought to be crucial in regulating certain aspects of hypothalamic

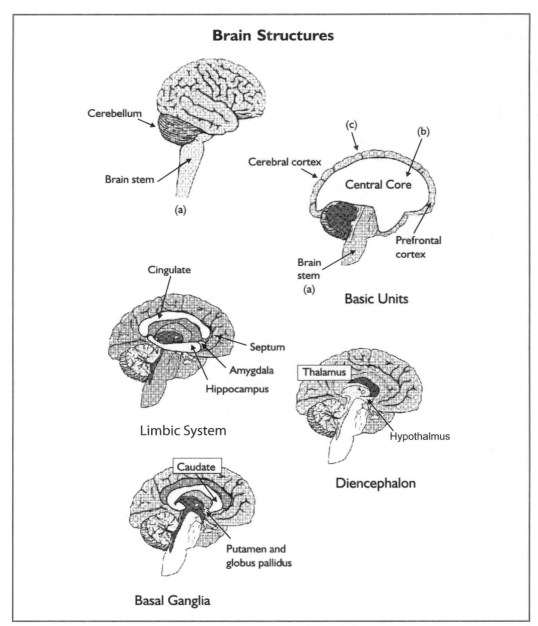

Brain Structures

Cerebellum

Brain stem

(a)

(c)

(b)

Cerebral cortex

Central Core

Prefrontal cortex

Brain stem

(a)

Basic Units

Cingulate

Septum

Amygdala

Hippocampus

Limbic System

Thalamus

Hypothalmus

Diencephalon

Caudate

Putamen and globus pallidus

Basal Ganglia

Figure 3-C

functioning. The hypothalamus is intimately connected to the structures of the limbic system and to the pituitary gland.

The Limbic System: The "Emotional Brain"

The structures of the limbic system (amygdala, septum, cingulate, and hippocampus) are common to all mammals (see figure 3-C). The limbic system is involved in three primary functions: the appraisal of emotional stimuli, initiation of emotional responses (e.g., the "fight-or-flight" response), and, finally, shutting down reactivity

Neuroanatomy, Psychological Functions, and Psychopathology

Brain Structure	Functions	Psychopathology
Cortex	Higher cognitive processing	Dementia, confusional states
Prefrontal cortex	Impulse control, attention, behavioral monitoring, organization of complex information processing	Attention-deficit disorder, schizophrenia, obsessive-compulsive disorder, depression
Diencephalon		
thalamus	Many nerves pass through this brain structure	Not implicated in major psychiatric disorders
hypothalamus	Regulates sleep cycles, hunger, sex drive; controls endocrine and autonomic nervous system; influences immune system	Depression, anxiety disorders, sleep disorders
Limbic system		
amygdala	Elicits and controls aggression, primitive threat appraisal	Impulse control disorders, depression, borderline personality disorder,* anxiety disorders
septum	Emotional and stimulus "gate," pleasure centers	Schizophrenia, impulse control disorders, addictive disorders
cingulate	Neuronal pathways connecting limbic system structures and prefrontal lobes; affect regulation	Obsessive-compulsive disorder, anxiety disorders
hippocampus	Recent memory, new learning, impulse and emotional control	Alzheimer's disease, postconcussion syndrome, depression
Basal ganglia	Controls aspects of motor behavior; obsessive-compulsive disorder	Parkinson's disease, antipsychotic medication side effects (extrapyramidal symptoms [EPS])
Brain stem		
reticular system	Neuronal pathways connecting limbic system and prefrontal lobes; stimulus filter or "gate"	Attention-deficit disorder, schizophrenia

* likely, but not proven

Figure 3-D

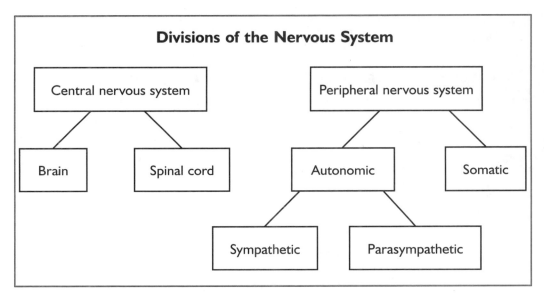

Divisions of the Nervous System

Central nervous system

Peripheral nervous system

Brain

Spinal cord

Autonomic

Somatic

Sympathetic

Parasympathetic

Figure 3-E

after external stressors subside (and restoring the nervous system and body to a state of homeostasis).

A highly detailed discussion of the limbic system is beyond the scope of this book, although we will address several basic issues here.

Information Processing

Incoming sensory information is appraised by way of two main processing centers in the brain. The cerebral cortex (the most highly evolved part of the brain) is capable of complex information processing and critical thinking. A parallel system exists subcortically. The amygdala (there are two amygdalae in the brain; one in each temporal lobe) has the capacity to register, perceive, and analyze sensory data also. However, the appraisal of environmental stressors, at the level of the amygdala, is crude. This brain structure is able to engage in gross pattern recognition, and if such patterns resemble objects or events previously associated with danger, neuronal impulses exiting the amygdala elicit a fight-or-flight response (independent of the cerebral cortex). Since perception at the amygdala level is often rapid, crude, and inexact, there are many false alarms (for example, misperceiving a piece of rope as a snake). However, this primitive fear-appraisal system is believed to be adaptive and ultimately aids or facilitates survival (Le Doux 1996).

Igniting the Fight-or-Flight Response

When a person is confronted with a stressor, as noted above, this is perceived and interpreted on two levels (cortical and subcortical), and an emotional response is initiated. The main pathway for this involves neuronal activation of the hypothalamus by the amygdala.

At the level of the hypothalamus, three primary stress-response pathways are activated (these are illustrated in more detail in figures 9-B and 9-C in chapter 9). The first, and most immediately felt response to a perceived danger, is evoked by the sympathetic nervous system (SNS). Nerves of the SNS go to almost all areas of the body and immediately release norepinephrine. This readily activates adrenergic receptors and causes increased heart rate, increased blood pressure, and sweating. SNS nerves also penetrate to the core of the adrenal gland (the adrenal medulla), which then discharges norepinephrine and adrenaline into the bloodstream.

The two additional pathways are termed neuroendocrine (i.e., brain activation of endocrine glands). The hypothalamic-pituitary-adrenal pathway (commonly called the HPA axis) results in the release of steroid hormones from the adrenal gland (this class of hormones includes glucocorticoids, which facilitate the release of glucose into circulation). In humans, the main glucocorticoid is cortisol.

The second neuroendocrine pathway is the hypothalamic-pituitary-thyroid axis. When activated, it causes the release of the two thyroid hormones: thyroxine (T4) and triiodothyronine (T3). The combined effect of these primary stress hormones, along with SNS activation, is to quickly mobilize the body to take action to avoid danger (fight or flight).

Return to Baseline

Finally, the various stress hormones, which are circulated throughout the bloodstream, reenter the brain and trigger a shutting down of the stress response. This process of hormonal feedback allows the nervous system to regulate itself and, when danger subsides, to return to a state of homeostasis.

The hippocampus is one of the most important limbic structures that reduces arousal; in a sense, it turns off the stress response (specifically, it shuts off the HPA axis). The hippocampi (again, one in each temporal lobe) are densely populated with glucocorticoid receptors (GR). When cortisol molecules reach the hippocampus and bind to the GRs, that activates the hippocampus, which then exerts inhibitory control over the hypothalamus and thus deactivates the stress response. Feedback and inhibition also take place at the levels of the hypothalamus and pituitary. Additionally, some evidence exists suggesting that the anterior (i.e., most frontal aspect) cingulate gyrus also plays a role in reducing emotional arousal (Mayberg 1997).

Peripheral Nervous System

As figure 3-E indicates, in addition to the CNS (brain and spinal cord), the nervous system contains a further division, the peripheral nervous system (PNS). Within the PNS is the somatic division, which controls voluntary action of the skeletal muscles and carries information from sensory organs to the CNS.

A second branch of the peripheral nervous system is the autonomic nervous system (ANS). The ANS innervates involuntary organs, such as the heart, smooth muscles, and glands. Further divisions of the peripheral ANS are the sympathetic and parasympathetic systems. These systems generally can be thought of as antagonistic, although this is not absolute for every activity. Most organs are innervated by both systems, and regulation is established through opposing functions.

The sympathetic nervous system (SNS) plays a role in the fight-or-flight response. Set in motion by activity in the limbic system and hypothalamus, the SNS mobilizes the body to take action in response to dangerous situations. Conversely, the parasympathetic system, which is activated at times of relaxation and quiescence, acts to reduce heart rate and blood pressure in an overall attempt to conserve energy (see figure 3-F).

Effects of SNS and PNS Activity on Target Organs

Organ or Gland	Sympathetic Actions	Parasympathetic Actions
Pupils	Dilate	Constrict
Salivary glands	Reduce secretions	Secrete
Lungs (bronchi)	Dilate	Constrict
Heart	Increase rate	Slow rate
GI tract	Interrupt digestion	Digest
Adrenal gland	Secrete	—
Bladder	—	Empty fluids
Arteries	Constrict	Relax

Figure 3-F

Side Effects Affecting Autonomic Nervous System

Parasympathetic System—Anticholinergic Effects	Sympathetic System—Adrenergic Effects
Blurry vision	Hypotension (low norepinephrine)
Dry mouth	Rapid heart rate (elevated norepinephrine)
Constipation	
Urine retention	

Figure 3-G

Many psychotropic medications can, unfortunately, affect the parasympathetic and sympathetic nervous systems, thus producing side effects. The parasympathetic system is mediated by the chemical acetylcholine. As we shall see in subsequent chapters, many psychiatric medications have anticholinergic effects (that is, they block acetylcholine) with resulting side effects (see figure 3-G).

The sympathetic system is mediated primarily by norepinephrine. (Nerve cells activated by norepinephrine, epinephrine, and related compounds are called adrenergic nerves.) Certain psychotropic medications either block or activate adrenergic neurons in the SNS, again producing undesirable effects.

Pathways to Psychopathology

Certainly a number of psychiatric disorders do not appear to involve gross dysfunction in underlying neurobiology or neurochemistry. Such disorders may aptly be seen primarily as either psychological reactions to psychosocial stressors and/or characterological or temperamental difficulties. However, an increasing number of psychiatric disorders are being found to have neurobiologic aspects; either a primary biological problem is the sole cause, or brain changes have resulted from encounters with stressful life events.

Among those disorders that have a biologic element, let us consider the following:

- Genetically transmitted vulnerability, which may manifest in psychiatric disorder. This includes disorders such as schizophrenia, bipolar disorder, major depression, and attention-deficit disorder. Other conditions that may be related to genetic factors include these: obsessive-compulsive disorder, panic disorder, and some substance abuse disorders.

- Nonneurologic medical illnesses that ultimately affect neurochemistry (e.g., thyroid disease).

- Acquired brain dysfunction, due to multiple causes such as brain trauma, toxins, chronic effects of substance abuse, primary brain diseases (e.g., brain tumors, Alzheimer's disease, and so on), prenatal factors that have caused abnormal brain development, for example, fetal alcohol exposure, and so on.

- Abnormal brain development due to excessive stress. Considerable research strongly suggests that very severe stress can alter brain functioning in more or less permanent ways. Most notable are the effects of severe neglect or abuse early in life (this will be explored in greater detail in chapter 12 on post-traumatic stress disorder) (Nemeroff 1997; Lewis, Amini, and Lennon 2000).

- Brain damage caused by exposure to excessively high levels of stress hormones (e.g., abnormally high levels of cortisol, often seen in major depression, may damage nerve cells in the hippocampus). For details see chapter 7 on depression (Sapolksy 1996).

What has become abundantly clear is that the older and more categorical model of *"either* biological *or* psychological" etiology is no longer a relevant schema. Primary biological disorders do exist, but whether or not they become manifest may be highly dependent on the effects of psychological stress. Conversely, severe and prolonged stress can often transform a rather pure "psychological disorder" after weeks or months, until we see changes in brain chemistry and stress hormones emerge.

Psychological treatments are often effective in treating many psychiatric illnesses and (as some research is beginning to show) may in fact alter or improve underlying neurobiology (Gabbard 2000). However, when significant abnormalities in brain functioning exist, biologic interventions such as pharmacotherapy may be necessary.

4

Pharmacology

Psychiatry, perhaps uniquely in health care, operates from an established multidisciplinary approach. The opportunity, as well as the responsibility, exists for all clinicians to be involved in medication decisions as appropriate to their discipline. As treatment approaches in mental health continue to evolve, it is likely that current practices will expand and demand participation from knowledgeable therapists.

From a practical standpoint, possessing fundamental knowledge is critical in the rapidly changing field of psychopharmacology, along with the attendant challenge of understanding emerging treatments, new applications of existing medications, and multiple drug regimens. Additionally, medical comorbidity in psychiatric patients (coexisting medical illness and psychiatric disorder) mandates at least a familiarity with psychotropics' potential actions and interactions with various nonpsychotropic therapeutic agents.

In your practice as a psychotherapist, it is not essential to become an expert in the area of physiology, pharmacology, or biochemistry. However, it is important to become generally familiar with a few preliminary concepts, which will lay a groundwork for the clinical chapters that follow. This chapter presents basic pharmacologic principles, defines terminologies commonly found in later chapters of this book (and in standard medical or medication texts), and integrates factual information about medication effects on organ systems and at the cellular level.

Basic Principles of Pharmacokinetics

The broad definition of a drug as "any substance that brings about a change in biologic function through its chemical actions" (Katzung 2001) is helpful in understanding the relationship between the body and administered medications. This is a fluid and interactive process, composed of two elements: *pharmacodynamics* and *pharmacokinetics*.

Pharmacodynamics can be viewed as the drug's effect on the body (discussed in detail for specific drugs in part three of this book). Conversely, pharmacokinetics can be considered the body's effect on the drug. There are four basic pharmacokinetic factors: *absorption, distribution, biotransformation,* and *excretion* (see figure 4-A). Every drug will exhibit a unique kinetic profile (like a fingerprint) composed of these factors. This chapter provides a general description of pharmacokinetic principles and their significance in clinical practice. (Expanded discussion for each area of pharmacokinetics is provided in appendix A.)

Absorption

Most drugs are initially, and predominantly, absorbed in the stomach or small intestine. The degree of absorption in the digestive tract can be affected by patient-dependent factors, such as whether the medication is taken with or without food. Further, as a drug proceeds to its ultimate destination, it may have numerous barriers to cross, depending on the absorption characteristics of the drug itself. For instance, in the central nervous system (CNS), the blood-brain barrier allows passage of only certain molecules into the brain. Penetration of medication into the CNS is restricted by a host of factors that protect the CNS from exposure to toxins, although this barrier is not absolute or impenetrable. (See appendix A for discussion of related factors of bioavailability and first-pass phenomena.)

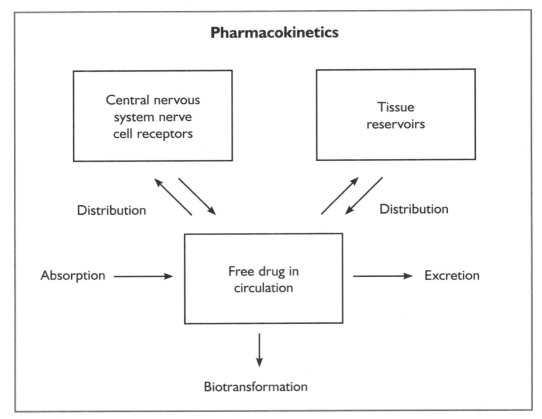

Figure 4-A

Case 6

Patricia A. is a forty-five-year-old female referred to the day treatment program at your hospital. She is an intelligent, energetic woman whose chief complaint is "difficulty remembering things." She is moderately anxious about this symptom, since she is expecting to return to work in two weeks after a six-month medical leave of absence. She was diagnosed with breast cancer seven months ago, for which she received chemotherapy and radiation treatment. Tests indicate that her cancer has not spread, and her physician reports an excellent prognosis.

Patricia is a member of a support group for cancer survivors, which has helped her "tremendously." She hopes someone in your program can help her "get a handle on this memory thing." Her job requires that she retain and recall detailed numerical data, and she does not want to return to work at "less than 100 percent." You will provide psychotherapy to her on a daily basis for the next ten days.

During your initial session with her, she tells you that she is sure that her memory loss is related to the effects of her chemotherapy, and is therefore somewhat doubtful that you will be able to help her. You find that this might be a reasonable question to pursue before proceeding too far in therapy with her. Your program relies heavily on interdisciplinary treatment, so you request psychological testing from the psychologist and a medication review from the pharmacist. Psychological testing results show Patricia to be above average in intelligence with no evidence of organicity or personality disorder. The pharmacist reports that none of the chemotherapeutic agents that Patricia received crosses the blood-brain barrier appreciably or affects healthy brain tissue.

Typical memory loss secondary to cancer treatment is short term and is usually attributable to pretreatment antianxiety medications. Based on these reports, you feel confident in moving ahead with therapy and exploring Patricia's anxiety and memory loss from a nonorganic focus.

Distribution

Once a drug has been absorbed and reaches the bloodstream, it is then distributed to various organs or sites of action throughout the body. Certain medications have characteristic distribution patterns, which are extremely important in understanding response to treatment. A critical example in psychiatry is the extensive depositing of tricyclic antidepressants and antipsychotic medications in fat and muscle cells. In effect, these areas act as reservoirs or holding tanks. In some instances, concentrations of a drug in reservoir areas will exceed levels in the bloodstream. This explains why serum levels of antidepressants are not absolutely indicative of total body concentration. (See appendix A for a detailed description of distribution phases and protein binding.)

Case 7

Helen P. is an obese twenty-seven-year-old woman who has been taking the antidepressant desipramine. She was started on a low dose and gradually increased to a dose of 300 mg daily, which she has been taking for the past three months. Even though Helen has only in the last two months been able to notice an effect, she now reports a significant improvement in her depression and no side effects. Her physician has forwarded results of periodic desipramine blood levels to you, and all are within therapeutic range. However, Helen recently discovered that a coworker also takes this medication, in a dose of 150 mg daily, and is doing well. She reveals to you that, without consulting her physician, she has cut her dose in half over the last two weeks because she thinks her dosage was too high.

You firmly encourage Helen to discuss this matter with her doctor, and point out to her that a dose of 300 mg is still within the standard accepted dosage range and that blood-level monitoring has shown this dose to be right for her. You further remind her of the risk and consequences if her depression should recur. Because you are aware that this tricyclic antidepressant is probably extensively stored in her fat tissue, you are able to provide needed reassurance that her treatment is reasonable and being safely monitored.

Biotransformation

The body's reaction to drugs as foreign substances results in several processes of elimination, one being metabolism (biotransformation) and the other excretion. Metabolism occurs primarily in the liver, via specific action of enzymes that change the original chemical into compounds that are more easily excreted by the kidneys. Biotransformation is a complex process. Understanding metabolic activity is crucial in medication management, especially when medication treatment is not working adequately.

When medications are chemically altered by the process of biotransformation, the results are the production of numerous chemical by-products, called *metabolites*. Some metabolites are useful and desirable, in that they produce desired effects; for instance, the reduction of psychiatric symptoms. Unfortunately, some metabolites affect various bodily tissues and result in undesirable side effects. In addition, since most medications undergo significant metabolism, the risks of drug *toxicity* (poisoning due to excessively high levels of a drug) must be considered whenever metabolism is impaired. Antidepressants, antipsychotics, and anticonvulsants are all extensively metabolized by liver enzymes. Thus, impaired liver functioning can result in abnormal metabolism of these medications. Conversely, increased activity of liver enzymes can cause excessive metabolism, resulting in a decreased drug level and an inadequate response to treatment. (Appendix A contains additional information regarding metabolic enzymes and drug metabolites.)

Case 8

Susan is a forty-five-year-old woman whom you have seen in therapy, off and on, for several years. You have diagnosed her with dysthymia, and currently she meets the criteria for major depression. In the past, you and her primary care physician have recommended antidepressant treatment, which she has declined. She is motivated to "manage her moods" without chemicals, and maintains a regular exercise regimen and stays in close contact with friends when she feels sad. However, she reports recent worsening of insomnia and daytime fatigue and is finding it harder to keep herself "under control." Her doctor has suggested she may be perimenopausal, which can be associated with sleep disturbance and mood lability.

Due to her worsening symptoms, she reluctantly agreed to antidepressant treatment. Six weeks ago her doctor prescribed paroxetine (Paxil), 20 mg daily, with an upward titration from 10 mg daily for the first five days. Susan experienced extreme drowsiness, dry mouth, and constipation, and stopped the medication after two weeks. Her physician then prescribed venlafaxine (Effexor), at a very low starting dose, but again, after several weeks, Susan continued to experience intolerable side effects of dizziness, blurred vision, and profuse sweating. She agreed to one more trial of an antidepressant, although she expressed her frustration with this aspect of treatment. She is currently taking sertraline (Zoloft), 75 mg daily and, after two weeks, has tolerated the medication well. She is encouraged by the lack of side effects compared to the other antidepressants and is willing to continue taking it as long as necessary.

You are curious as to the pattern of side-effect response that Susan experienced and confer with her doctor. Her physician speculates that Susan may be a slow metabolizer of medications metabolized by the CYP2D6* system, which is the case for paroxetine and venlafaxine. Slow metabolizers often experience severe side effects to low or average doses of medications. This assumption is supported by Susan's tolerability of sertraline, which is metabolized by the CYP2C9* and CYP3A* systems.

Excretion

Excretion is the process by which drugs are eliminated from the body. Excretion occurs primarily via the kidneys, although other routes include the gastrointestinal tract; the respiratory system; and sweat, saliva, and breast milk. Adequate excretion is dependent on effective kidney function. Disease- or drug-induced damage to the kidneys can lead to kidney failure, resulting in a toxic accumulation of medications in the bloodstream.

An important characteristic of medications is the *half-life* ($t_{1/2}$), which is defined as the amount of time required for the serum concentration to be reduced by 50 percent (Benet, Mitchell, and Sherner 1990b). Half-life is used to determine dosage amounts and intervals for most medications.

Half-life measurements are used to estimate the time required for a drug to reach what is called *steady state*. Steady state occurs when concentrations of a medication in the bloodstream have reached a plateau so that the amount administered is equal to the amount being eliminated. It is generally accepted that for most drugs, steady state is attained after four half-lives; for example if the half-life is twenty-four hours, then steady state is usually reached in four days. It is important to remember that reaching steady state does not always correspond to a drug's onset of desired action. With antidepressants, for instance, steady state will be reached long before a therapeutic effect is noted. (See figure 4-B; also see appendix A for discussion of a related topic, the therapeutic index.)

---

* These are specific classes of liver enzymes (see appendix A).

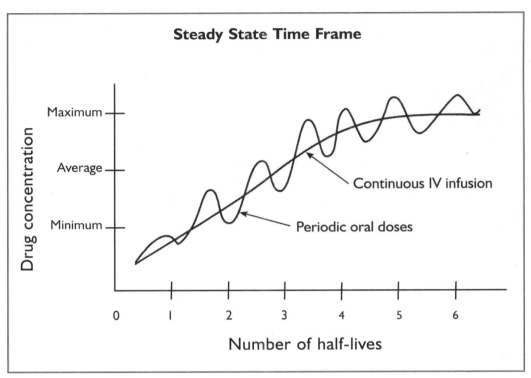

Figure 4-B

Case 9

Frank is a twenty-four-year-old honor student, majoring in engineering, whom you have been seeing for four months through the student counseling center. He initially presented with major depression, although he has never been suicidal. He has significant narcissistic and passive-aggressive traits. He began treatment with Prozac, 20 mg daily in the morning, two weeks ago. His agreement to take medications came after much discussion with you and the psychiatrist, including detailed information regarding dosage range, onset of action, and side effects.

During today's session, he angrily informs you that the medication is not working and challenges you to answer some questions he has formulated after extensive online research. His opinion, based on mathematical calculations, is that the drug has had plenty of time to reach a therapeutic level. He concludes that "the whole idea is some sort of placebo experiment" and threatens to terminate treatment.

This behavior is characteristic of Frank, and you respond in a calm and nondefensive way. You acknowledge his need to thoroughly understand the medication and that it can be frustrating to wait for indicators that the drug is working. However, you remind him that the typical response time for most antidepressants is three to four weeks and is not absolutely related to serum level of the medication. You suggest other sources of information, written for patients, which may more specifically address his needs. You also offer encouragement that he has tolerated the medication without significant side effects.

Medication Effects

When medications are chemically reorganized into various metabolites, these resulting compounds produce a variety of effects—some desirable, some undesirable. All medications, including psychotropics, typically have five primary effects:

- *Pharmacological effect*—the desired therapeutic effect, such as antipsychotics reducing hallucinations.

- *Side effects*—typically considered to be undesirable effects, such as constipation, dry mouth, blurry vision, and so on. Occasionally, side effects can be used to benefit the patient; for example, using a medication's sedating side effect to help an anxious patient fall asleep at night. Side effects, although generally undesirable, are by definition fairly common and predictable and may be somewhat preventable. Side effects are generally considered extensions of the pharmacological properties of a drug and account for 70 to 80 percent of adverse drug events (Glazener 1992).

- *Idiosyncratic effects*—extremely rare, adverse effects that are difficult to predict. They are often specific to an individual or to certain groups of patients who share common genetic or biologic features.

- *Allergic reactions*—some individuals have an immune response to medications, generally a skin rash or hypersensitivity. The body may respond to the medication as if it were a foreign substance or organism, and produce allergic symptoms. A severe type of allergic reaction, called *anaphylaxis*, can include difficulty breathing, fever, and irregular heart beat. Anaphylactic reactions are potentially fatal, as is, for example, an allergy to penicillin.

- *Discontinuance syndrome*—response to stopping or interrupting medication treatment. Examples are narcotic withdrawal or "cholinergic rebound" when tricyclic antidepressants or antipsychotics are abruptly stopped.

Drug Interactions

Basic pharmacologic principles apply as much to drug *interactions* as to drug actions. Each kinetic property—absorption, distribution, metabolism (biotransformation), and excretion—is potentially affected by the presence of coadministered medications. Drug interactions involving metabolism are of particular clinical significance. The reader is referred to appendix A for an expanded discussion on this topic. Drug interactions follow a variable time-course pattern, from immediate to delayed. Consequently, it is important to remember that several weeks may elapse before the effects of an interactive combination are evident.

And the comorbidity of medical and psychiatric disorders requires at least some degree of multiple drug prescribing. For example, many patients suffering from serious physical disorders as well as depression will require medication treatment for both conditions. Examples include diabetes mellitus, cancer, and cardiovascular disease. Familiarity with drug interactions can be an important addition to diagnostic skills.

Although significant interactions for specific drugs will be addressed in subsequent chapters, case 10 illustrates the most frequently encountered of all drug interactions, enzyme inhibition (Hansten and Horn 1990). This interaction occurs when two drugs rely on the same enzyme system for metabolism. In this "competition," one drug usually wins over the other and is preferentially and completely metabolized. Conversely, metabolism of the other drug is inhibited, leading to an increased serum level. This increase can at times produce greater effectiveness than anticipated from a given dose, or it can produce serious adverse effects, such as toxicity.

Case 10

Eugene is a sixty-year-old man who is being treated for a first episode of major depression. Eugene's wife died unexpectedly a year ago, and he has had difficulty "coming to terms" with life alone. He reports decreased appetite, sleep disturbance, tearfulness, and anhedonia. He began taking 10 mg of fluoxetine daily one week ago and is scheduled to increase his dose tomorrow to 20 mg daily. This is his first psychiatric treatment. Eugene has a history of hypertension, which has been well controlled for many years with metoprolol, a beta-blocker.

This week, during your session with Eugene he appeared fatigued and complained of shortness of breath and light-headedness. His blood pressure, taken at home the morning you saw him, was 100 over 60. He asked you if the antidepressant could be causing these side effects. You recommended that Eugene see his doctor that same day. You called and arranged for an appointment after your session was over. Eugene's physician called you later that day to report that Eugene's blood pressure and pulse were both dangerously low, which she suspected was due to a drug interaction between fluoxetine and metoprolol, causing an increased level of the latter. Eugene's doctor changed his antidepressant to citalopram (Celexa), which he tolerates without problems.

There is a likelihood that psychiatric patients (especially older people) will receive multiple medications. People with clinical syndromes that include associated physical symptoms, such as anxiety disorders and depression, are often initially treated by a nonpsychiatrist prescriber. The medications prescribed can include gastrointestinal agents, antihypertensives, analgesics, and sedative-hypnotics. Subsequent referral to a psychiatrist may result in the addition of a psychotropic medication. Thus the psychotherapist may ultimately inherit this patient with the attendant possibilities of drug interactions.

The presentation of this material does not suggest that psychotherapists are responsible for identifying and monitoring drug interactions. That is a job best left to physicians and pharmacists. However, in certain cases the effects of interactive drugs will be evident in therapy. For example, when a previously good medication response has abated, or when the intensity of side effects is inconsistent with dosage, ruling out drug interactions is helpful. Also, psychotherapists often have more complete information about a client's treatment than do individual physicians, each of whom may be independently prescribing potentially interactive medications. In these situations, it is the psychotherapist who often sounds the initial warning.

Medication Effects on a Cellular Level

For most psychiatric medications to have an effect on symptoms, they must first gain entrance to the brain. (Notable exceptions are most beta-blockers, which have an effect primarily in the peripheral, not in the central nervous system. See chapter 1.) The central nervous system is protected by dense membranes and tightly packed capillaries, collectively referred to as the *blood-brain barrier*. The blood-brain barrier controls chemical access to the brain, preventing the entry of a host of molecules that could be potentially toxic to the brain. Drugs that are *lipophilic* are generally better able to penetrate the blood-brain barrier, and most effective psychiatric medications are highly lipophilic. Once in the brain, the next step is for medications to have an effect on individual nerve cells.

As noted in the previous chapter, the functioning of nerve cells is maintained or altered by the effects of various molecules, which are able to bind to receptors located on the surface of neuronal cell bodies, dendrites, and nerve terminals. (Note: Some receptors are also found in the interior of nerve cell bodies.) Molecules that are able to bind to a receptor are referred to as ligands. Ligands include neurotransmitters, hormones, and certain exogenous agents such as drugs, or trace elements (e.g., lithium), and some chemicals found in foods and herbs.

For a ligand to bind to a receptor, it must have a highly specific molecular shape, much in the same way that a key must precisely fit a lock in order to open it.

Cellular response to ligand binding: There are two fundamental ways to understand the cellular response. The first involves an *agonist* effect, where a ligand activates the receptor. The second involves an *antagonist* effect, which occurs when a ligand occupies a receptor site but does not activate it. The process of *antagonism*, also known as *blocking*, prevents other molecules from activating the receptor. This has been likened to the lock-and-key metaphor again, in that some keys can be inserted into a lock, but if it is not the right key, it cannot open the lock. However, as long as it occupies the lock, other keys cannot be inserted; that is, it blocks the lock.

The nervous system must be capable of making adaptive responses to changes in the external environment (e.g., stressors) and to shifts in the internal biologic milieu. Receptors represent a physiological mechanism by which stimulation can influence the action of nerve cells. Via agonism or antagonism of receptors, a host of molecules (including psychiatric medications) can have an impact on cellular functioning.

Specific Receptors, Receptor Actions; Drug Effects and Side Effects

The ideal psychiatric drug would be a highly selective molecule that would be targeted to bind to a specific receptor on specific nerve cells in the brain *and* have no effect on other receptors or neurons. It would also be administered in the most direct and convenient way possible for the patient. Such drugs do not exist, but are highly sought after by pharmaceutical companies. Three major problems stand in the way of development of such ideal drugs.

First, many molecules, owing to their unique molecular shape, inadvertently bind to more than one receptor. For example, a number of antipsychotics bind not only to postsynaptic dopamine receptors (which creates a dopamine blockade and presumably accounts for antipsychotic effects), but also lock onto acetylcholine muscurinic receptors (this can result in a number of side effects, including memory impairment, blurry vision, and constipation, to mention but a few of the common anticholinergic side effects).

A second problem is that a particular drug molecule, for example, binds to some dopamine receptors in the limbic system, producing desired, antipsychotic effects. However, it simultaneously binds to other dopamine receptors, but they are located in the basal ganglia, where it produces significant extrapyramidal side effects (such as tremors). Such drug molecules cannot be delivered to just one part of the brain and be sequestered there, but rather, they are disseminated to numerous brain regions.

The third problem is that, among classes of receptors, numerous subtypes have been discovered and drug molecules typically do not just interact with one subtype. For example, currently fourteen different serotonin receptors have been identified. Drugs that, in a global sense, increase brain serotonin levels, have multiple effects since some serotonin receptors are inhibitory and some are excitatory.

The pharmacologist may want to target serotonin (abbreviated 5-HT) 5-HT1a receptors to have an antidepressant effect, but also can't help but activate all other 5-HT receptor subtypes, provoking numerous side effects. Thus, the development of highly selective molecules that potentially could target particular receptor subtypes, and leave others alone, is the dream and the challenge for many pharmaceutical company chemists. An important perspective for understanding medication effects and side effects requires a knowledge of the various types of receptors that are found on the surfaces of particular nerve cells in the brain; it also requires becoming familiar with the assortment of actions that drugs have on the receptors. Many hundreds of receptors have been identified, but a smaller and more manageable list of those most relevant to psychopharmacology are outlined next (see figure 4-C).

Identification and classification of serotonin receptors is a complex and rapidly changing field. Seven families of serotonin receptors (5-HT1 through 5-HT7) and at least fifteen subpopulations have been identified. No pharmacologic agent exhibits single-receptor specificity, making it difficult to attribute effects and side effects to a single serotonin receptor subtype. Functional receptor activity does not necessarily translate to clinically relevant pharmacological properties. Any attempt to describe the full array of known, or hypothesized, serotonin receptors and effects is beyond the scope of this book. Figure 4-D summarizes the 5-HT receptor types presumed to be dysregulated in various psychiatric disorders. Figure 4-E provides currently suggested properties of serotonin receptors and psychiatric drugs.

Specific Receptor Actions

Receptors[a]	Action	Drugs That Can Produce This Action	Desired Effects	Adverse Effects
NE (in general)	Activate	Antidepressants	Antidepressant	Sympathomimetic (increase heart rate, blood pressure, sweating, tremors, jitteriness, and anxiety)
NE α-1	Activate	Antidepressants	Increase alertness	Increase blood pressure
NE α-2[b]	Activate	Clonidine	Decrease aggression; reduces hyperactivity	Decrease blood pressure, causes light headedness
NE α-2	Block	Yohimbine	Combats sexual dysfunction	Sympathomimetic
DA	Block	Antipsychotics	Antipsychotic	Counters extrapyramidal effects, apathy, emotional blunting; increases prolactin secretion
DA	Activate	Cocaine, stimulants, Wellbutrin	Antidepressant, reduces hyperactivity	Psychosis, anxiety
HI	Block	Benadryl, tricyclics, some antipsychotics	Sedation (to promote sleep)	Sedation, weight gain, hypotension
ACH	Block	Tricyclics, some antipsychotics, Paxil	Reduces acute extrapyramidal effects	Constipation, urinary retention, blurred vision, increased heart rate, memory impairment, confusion, dry mouth

(a) Receptor abbreviations: NE (norepinephrine), 5-HT (serotonin), DA (dopamine), H-I (histamine), Ach (acetylcholine/muscurinic).

(b) NE α-2 receptors are inhibitory and thus stimulating them, in essence, activates a braking mechanism and reduces arousal.

Figure 4-C

Symptoms/Conditions	Possible 5-HT Receptor(s) Involved
Anxiety	5-HT1A, 5-HT2A
Depression	5-HT1A, 5-HT2
Psychosis	5-HT1A, 5-HT2A/C, 5-HT6, 5-HT7
Aggression, Impulsivity	5-HT1A
Craving	5-HT1A, 5-HT3, 5-HT4
Depression	5-HT1A, 5-HT2
Memory, Cognition	5-HT3, 5-HT4, 5-HT5, 5-HT6
Pain	5-HT2A

Figure 4-D

Specific Receptor Actions

Receptor	Action	Drugs That Can Produce This Action	Physiological Effects	Side Effects
5-HT1A	Activate	Buspirone	Antianxiety	Sedation, headache, low blood pressure
5-HT1A 5-HT2A/2C	Activate	SSRIs	Antidepressant	GI symptoms, headache, insomnia, restlessness, sexual dysfunction
5-HT2A	Activate	LSD	Hallucinogenic	
5-HT2A/2C[a]	Block	Antipsychotics, especially second generation	Antipsychotic	Sedation, weight gain, low incidence of EPS

(a) 5-HT2 inhibitory are receptors on the surface of dopamine neurons. Thus when stimulated (i.e., activates the brake), it reduces dopamine activity. When this happens in the basal ganglia, it can cause extrapyramidal effects and amotiviation. If 5-HT2 receptors are blocked on dopamine nerve cells in the frontal cortex, it can reduce apathy and amotivation (i.e., reduce the negative symptoms of schizophrenia).

Figure 4-E

5

Medication Nonadherence

Both in general medicine and psychiatry, the number one cause of treatment failure is not taking medications as prescribed. In numerous studies people with chronic illnesses often discontinue their medications or do not take them as prescribed (Shea, 2006). A preeminent writer on the topic of noncompliance (nonadherence) is psychiatrist Shawn Shea. Many of his insightful ideas are mentioned in this chapter. There are a number of reasons for nonadherence. Those commonly seen in patients treated with psychiatric drugs include the following.

Many psychotropic medications require weeks of treatment before the first signs of clinical improvement are experienced. Most psychiatric disorders (most notably, depression) result in pessimistic and hopeless feelings in the patient. Even if they have been told about the need to wait in order to see improvement, patients frequently conclude that the drug is not working out, and they discontinue the medication. They also may drop out of treatment altogether. What makes this especially difficult to deal with is that they often do not share their feelings and concerns with the treatment provider. Thirty percent of depressed patients never fill the first prescription, which is a testament to the impact of feelings of hopelessness interfering with treatment.

Side effects often lead to discontinuation of medication. At times, side effects are intense and unpleasant enough to frighten the patient. A common example is when the side effect *activation* (acute onset anxiety) occurs after the first dose of an antidepressant that was prescribed for a person suffering from an anxiety disorder. Intense anxiety may not only lead to medication discontinuation, but also leave the patient traumatized to the point of deciding never to seek psychiatric treatment again. This decision (especially for those with chronic mental illnesses) can lead to lifelong consequences (i.e., never again seeking treatment that could potentially do a lot to reduce their suffering). Often side effects such as weight gain or sexual dysfunction are the cause of patient-initiated discontinuation.

Missing doses is another contributing factor to nonadherence. This is more likely to occur when a patient is taking medications that require multiple dosing during the day (e.g., twice-a-day dosing). This certainly occurs for many people in general who

Medications and Side-Effect Sensitivity

Extreme sensitivity to any drug may foster noncompliance. There are three important issues to explore when this problem emerges.

Sensitivity and significant side effects may be due to pharmacokinetics. Patients who metabolize poorly (slowly) may experience high blood levels of a medication, which can result in excessive side effects. Initial low doses and gradual titration often solve this problem. However, some people continue to experience intolerable side effects. The two options are to switch to another medication or to "microdose." Here the patient is given very low doses of a medication (e.g., 1 mg Prozac). Some tablets can be cut into smaller pieces (note: caution is warranted here when the medication is a sustained-release formulation, because in these cases, cutting the pill may create problems with drug delivery). Many medications are available in liquid form, allowing for microdosing. Or *compounding pharmacies* can formulate medicines that deliver tiny doses of a drug. Some patients who report, "I have always been too sensitive to side effects," have never been treated via microdosing. It often is an effective strategy.

The following may be helpful when patients are overly sensitive to what might be considered a minor side effect. One of the authors (J. P.) recalls when—especially in the days of tricyclic antidepressants—very severely depressed patients would be given a prescription for a tricyclic. At the next appointment, a week later, the patient would be asked how it was going with the medication and would respond,

are being treated for a variety of medical illnesses, but it's often even more pronounced in psychiatric patients. Impaired memory (seen in many mental illnesses) may be a significant factor. Complex dosing—for instance, taking a number of different medications—can also be a factor contributing to missed doses.

Fears and worries about adverse medication effects, such as addiction, are not uncommon. (These fears exist not only for patients, but also for parents who have their child in treatment.) Another common and very understandable fear has to do with possible increases in suicidality in those taking antidepressants. Antidepressant advertisements on television always state that increased suicidality may occur with antidepressants (this issue is addressed in detail in chapter 23). One of the biggest problems is when such fears go unexpressed; patients may, for various reasons, not tell their doctors. If the concerns are brought to the prescriber's attention, it is generally addressed by providing information from studies that show, for instance, that stimulant treatment for ADHD actually decreases rates of substance abuse in teens with ADHD. Or it may be addressed through discussion of the complex issues anticipated with antidepressant treatment and possible increases in suicidality. However, often, providing this kind of information is not effective. What patients and parents need first is to really be heard. There is a time and place to provide information about these risks, but until our patients have had a chance to truly discuss their fears, such information may fall on deaf ears.

Financial concerns (e.g., unaffordable medications) also contribute to nonadherence. Some people with a limited income feel uneasy or embarrassed discussing this with their doctors. Again, such issues need to be discussed in a straightforward and empathetic way.

Psychological dynamics are also a contributing factor. The list of possible adherence problems due to psychological issues is long and complex. Here are a few of the issues most commonly encountered in clinical practice:

- Some medications induce sedation or other side effects that may leave the patient feeling out of control. The experience of loss of control accompanies many psychiatric disorders. Medication side effects can, at times, exacerbate this feeling.

- Patients perceive that prescribers see their problems only from a biological perspective without taking into consideration their emotional and psychological issues.

- There may be *secondary gain* from continuing to be "sick." For example, a woman who is depressed in the aftermath of her husband's affair says she wants to get better. However, noncompliance and ongoing depressive symptoms may be, in essence, a way of saying, "Look what you have done to me." It is a way for her to punish her husband or elicit caring and compassion from others. Secondary gain may be conscious, but it also can be unconsciously motivated.

- Sometimes, defeating the doctor is gratifying. Consciously or unconsciously, nonadherence leads to repeated medication failures. Often this dynamic is seen in people who have a history of significant child abuse. They may sincerely ask for help to reduce painful symptoms. However, the unconscious need to control, punish, or in other ways render the prescriber impotent, may drive nonadherence. This dynamic does not go away unless it is unearthed and explored in therapy.

- Feeling overwhelmed, patients cannot adequately take in and process what the doctor has told them about medication treatment and what to expect from this treatment. Many people leave an appointment with their primary care doctor and begin to take antidepressants. The prescriber may have done a good job of informing the patient about the fact that antidepressants often require two to four weeks before they begin working. Depressed patients often have difficulty with memory, owing to decreased capacity for maintaining attention and concentration. After three days of taking their medicine, they notice no signs of improvement and forget the information the doctor provided. They conclude that the antidepressants don't work, and therefore discontinue them.

- Negative stigma regarding mental illnesses certainly still persists. Taking a medication

"I stopped taking it after one day." "How come?" the prescriber would ask. "I got a dry mouth," would be the response. Faced with horrible depression and escalating suicidal ideas, patients bailed out due to dry mouth. Why? Because they were depressed. Severely depressed patients already are feeling overwhelmed and hopeless. Whereas many people would well tolerate a dry mouth, it is just another negative thing that happens to people with depression, so they give up. All clinicians know that hopelessness and pessimism are cardinal symptoms of depression. Many a straw has broken the psychotropic camel's back for those suffering from depression.

Finally, some side effects, even if mild to moderate, may cause special problems for individuals given their unique lifestyles and medical status. For example, a bus driver may not safely work if a drug causes sedation. An obese patient with type II diabetes may not be able to take certain atypical antipsychotics or mood stabilizers, owing to a common side effect of weight gain. In these cases, pros and cons must be assessed before initiating treatment, and choices of medication will be based on an inventory of personal factors (e.g., medical status). It is all too common for people who have struggled with side effects (e.g., sedation) when taking a number of drugs to be told, "Well, you'll just have to tolerate the side effects." In some cases this may be unavoidable. However, every effort should be made to try new medications or combinations of medications before concluding that particular side effects are, in fact, unavoidable.

is a concrete reminder: *I have a psychiatric disorder*. This is a significant issue that can lead to nonadherence.

■ Finally, messages from close friends and family may undermine treatment: for example, "Hey man, I heard that that drug can make you suicidal," "You don't need medicine; if you just try harder, you can pull yourself out of this," or "People get addicted to those drugs. I wouldn't take them." In *some* 12-step programs, pressure is put on members to stay away from all "mind-altering" drugs. Certainly some classes of drugs (e.g., minor tranquilizers) do pose real dangers of addiction in those who are vulnerable to substance abuse; however, most classes of psychiatric drugs are not addictive. Some religious groups also may strongly discourage psychiatric treatment. The impact of these social and interpersonal pressures can be substantial.

All of these reasons for nonadherence should be kept in mind, especially when the patient isn't getting better. According to Shawn Shea (2006), patients always weigh the pros and cons of any medication that they are taking. Often this is done in a nonsystematic way, and the decision "to take or not to take" is not shared with their doctors. Dr. Shea advises that it is always important to bring up the topic in a preemptive way, at the time when the prescription is first written:

■ Consider the pros and cons, such as effectiveness of the drug, side effects, the cost of the medicine, and any psychological issues, as discussed previously.

■ Anticipate side effects. Share with the patient, "I'm sure you know that some medications have side effects, and you may experience this. It matters a lot to me to make sure this therapy is effective, so please don't hesitate to tell me if you encounter any side effects. If you do, we'll find a way to deal with it." The weighing of pros and cons is best done in the doctor's office, where both the patient and the prescriber can systematically evaluate things.

■ Periodically ask patients for an assessment of their medications: "How well would you say you are doing on the medicine?"

■ Ask what family members are saying about the patient's medical treatment (this often matters a lot).

When side effects do emerge, it is important to evaluate how severe they are. Are they tolerable? Are they disabling, or do they interfere with important life activities? Might the side effects diminish with time?

An important key to good treatment outcomes is to give patients (and parents) time to really explore any concerns or worries that they might have about the psychiatric medication being recommended. For instance, patients may express fears of addiction if they take an antidepressant. As noted previously, often, just giving patients the information that the drug is nonaddictive is not effective. It is considerably more helpful to explore in some detail with patients how they feel about it and what they have been told about the drug. Truly hearing the patient's concerns is, first and foremost, a decent way to interact with a fellow human being. It also may flesh out worries that have gone unspoken. This thoughtful way to address fears and worries not only helps reduce nonadherence, but also can contribute to establishing a positive therapeutic alliance.

Part Two

Clinical Syndromes:
Etiology, Diagnosis,
and Treatment Implications

In part two of this book we address in some detail the biological etiology and differential diagnosis of major clinical syndromes. In our approach to diagnosis, we incorporate some *DSM-IV-TR* criteria. However, at times alternative classifications and criteria are employed. Our aim is to provide a useful and clinically relevant approach that will help the therapist in decision making, particularly with regard to referral issues and medication treatments.

This section of the book begins with a chapter on preliminary diagnostic considerations. Following this are chapters addressing the most common clinical syndromes. The specifics of medication treatment (dosing, effects, side effects) will follow in part three.

6

Preliminary Diagnostic Considerations

Before launching into a detailed discussion of major psychiatric disorders, it is important to explore some preliminary diagnostic issues. These issues should be considered in the initial workup of any client for whom medications are being considered.

The most common approach to diagnosis (that of the *DSM*), and the approach we present in this book, is based on the identification of specific target symptoms that make up a particular disorder or syndrome. Such an approach certainly has merit. Yet it is crucial to keep in mind that any particular behavior, symptom, or trait *may* have diverse etiologies. That is, identical symptomatic behaviors may spring from biochemical dysfunctions, social learning experiences, or characterological sources. The three most common sources of etiologic confusion will be discussed in this chapter: the interaction between Axis I and Axis II; substance abuse and psychiatric symptomatology; and, finally, physical illnesses that present with cognitive, emotional, and behavioral disturbances. Successful pharmacologic treatment often depends on a thorough understanding of these important issues.

Axis I and Axis II: Complex Interactions

DSM-IV employs a multiaxial diagnostic system. Axis I includes major psychiatric symptom disorders and syndromes, and Axis II is reserved for long-standing personality styles and disorders. This distinction between the more acute, episodic, symptomatic disorders (Axis I) and more traitlike, pervasive, and enduring personality problems (Axis II) is a useful and important advance over earlier diagnostic systems. Differentiating state and trait variables has helped researchers and clinicians alike to identify more clearly and reliably a host of psychiatric disorders. The distinction also

Key Terms

Agonist. Drug or chemical that acts on a receptor to mimic the effects of a naturally occurring substance (such as a hormone or neurotransmitter), or of another chemical; for example, beta adrenergic agonist medications mimic epinephrine and produce relaxation of bronchial (lung) muscles to treat asthma.

Antagonist. Substance or drug capable of blocking (at the receptor) the activity of an agonist without exerting any effect itself. For example, antipsychotics are dopamine receptor antagonists.

Differential diagnosis. The process of considering diagnostic possibilities based on a comparison of signs and symptoms of two or more disorders or diseases.

Egodystonic. Symptoms subjectively experienced by the patient as being aversive, undesirable, or alien.

Egosyntonic. Signs or symptoms judged to be pathological by others but not experienced as distressing by the patient.

Etiology. The study of the causes of disorders and diseases.

Pathophysiology. The underlying physiological dysfunction or disease that contributes to the manifest symptoms of a disease.

Target symptoms. In this book, the distinctive symptoms that are the focus (target) of medication treatment.

Toxicity. Serious medication-related adverse effects associated with actual or potential damage to tissues, organs, or the entire body system. Toxicity may be directly related to critically elevated blood levels of a drug and may be acute (as in a

has been useful in planning therapeutic interventions, in understanding treatment outcomes, and in making predictions about the course of disorders and their prognoses. Yet, in many respects, the boundaries between Axis I and Axis II are not entirely clear-cut. Understanding the complex interactions between Axis I and II is as important in pharmacological treatment as it is in psychotherapy. Axis I and II disorders influence one another in four common ways:

- Axis I disorder evokes or intensifies Axis II characteristics.

- Axis II dynamics predispose to Axis I disorders.

- Axis II characteristics reflect atypical or mild chronic Axis I disorders.

- Axis II dynamics influence Axis I treatment response.

Let's take a look at each of these interactions.

Axis I Disorder Evokes Axis II Characteristics

Axis I disorders oftentimes enhance or exaggerate preexisting personality traits. For example, sometimes an Axis I disorder unearths behavior that was not at all evident prior to the clinical episode. The clinician may conclude that a patient has a major depression and a personality disorder, only to discover that the personality disorder disappears with successful treatment of the Axis I disorder. This is frequently seen in individuals diagnosed as borderline personalities in which the impact of serious depression or panic disorder results in psychological regression. During the Axis I episode there are, in fact, features verging on borderline. However, in as many as a third of such patients, with resolution of the major symptom disorder, their level of functioning resumes its normal or (more often) neurotic preclinical level. Since borderline characteristics were not evident prior to the major episode of depression or panic, and the history was not one of "stable instability," to call such a patient borderline is technically inaccurate.

Case 11

Barbara M., thirty-five, was admitted to an inpatient psychiatric unit after she developed suicidal ideas and incidents in which she repeatedly sliced the inside of her calf. Her admitting diagnosis was major depression and borderline personality disorder. The borderline diagnosis was based on the rather bizarre self-mutilation. The treating psychiatrist informed the patient's family that her acute depression could indeed be treated but that the apparent personality disorder would likely be a serious, ongoing problem and the prognosis was more guarded.

tranquilizer overdose) or chronic (as in prolonged, moderately elevated lithium level). A drug may also produce "toxic effects" at therapeutic doses (such as phenothiazine's potential for inducing bone marrow damage, which in turn causes decreased production of white blood cells).

Barbara's history, however, failed to reveal any previous signs of psychiatric problems. She was a very successful owner of a small print shop and had a history of solid interpersonal relationships. Her depressive disorder occurred after her best friend had been tragically killed in a boating accident. After five days of hospitalization, she was discharged. Five weeks later, after twice weekly psychotherapy and antidepressants, she was virtually symptom-free. There was no hint of the primitive personality disturbance evident when she was first hospitalized.

Another common example is when a very severe depression or anxiety disorder pulls the rug out from under a person. As a result, we may see the emergence of helplessness and overly dependent behavior. This *may* be an exaggeration of preexisting dependent traits, but it may also be the kind of regressive behavior seen across many personality styles when one is laid low by a serious, debilitating illness.

Axis II Dynamics Predispose to Axis I Disorders

Certain personality disorders may predispose an individual to increased risk of developing an Axis I disorder. We can see this emerge in at least two ways. First, people with personality disorders often, if not always, experience particular, unique areas of emotional vulnerability. For example, histrionic, dependent, avoidant, and many borderline patients have strong dependency longings and an exquisite sensitivity to separation stresses. As a group, these people are at higher risk for developing major depressions, serious anxiety reactions, or both in the wake of interpersonal losses. For these patients, relatively minor social rebuffs, rejections, or losses may precipitate significant depressive reactions. In a parallel manner, obsessive and paranoid personalities highly value being in control. Even minor life stresses that decrease one's sense of control or predictability can plunge these people into states of high anxiety, hypervigilance, and ruminative self-doubt.

A second way Axis II problems can increase risk is that repetitive maladaptive behavior patterns can result in recurring interpersonal stressors. For example, the clinging, overly dependent personality may, by his or her interpersonal style, repeatedly drive people away. Here the maladaptive behavior provokes numerous rejections, which in turn can lead to episodes of depression.

Thus, when medications are used to treat various Axis I disorders, it is wise to keep in mind that, despite the success of drug treatment, ultimate therapeutic success and relapse prevention may depend heavily on the role Axis II factors play.

Axis II Characteristics Reflect Axis I Disorder

It is possible that what initially appear to be characteristic symptoms of personality disorder may reflect some form of mild, chronic, or atypical Axis I disorder. Let's consider several examples. For years clinicians described certain patients as suffering from masochistic or depressive personalities. These people were often seen as chronically pessimistic, bitter, irritable individuals, and the implication was that the low-grade depressive traits were manifestations of personality—that is, etched into the character of the individual. Although certainly this is the case for some people, in recent years a significant number of dysthymic patients have experienced very positive results when treated with antidepressants.

These so-called depressive characters likely have suffered from a form of chronic, low-grade biological depression. Similarly, recent reports of successful treatment of social anxiety in "avoidant personalities" using MAO inhibitors or SSRIs may indicate another group of patients whose character pathology seems to be rooted in a type of biochemical disturbance.

Undoubtedly, many people presenting with personality problems are best understood as exhibiting true disorders of character, and for these people medication treatment is not appropriate. However, it is very important not to conclude automatically that such behaviors are solely attributable to character pathology (see figure 6-A). Certain behavioral characteristics or traits seen in various personality disorders *may* be due to subtle neurochemical malfunction, which may respond to medication.

Just because a trait is long-standing, it is not appropriate to automatically assume that it is truly characterological. Figure 6-A can serve as a reminder to consider the *possibility* that certain characteristics may be due to chronic biochemical dysfunction. (See interesting discussions of this topic in Peter Kramer's best-selling book, *Listening to Prozac*, 1993.)

Axis II Dynamics Influence Axis I Treatment Response

As mentioned in chapter 2, individuals' particular personality styles and unique psychodynamics will often dramatically influence how they respond to pharmacotherapy. Robert Michaels (1992) has commented that in general clinical practice, two-thirds of patients with Axis I disorders appear to respond quite well either to medication treatment or to brief, targeted psychological interventions, such as cognitive-behavioral or interpersonal therapy. However, a significant minority of patients with clear-cut Axis I disorders don't respond well to such treatments, primarily due to serious comorbid character pathology. In treating these people, at the very least the clinician must be alert to how personality factors influence treatment outcome; often medication treatment must be accompanied by more intensive psychotherapy that addresses the personality disorder.

Personality Traits That May Reflect Biochemical Disorders

Axis II Traits	Medication-Responsive Axis I Disorder	Psychotropic Medication Options
Chronic boredom; emptiness; irritability; hypochondriasis; low energy; chronic fatigue; pessimism, negative thinking; feelings of shame, humiliation	Depression	Antidepressants
Easily hurt by criticism; helplessness, dependency; difficulty making decisions	Depression, anxiety disorders	Antidepressants
Social anxiety; avoidance	Social phobia, panic disorder	Antidepressants, beta blockers, benzodiazepines
Magical thinking; odd speech	Psychotic disorders	Antipsychotics
Excessive worry	Generalized anxiety disorders	Antidepressants, buspirone, benzodiazepines
Impulsiveness; stimulus-seeking; affective instability	Attention-deficit disorder, bipolar disorder	Stimulants, mood stabilizers
Separation stress; nonassertivenes	Anxiety disorders	Antidepressants, benzodiazepines
Perfectionism; preoccupation with rules, order, details, lists, or cleanliness; workaholic	Obsessive-compulsive disorder	Antidepressants (SSRIs)

Figure 6-A

Substance Abuse

Substance abuse can directly cause or contribute to a wide array of psychiatric symptoms: depression, anxiety disorders, psychosis, mania, and so on. Not only can the use of recreational drugs produce psychological symptoms, but frequently such substances markedly interfere with psychological or psychiatric treatment. A common example of this occurs when moderate-to-heavy alcohol use adversely affects liver functioning, causing prescribed psychotropic medications to be inadequately metabolized. The result can be inadequate blood levels of the medication, as in the following case.

Case 12

Jerry H. was first seen for psychiatric consultation six months ago. He presented with a classic major depression, which had emerged during an especially difficult marital separation and divorce. Jerry had initially reported only occasional social drinking, "a few times a month." After five months of psychotherapy and aggressive antidepressant treatment, he was still quite depressed. Three antidepressant medications had been tried in conjunction with cognitive-behavioral psychotherapy, with little improvement. It was eventually learned that Jerry actually had been consuming four to six beers every night. Three weeks after the alcohol use had been curtailed, he began to show his first positive response to the antidepressant. The alcohol use (unknown to the therapist for five months) had been the main culprit in preventing antidepressants from ever reaching adequate blood levels.

Although a very wide range of prescription and nonprescription drugs can cause psychiatric symptoms, the two most commonly encountered in clinical practice are alcohol and caffeine. (In subsequent clinical chapters, additional specific drugs will be listed as they contribute to particular psychiatric disorders.) It is always important to get a complete drug history on each person being evaluated.

In general, more than 1.5 ounces of alcohol (or the equivalent: one beer or one glass of wine) per day, may directly contribute to psychiatric symptoms, may interfere with proper metabolism of psychotropic medications, or both. Obviously, excessive use often leads to two additional complications: addiction or dependence and the use of the drug as a means of acting out (emotional numbing), which can interfere with the process of self-exploration, abreaction, or "working through" in psychotherapy. Appropriate psychotherapy and pharmacotherapy can (and often do) fail because of ongoing and often unrecognized substance abuse.

In general, over 250 mg (especially amounts over 500 mg) of caffeine per day can cause or contribute to psychiatric symptoms, especially anxiety, irritability, sleep disturbance, and agitation. Figure 6-B provides a guideline for a caffeine history—which should be done on every person being evaluated.

Physical Illness

A number of investigators have found that a rather substantial minority of people seeking psychiatric services are actually suffering from undiagnosed physical illness. The primary medical disorder either causes or contributes to the emergence of psychiatric symptoms. Let's sample a couple of studies: Hall et al. (1978) carefully evaluated 658 consecutive psychiatric outpatients. These researchers found that 9 percent had medical disorders that were the primary cause of psychiatric symptoms. Koran and colleagues (1989) found an even higher number of psychiatric patients with underlying medical disorders—17 percent.

Robert Taylor (1990) has aptly referred to such cases as "psychological masquerade." Here, unrecognized medical disorders either directly or indirectly affect the biochemistry of the brain and produce a host of emotional, cognitive, and behavioral symptoms.

Caffeine Content of Common Substances

Beverages		
Coffee	6 oz	125 mg
Espresso	1 oz	35 mg
Decaf coffee	6 oz	5 mg
Tea	6 oz	50 mg
Green tea	6 oz	30 mg
Hot cocoa	6 oz	15 mg
Soft drinks	12 oz	46–60 mg
(colas, Mountain Dew, Mr. Pibb, Mello Yello, Dr. Pepper, Big Red)		
Energy drink	12 oz	250 mg

Prescription Drugs

Cafergot	100 mg
Fiorinal	40 mg
Fioricet	40 mg

Over-the-Counter Drugs

Appetite-control pills	100–200 mg
NoDoz	100 mg
Vivarin	200 mg
Anacin	32 mg
Excedrin	65 mg
Midol	60 mg
Vanquish	33 mg
Triaminicin	30 mg
Dristan	16 mg
Extra Strength Excedrine	65 mg

Source: FDA National Center: Drugs and Biologics (as cited in Avis 1998).

Figure 6-B

It is crucial to identify those people suffering from psychological masquerade for two reasons: First, various medical illnesses need to be treated early. Failure to recognize and treat them may result in prolonged suffering, permanent impairment, progressive physical decline, and, at times, death. Second, one's best efforts at providing psychological treatment may be in vain if the underlying medical condition goes unrecognized. However, nonmedical therapists are not trained in medical diagnosis. So what steps can they take to identify those patients who have a physical illness?

The role of the nonmedical therapist is not to make definitive medical diagnoses, but rather to be alert to certain warning signs that may signal the presence of a physical illness or that at least increase one's index of suspicion. Obviously, when a medical illness is suspected, a referral to a physician or emergency medical facility is in order.

For practical purposes we can divide medical illnesses with psychiatric symptomatology into three categories:

- Illnesses and conditions that do not directly affect the CNS but can lead to secondary (reactive) emotional responses. These conditions are generally recognized and reported by the patient. Examples are a person who develops a serious reactive depression after sustaining a spinal cord injury and paralysis, and an individual who is diagnosed with glaucoma and may be facing blindness.

- Illnesses and conditions that affect the CNS and impair cognitive functioning. These conditions are of greatest importance—where the medical problem may go unnoticed and what predominates are psychiatric symptoms.

- Illnesses and conditions that affect neurochemistry but do not affect cognitive functioning. The latter two conditions include some primary disorders of the nervous system (such as brain tumors and certain degenerative diseases) and a host of systemic illnesses that indirectly influence brain chemistry.

Illnesses and Conditions Affecting Cognitive Functioning

Disorders affecting cognitive functioning can be further subdivided into acute and chronic or insidious categories. Acute disorders tend to have a more profound effect on brain functioning and have an impact on the following cognitive functions:

- Patients may appear to be drowsy and suffer from what is called "clouding of consciousness."

- Attention and concentration may be impaired.

- Speech may be slurred.

- Content of speech may reveal confused and disorganized thinking.

- Gait may be unsteady.

- The person can become disoriented.

- Recent memory (the ability for new learning and recall) is impaired.

- There may be agitation and/or labile emotions.

These areas of functioning can be evaluated by the use of a brief neurocognitive mental status exam (see appendix E). Acute disorders affecting the CNS have multiple etiologies (see figure 6-C). Many of these conditions can be potentially life threatening, thus immediate medical attention is indicated.

Acute Organic Brain Syndromes

- Anoxia
- CNS infections
- CVA (strokes), hemorrhages
- Head injuries
- Metabolic disorders, such as hypoglycemia, adrenal disease, vitamin deficiencies, electrolyte imbalances
- Organ diseases, such as hepatic encephalopathy
- Pernicious anemia
- Toxic reactions, such as drug interactions or overdoses

Figure 6-C

Causes of Chronic Organic Brain Syndromes

- AIDS or HIV dementia
- Alzheimer's disease
- Chronic sequelae of head injury
- Cognitive disorders associated with chronic substance abuse
- Huntington's chorea
- Hydrocephalus
- Lewy body dementia

- Multi-infarct disorder
- Multiple sclerosis
- Neoplasms (CNS tumors)
- Parkinson's disease
- Pick's disease
- Wilson's disease

Figure 6-D

Chronic, insidious brain syndromes usually do not present with a clouding of consciousness; patients appear fully awake. Also, disturbances in gait and slurred speech are *generally* not seen. (Exceptions do exist, however. For instance, in Parkinson's disease there is a gait disturbance.) The onset of symptoms is gradual. Hallmark symptoms usually include impaired recent memory, poor ability to reproduce geometric designs, impaired concentration, and an erosion of higher-level cognitive abilities (such as impaired reasoning and judgment). These disorders can also be evaluated using the brief neurocognitive mental status exam in appendix E, and by taking a complete history from the patient and an informed relative. If a chronic brain syndrome is suspected, a medical referral is indicated. Figure 6-D lists causes of common chronic brain syndromes.

Illnesses and Conditions Affecting Neurochemistry

There are a number of medical disorders that have little or no effect on cognitive function but can adversely affect the biochemistry of the limbic system and other subcortical brain areas. Thus, although individuals suffering from these conditions may appear intact on the brief neurocognitive mental status exam, they may exhibit pronounced psychiatric symptoms as the systemic medical illness dysregulates the chemistry of the brain.

How might the nonmedical therapist detect the presence of such medical disorders? We will look at two approaches: to evaluate for global warning signs (see figure 6-E), and to ask about particular physical symptoms (see figure 6-F). In each case, the clinician should do a brief overview of various signs and physical symptoms. The goal again is not to make a medical diagnosis but rather to either raise or lower one's index of suspicion. If a medical condition is suspected, a referral for appropriate medical care is indicated.

Many of the symptoms listed in figure 6-F are fairly nonspecific and may be elicited from many patients, but some particular physical symptoms should raise your index of suspicion, such as when there are several physical complaints, not just a simple nonspecific complaint like fatigue. When in doubt, refer for evaluation. In fact, it is probably advisable that anyone with a significant psychiatric disorder have a medical evaluation.

Keep in mind that medications and other drugs are a very common cause of emotional symptoms—this includes prescription, nonprescription, and other recreational drugs and alcohol. Obtaining collateral history from family members may be helpful, as well as conducting the "bag test": having the person bring in all (this cannot be stressed too much) medications he or she is taking for the therapist to see and make a record of.

In summary, after assessing for the presence of Axis II characteristics and understanding how these may influence the primary symptom disorders, and after ruling in or out substance abuse and coexisting medical illnesses, the clinician is ready to formulate a clinical diagnosis. The following chapters address major diagnostic groups with a focus on clinical presentation, differential diagnosis, etiology, and treatment decision making. In each area we pay particular attention to which diagnostic characteristics indicate the need for psychotropic medication treatment.

Medical Illness Checklist

- Onset of psychiatric symptoms has "come out of the blue"—not precipitated by identifiable psychosocial stressors.
- The patient is over fifty-five, thus at increased risk for a host of medical illnesses.
- The patient takes multiple medications—which may interact adversely.
- No personal or family history of similar psychiatric symptoms.
- Recent history of head injury.
- Hallucinations or illusions—especially visual, olfactory, tactile, or gustatory (such perceptual disturbances are generally indicative of neurologic disease).
- The patient looks physically ill or has abnormal vital signs (such as very low blood pressure, fever, weak pulse).

Source: Taylor (1990)

Figure 6-E

Specific Physical Symptoms Checklist

Physical Symptoms	Psychiatric Symptoms	Possible Disorder
Abdominal pain, jaundice, constipation	Depression	Pancreatic cancer
Weight gain, cold intolerance, dry skin, hair loss, puffy face, fatigue	Depression, psychosis	Hypothyroidism
Weight loss, heat intolerance, sweating, tremors, wide-eyed state	Anxiety, agitated depression	Hyperthyroidism
Bad breath, urine odor, frequent urination	Depression	Diabetes mellitus
Weakness, dizziness, light-headedness, sweating, tremors	Anxiety (acute onset)	Hypoglycemia
Muscular weakness, fatigue	Depression	Myasthenia gravis
Sensory disturbances, paresthesia, transient motor disturbances	Depression, euphoria, conversion symptoms	Multiple sclerosis
Weakness, fatigue, diffuse pain, incoordination	Depression, impaired memory	Pernicious anemia
Abdominal pain, weakness, confusion after ingestion of alcohol or barbituates	Anxiety	Porphyria
Increased skin pigmentation, weight loss, diarrhea, muscle cramps, low blood pressure	Depression	Hypoadrenalism (Addison's disease)
Muscle weakness, moon face, hirsutism, hypertension	Irritability, euphoria, depression	Hyperadrenalism (Cushing's disease)
Hypertension, headache	Anxiety	Pheochromocytoma (adrenal gland tumor)
Fever, malaise	Depression, agitation	Viral or bacterial infection
Fatigue, joint pain	Depression	Various rheumatoid disorders (e.g., fibromyalgia), chronic fatigue syndromes
Headaches, weakness, changes in vision	Depression, mania, personality changes	Brain tumor
Any physical symptoms	Any psychiatric disorder	Drug effects or side effects

Note: This list does not cover all possible medical disorders that may cause psychiatric symptoms; however, these do represent those most commonly encountered in clinical practice.

Figure 6-F

7

Depressive Disorders

Depressive disorders (also often referred to as affective or mood disorders) represent an extremely broad, heterogeneous group of disorders. These clinical syndromes share some common symptoms (especially dysphoria) but, in fact, reflect a number of disorders that have diverse etiologies: characterological, acute reactive, and biologic. (Note that bipolar disorder is covered separately, in chapter 8.) The symptoms, course, prognosis, and response to treatment vary considerably depending on the particular type of depressive disorder seen clinically; thus a solid understanding of the differential diagnosis is crucial for treatment-oriented decision making.

Differential Diagnosis

It is helpful to first view depressive disorders as falling broadly into three primary groups: reactive dysphoria, grief, and clinical depression.

Reactive dysphoria is characterized by relatively low-grade mood changes—sadness, disappointment, despair—that occur in response to minor losses and disappointments. The emotional responses are considered to be normal and appropriate. They are transient, and most importantly, these mood disturbances do not typically interfere with functioning; that is, they have little impact on academic, occupational, or social or interpersonal functioning.

Grief, or uncomplicated bereavement, can be a much more prolonged and intensely painful experience. Grief is a normal and emotionally necessary response to major losses, such as death of a loved one or divorce. Most normal grief reactions result in significant degrees of emotional distress for a period of six to twelve months, and continued, albeit less intense, grieving often lasts for an additional one to three years. Social and occupational functioning can be derailed for a while, although most people experiencing a grief reaction do continue to work and socialize.

There are two important features that distinguish grief from clinical depression. First, as noted in Freud's classic, "Mourning and Melancholia" (1917), with grief, self-esteem remains relatively intact, despite significant dysphoria. Second, as painful as it is, the grieving process is healthy and adaptive; it is an active process of mourning that eventually leads to emotional healing. In clinical depressions self-esteem almost always erodes, and true depression is a clearly pathological condition.

Certainly, what appears initially to be a grief reaction can disintegrate into a true clinical depression, so the boundary between these disorders is not always sharply defined. When the following symptoms emerge in the wake of a serious loss, this signals that normal grief has evolved into a clinical depression:

When Grief Becomes Clinical Depression

- Marked erosion of self-esteem
- Agitation*
- Early morning awakening*
- Serious weight loss*
- Suicidal ideation or attempts
- Anhedonia (loss of the ability to experience any pleasure)*
- Marked impairment of social, interpersonal, academic, or occupational functioning

* When this clinical picture emerges, psychotherapy, psychotropic medication treatment, or both become necessary. These symptoms marked with an asterisk are targets for antidepressant medications.

The vast majority of individuals encountering uncomplicated bereavement do not need psychological or psychiatric treatment. However, it is estimated that 25 to 30 percent of individuals do in fact develop a clinical depression following a major loss.

Clinical depressions are characterized by their intensity, duration, impact on functioning, and a host of symptoms. Most true clinical depressions result in tremendous personal suffering, can last for months to years (left untreated), and severely affect normal daily functioning.

We can further divide clinical depressions into the following categories:

Types of Clinical Depression

- *Major unipolar depressions*: reactive, biological, reactive-biological, atypical
- *Bipolar disorder*: manic and depressive episodes (see chapter 8)
- *"Minor" depressions*: dysthymia, chronic residuals of partially recovered major depressions

---

Major Unipolar Depressions

For practical purposes and to aid in treatment decision making, it is useful to conceptualize three primary types and one atypical version of major depression. All have in common marked impairment in functioning, a typically long duration, and one or all of the core symptoms listed below:

Core Symptoms Common to All Depressions

- Mood of sadness, despair, emptiness
- Anhedonia (loss of the ability to experience any pleasure)
- Low self-esteem
- Apathy, low motivation, and social withdrawal
- Excessive emotional sensitivity
- Negative, pessimistic thinking
- Irritability
- Suicidal ideas

Note: Some degree of decreased capacity for pleasure (anhedonia) may be seen in all types of depression. In depressions that involve a biochemical disturbance, this loss of ability to experience pleasure can become so pronounced that the patient has almost no moments of joy or pleasure. Such people are said to have a "nonreactive mood," which means that they are unable to get out of their depressed mood even temporarily.

Reactive depressions

Classic reactive depressions (sometimes referred to as psychological depressions) can range in intensity from mild or moderate (for example, adjustment disorders with depressed mood) to severe (major depression). These disorders occur in response to identifiable psychosocial stressors. These stressors may be acute and intense (such as loss of a loved one), insidious (as in the case of a gradual deterioration in the quality of marital relationship), or in the distant past (for example, the emotions experienced by a survivor of child abuse who in adulthood begins to recall long-forgotten abusive events).

In its pure form, reactive depression can present with severe levels of symptomatology, yet basic physical functions (sleep, energy levels, and so on) are relatively unaffected. Note that many, if not most reactive depressions do take on biological features, as will be described next, but the pure reactive disorder noted here is seen without major physiological symptoms.

Biological depressions

Biologically based depressive disorders, in their purest form, are not seen as a reaction to stressors. In fact, they can emerge apparently spontaneously, "out of the blue"—in individuals encountering little in terms of

Depression Facts

- Lifetime prevalence for depressive disorders is 17 percent.
- Suicide rate for patients with major depression is 9 percent.
- Eighteen million people per year suffer from major depression in the United States. Another 7.5 million experience chronic low-grade depression.
- The incidence of depression ratio of women to men is 2:1.
- Only 50 percent of Americans who suffer a bout of major depression will seek treatment. Yet treatment can be effective in up to 80 percent of depressed patients—even those suffering with very severe depressions.

Medical Disorders That Can Cause Depression

- Addison's disease
- AIDS
- Anemia
- Asthma
- Chronic fatigue syndrome
- Chronic infection (mononucleosis, tuberculosis)
- Chronic pain
- Congestive heart failure
- Cushing's disease
- Diabetes
- Hypothyroidism
- Infectious hepatitis

- Influenza
- Lyme disease
- Malignancies (cancer)
- Malnutrition
- Multiple sclerosis
- Parkinson's disease
- Premenstrual dysphoria
- Porphyria
- Rheumatoid arthritis
- Sleep apnea
- Syphilis
- Systemic lupus erythematosus
- Ulcerative colitis
- Uremia

Figure 7-A

Drugs That Can Cause Depression

Type	Generic name	Brand name
Alcohol	Wine, beer, spirits	Various brands
Antianxiety drugs	Diazepam	Valium
	Alprazolam	Xanax
	Lorazepam	Ativan
Antihypertensives (for high blood pressure)	Reserpine	Various brands
	Propranolol hydrochloride	Inderal
	Methyldopa	Various brands
	Guanethidine sulfate	Ismelin sulfate
	Clonidine hydrochloride	Catapres, Kapvay
	Hydralazine hydrochloride	Various brands
Antiparkinsonian drugs	Levodopa carbidopa	Sinemet
	Levodopa	Various brands
		Dopar, Larodopa Symmetrel
	Amantadine hydrochloride	
Birth control pills	Progestin-estrogen combination	Various brands
Corticosteroids and other hormones	Cortisone acetate	Cortone
	Dexamethasone	Decadron
	Prednisone	Various brands
	Estrogen	Premarin, Ogen, Estrace, Estraderm Provera,
	Progesterone and derivatives	DepoProvera, Norlutate
Dermatological	Isotretinoin	Sotret, Amnesteen
Gastrointestinal	Metroclopramide	Reglan
Antiviral	Interferon	Roferon-A, Intron-A, Reberon, and various others

Figure 7-B

life stress. The trigger for biological depressions can be traced to any of a number of conditions that alter neurotransmitter function in key areas of the limbic system. The conditions responsible for biological depressions fall into four categories:

1. Medical illnesses that lead to systemic changes and ultimately to brain dysfunction (see figure 7-A). It should be noted that recently it has been found that thyroid dysfunction is a common disorder underlying 5 to 10 percent of serious depressions (especially Grade II/subclinical hypothyroidism). Because of this high frequency, a thyroid panel (with a measure of TSH: thyroid stimulating hormone) is strongly recommended in all cases of serious depression.

2. Female sex-hormone fluctuation, especially noted postpartum, during menopause, and premenstrually.

3. Medications and recreational drugs (see figure 7-B). (Note that alcohol and minor tranquilizers are often used or abused during times of emotional stress, and, almost invariably, eventually make depression worse.)

4. Endogenous biological depressions. These disorders appear to emerge spontaneously in certain at-risk individuals in the absence of stressful events. The prevailing theory (discussed below) is that such disorders likely reflect a genetically transmitted biologic vulnerability that leads to repeated dysfunction of selected neurons in the limbic system and resulting recurring depressive episodes.

In experimental settings, researchers have been able to identify some biological markers for these disorders, including reduced frontal cortex metabolic activity, abnormalities shown on sleep EEGs, particular genetic markers, and neurotransmitter metabolite irregularities in cerebral spinal fluid. However, for practical, economic, and safety reasons, such tests are not used in clinical settings. What have been and continue to be the most reliable markers of biological depression are the emergence of depression in the absence of identifiable psychosocial stressors *and* the presence of any of the following physiological symptoms:

Physiological Symptoms of Depression

■ Appetite disturbance—decreased or increased, with accompanying weight loss or gain

■ Fatigue

■ Decreased sex drive

■ Restlessness, agitation, or psychomotor retardation

■ Diurnal variations in mood—usually feeling worse in the morning

■ Impaired concentration and forgetfulness

■ Pronounced anhedonia—total loss of the ability to experience pleasure

■ Sleep disturbance—early morning awakening, frequent awakenings throughout the night; occasionally hypersomnia (excessive sleeping). Note that initial insomnia (difficulty in falling asleep) may be seen with depression but is not diagnostic of a major depressive disorder. Initial insomnia can be seen in anyone experiencing stress in general. Initial insomnia alone is more characteristic of anxiety disorders than of depression.

These symptoms are commonly referred to as *vegetative* or *neurovegetative* symptoms. Not only are these symptoms a marker of biological depression, but they also serve as our major target symptoms—alerting the therapist that the patient should be referred for antidepressant medication treatment.

Typically, for the diagnosis to be more definitive, the patient must have one or more of these symptoms on a sustained basis: present most days for a period of at least two weeks. Sporadic or occasional vegetative symptoms may hint at a neurotransmitter abnormality but do not suggest an entrenched clinical depression.

Reactive-biological depression

Sometimes referred to as endogenomorphic depressions, reactive-biological depressions represent a very large number of the depressions seen clinically. These disorders begin in much the same way as the more classic reactive depressions described above. However, with time, we see the emergence of various physiological symptoms. These disorders are not truly endogenous; however, at some point the effects of psychological stress appear to adversely influence brain functioning. What emerges is a sort of mixed depression—with both psychological-reactive and biologic symptoms.

Atypical depressions

Atypical depression is a subtype of major depression characterized by particular symptoms: see list below. Atypical symptoms (seen in 15 to 20 percent of major depressions) are very important to note, because most cases of bipolar depressions present with atypical symptoms. As will be noted in the next chapter, the use of antidepressants in bipolar depression is fraught with possible problems (e.g., cycle acceleration or provoking switches into mania). Thus, atypical symptoms should serve as a cue to carefully assess for bipolar disorder. In fact, when atypical symptoms are seen, one should consider the patient to have bipolar disorder until proven otherwise.

Symptoms of Atypical Depression

- Reactive dysphoria—sadness or despair comes and goes in response to psychological stressors
- Profound fatigue, low energy
- Hypersomnia (excessive sleeping)
- Increased appetite and weight gain
- Marked sensitivity to interpersonal rejection or separation

---

Efficacy of medication treatment

Major depressions can certainly occur once and never again. Yet, 80 percent of people experiencing a major depression encounter recurring episodes (on average, six per lifetime or chronic depression). Thus treatment and resolution of the current episode is crucial, but relapse prevention is also an important treatment goal. The eventual suicide rate for individuals with major depression is 9 percent. The economic burden to society is staggering: direct and indirect costs are estimated to be $44 billion per year in the United States, not to mention the incalculable personal suffering of patients and their families. Good patient education, especially focused on the early signs of recurrence, can go far to avert future episodes.

There is a large body of research supporting the finding that, when physiological symptoms are present, antidepressant medications are often effective. Presumably the presentation of the symptoms listed previously (physiological and atypical) signals the presence of an underlying dysregulation of particular neurotransmitters, especially norepinephrine, serotonin, and/or dopamine. More recent investigations have also implicated the role of cortisol, CRF (corticotrophin releasing factor), and substance P in the pathophysiology of depression. Physiological symptoms continue to be our most reliable behavioral markers of an underlying biological dysfunction. Thus very few people suffering from pure reactive-psychological depressions benefit from antidepressant medication treatment. However, improvement rates for the more physiologically based disorders (biological, reactive-biological, and atypical depressions), when treated with antidepressants, are as high as 80 percent.[1] Thus, the presence of the sustained physiological symptoms listed above can serve as primary target symptoms for antidepressant medication treatment.

It is very important to note that medical treatment of depression focuses primarily on restoring normal biological functioning (that is, improvement in physiological symptoms) and only secondarily affects mood, self-esteem, and so forth.

Psychotic Depressions

Major depression and bipolar illness (the subject of chapter 8) can, if extremely severe, manifest psychotic symptoms. Typically, the hallucinations and delusions seen in psychotic mood disorders are said to be "mood congruent," which means that the themes of these symptoms are congruent with the dominant mood. For example, a psychotically depressed patient might have delusions that she is the most disgusting or evil person in the world and should be executed. This delusional belief embodies the depressive themes of extremely low self-esteem and guilt. Compare this to schizophrenic symptoms, which most often are bizarre and unconnected to a dominant mood state, for example, the anxious man who believes a radio transmitter has been implanted in his thumb so that neighbors can hear broadcasts of his inner thoughts.

When symptoms of major depression and psychosis coexist, medication treatment is always warranted. (Often hospitalization, ECT, or both may also be necessary.) Psychotically depressed patients do not respond to psychotherapy alone, and they represent a very high suicide risk when actively psychotic. It has been firmly documented that treatment with antidepressants alone is not very effective (only 25 percent). Likewise, treatment with antipsychotics alone produce disappointing results (35 percent effective). However, combined antidepressant-antipsychotic treatment is significantly more effective (60 to 75 percent). Electroconvulsive treatment is really the gold standard in the treatment of psychotic mood disorders (90 percent effective). (See chapters 16 and 19, on treatment with antidepressants and antipsychotics, respectively.)

---

1. The high improvement rates are seen in those individuals for whom the diagnosis is correct and for whom treatment is appropriately managed. Diagnostic and treatment errors abound, and in general clinical practice, success rates usually fall far below 80 percent. Response rates are based on studies using combined depressants and psychotherapy.

Recurrent and Highly Recurrent Major Depression

Recurrent major depressions oftentimes involve two to six episodes in a lifetime. However, some individuals may have fifteen or more episodes per lifetime. There is increasing speculation that these cases of *highly* recurrent depressive episodes are likely to be a variant of bipolar disorder (i.e., bipolar III).

"Minor" Depressions

The depressive disorders described below are sometimes referred to as minor depressions because they do not reach the depths or intensity seen in major depression. However, the term "minor" may be a misnomer. Although these disorders are low-grade, they tend to be very long-term, often having their onset in late childhood or early adolescence and potentially lasting a lifetime. The cumulative toll such disorders exact on the quality of life and productivity over a lifetime are not minor at all! These chronic, low-grade depressions fall into two categories: dysthymia and chronic residuals of partially recovered major depression.

Dysthymia is characterized by the following symptoms:

Dysthymic Symptoms

Core Psychological Symptoms	Possible Biologic Symptoms
Chronic low-grade sadness	Low energy
Irritability	Decreased capacity to experience
Negative thinking	pleasure, enthusiasm, or motivation
Low self-esteem	

Unfortunately, dysthymic individuals can also suffer not only from chronic, low-grade depression but also from periods of major depression. As many as 80 percent of dysthymic patients will ultimately experience at least one major depressive episode. These more severe episodes are superimposed on the chronic depression, and often, upon recovery from the major episode, the patient returns to his or her preclinical baseline: low-grade depression. Such disorders have been termed *double depression* (see figure 7-C).

These minor depressions have long been seen as characterological and difficult to treat. However, during the past decade a large number of studies conclude that 66 percent of dysthymic patients do respond, and often respond well, to treatment with antidepressants (see Akiskal and Cassano 1997). It is likely, based on these findings, that approximately two-thirds of dysthymic patients may, in fact, be suffering from a type of chronic low-grade biologic depression. The other third may be experiencing more of a true characterological depression. For example, in unpublished data, Nicholas Ward (1992) finds that a history of serious early child abuse (emotional, sexual, or physical) in the context of dysthymia does not portend well for a good response to antidepressants. This finding should *not* preclude the use of antidepressants in survivors of child abuse, but rather serves to highlight the possibility that this version of dysthymia may issue more from pervasively tragic life circumstances and characterological problems than solely from disordered neurotransmitters.

A final type of minor depression is seen in those 15 to 20 percent of individuals who experience only a partial remission of symptoms following a major depressive episode. These people may clinically *look* dysthymic but are not. Typically, they do not have a lifelong history of low-grade or characterological depression. Usually these patients need ongoing and often more aggressive treatment to truly resolve the persistent depressive symptoms.

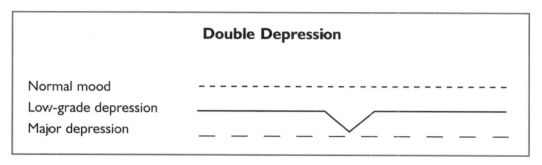

Figure 7-C

Seasonal Affective Disorder

Organisms evolve in ways that promote adaptation to the environment. Examples of this, seen in numerous species (both plant and animal), are the biologic functions influenced by photic stimulation (i.e., exposure to sunlight). Many hormones and neurotransmitters exhibit diurnal variations and are powerfully influenced by environmental stimuli, especially photic stimulation. The first five million years of human evolution took place in equatorial regions that experience a highly stable ratio of sunlight to darkness year-round (basically twelve hours of daylight, twelve hours of darkness). It was around these environmental stimuli that some fundamental biologic processes evolved and remain to this day.

About 150,000 years ago humans migrated to other geographic regions where seasonal changes in patterns of light and dark were first encountered (the farther away from the equator, the more pronounced changes are evident). As the human organism had to adapt to new environmental circumstances, this likely set the stage for difficulties. Apparently, many people manage this adaptation rather well, while others do not. Some of the more vulnerable people are hypothesized to suffer from seasonal affective disorder (SAD), a mood disorder that is ushered in by reduced exposure to bright light.

SAD is also seen in individuals who work at night (and sleep during the day)—some 20 percent of the workforce—and in people who live in areas that experience significant cloud cover and/or air pollution.

SAD can present with a full range of depressive symptoms with intensities varying from mild states of dysphoria to severe, major depression. Interestingly, the majority of people with SAD have symptoms that resemble *atypical depression*; that is, appetite increase, weight gain, fatigue, and hypersomnia. It is theorized that the basic underlying neurotransmitter dysfunction primarily involves serotonin, thus suggesting that if antidepressants are used to treat SAD, the drugs of choice are SSRIs or MAO inhibitors. Additionally, *high-intensity light therapy* has been found effective in treating SAD.

This involves daily exposure to bright light (either by way of a commercially available light box that provides between 2500 and 10,000 lux of light, or by encouraging the patient to go outside for at least one hour per day).

For more detailed information regarding SAD, the reader is referred to the book *Winter Blues*, by N. E. Rosenthal, Guilford Press (2006).

Premenstrual Dysphoric Disorder (PMDD)

Approximately 5 percent of women experience severe mood changes premenstrually. This may involve irritability, anxiety, and/or depression. When depressive symptoms are evident, they sometimes reach a level of severity suggestive of major depression. This disorder is characterized by the tremendous regularity in the onset and remission of symptoms. Mood symptoms generally occur for only a few days beginning several days prior to menses. Generally, there are no psychosocial stressors (i.e., it is best seen as an endogenous disorder). The limbic system contains estrogen receptors, and it is hypothesized that fluctuations seen in female hormones premenstrually may destabilize neurotransmitter functioning in key limbic areas. Clinical experience rather strongly supports the hypothesis that serotonin is the primary neurotransmitter underlying PMDD. The most effective pharmacological treatments currently available for PMDD are SSRIs.

Postpartum Depression

Subtle mood changes are seen in the majority of new mothers. The so-called "baby blues" occur in 50 to 80 percent of women following childbirth. However, such changes are not pathological and do not exclusively involve sadness. These mood changes involve increased sensitivity to the whole range of emotions, including happiness. Such enhanced sensitivity may enable new mothers to be even more attuned to the nuances of their child's emotions.

Postpartum depression is another story. It occurs in 10 percent of women and can have devastating effects. Generally, the onset is two to six weeks after delivery, and if left untreated, it may last from one to two years. Postpartum depressions are often severe and not only cause suffering for the woman but can also significantly interfere with crucial mother-child bonding.

Those most prone to postpartum depressions are women who also have experienced premenstrual dysphoric disorder and/or prior postpartum depressions. In addition, it is not rare that the stresses, the normal changes, and the sleep deprivation following delivery can precipitate a first episode of bipolar illness in a woman genetically predisposed to this disorder. Severe manias, obsessive-compulsive disorder, and psychoses may also develop following the birth of a child.

Why It's Important to Screen for Bipolar Disorder

Serious depressions come in two varieties: unipolar and bipolar. In the latter, depressions occur along with episodes of *mania* (extreme states of agitation, hyperactivity, racing thoughts, and sometimes psychotic symptoms) or *hypomania* (milder episodes of increased energy, euphoric mood, irritability, decreased need for sleep). More details regarding the diagnosis of bipolar disorder are covered in the next chapter.

For 60 percent of teenagers and adults, and 70 percent of children suffering from bipolar disorder, their first mood episode is serious depression. It has been well documented that antidepressant medications are risky drugs to use in treating bipolar depression. Most often they are generally ineffective in treating bipolar depression; they can cause the depressed person to switch from a state of depression to mania, and over time, they can worsen the course of bipolar disorder. It must be emphasized that manic episodes can be very problematic and sometimes dangerous (see chapter 8). The following clinical features may suggest a higher risk of bipolar disorder.

- Depressive symptoms that include *hypersomnia* (excessive sleeping), severe fatigue, increased appetite, carbohydrate craving, and weight gain. This group of symptoms, as noted earlier, is often referred to as "atypical symptoms."

- Psychotic symptoms (e.g., delusions or hallucinations).

- A family history of bipolar disorder.

It is very important for all people suffering with depression to be screened for possible bipolar disorder. The list above is helpful, and we also strongly recommend the self-administered Mood Disorder Questionnaire, which can be found on the following website: www.bipolarhelpcenter.com.

Etiology

It is easy to be seduced by surface symptoms and make assumptions about etiology and treatment. If all sore throats were treated with antibiotics, only about 10 to 15 percent would respond, because most sore throats are due to viral rather than bacterial infections. It is likewise with psychiatric disorders: common symptoms should not automatically lead to conclusions regarding common etiologies.

The causes of depression have been viewed from a number of developmental and psychological perspectives, including the following:

- Psychodynamic models focusing on retroflexed rage and inadequate psychological "metabolism" of aggression and the development of an overly punitive superego

- Attachment theories and the role that loss play in precipitating depression or mourning, in humans and in animals (Bowlby 1986)

- Object relations theory, which implicates faulty separation-individuation experiences and a failure to develop self-soothing introjects (Mahler et al. 1975)

- The learned helplessness model, in which depression is seen to emerge when people (or animals) perceive that "No matter what I do, I have no ability to influence aversive experiences" (Seligman 1990)

- The cognitive model, in which certain life experiences contribute to the development of pervasive cognitive schemas or cognitive distortions—negative mental sets and expectations that automatically influence ongoing perceptions, conclusions, and predictions about the future (Beck 1976)

Clearly, these models all have merit in helping to tease out complex factors that can contribute to the development of depression. These psychological causes also very likely influence much of what goes on in the so-called biologic depressions.

However, the focus of this section is limited to a discussion of current theories of biological causation—causes that either underlie or contribute to the development of the biologic-based depressions listed above.

The dominant theories of biologic causation draw from a diverse source of research, which will be highlighted only briefly here:

- Genetic studies (primarily derived from population, family, twin, and adoptive studies) suggest that certain depressive disorders may have a genetic loading, especially bipolar and recurrent unipolar depression.

- In both human and animal studies, exposure to two general classes of stress may result in the neurotransmitter abnormalities underlying depression. These include experiences of loss and exposure to highly stressful situations where no avoidance, escape, or coping is available (resulting in an eventual state of "learned helplessness").

- Certain medical illnesses can result in systemic biochemical and hormonal changes that affect the central nervous system (e.g., thyroid disease, viral infections, and so on; see figure 7-A).

- Numerous drugs have been shown to have a negative impact on 5-HT (serotonin), NE (norepinephrine), and DA (dopamine) in vulnerable individuals (see figure 7-B).

- Primary neurological disease may affect or destroy brain areas responsible for affect regulation (e.g., Parkinson's disease, Alzheimer's disease).

- Severe early neglect can result in persistent abnormalities in corticotropin releasing factor (CRF), which can result in exquisite vulnerability to depression (Nemeroff 1997).

- Decreased photic (bright light) stimulation can cause depression.

- Decreased physical exercise can cause or exacerbate depression.

- Very poor nutrition can result in a deficiency of certain amino acids that are essential for the production of neurotransmitters, resulting in depression.

Monoamine Hypothesis

The aforementioned data, coupled with numerous positive outcome studies of the effectiveness of antidepressants, has led to the development of the *monoamine* (or biogenic amine) *hypothesis* of depression. The theory holds that depressive symptoms are ushered in by a malfunction of norepinephrine (NE), serotonin (5-HT), and/or dopamine (DA) neurons, which play critical roles in the functioning of the limbic system and the adjacent hypothalamus. The basic neuronal malfunction is felt to be identical for NE, 5-HT, or DA neurons. Interestingly, it is possible to transiently deplete these neurotransmitters (using drugs and/or manipulating diet to exclude certain amino acids), yet most people who do not have a history of depression do not become clinically depressed. It is hypothesized that neurotransmitter depletion leads to depression only in the presence of a genetic predisposition to mood disorders.

Recall the discussion in chapter 3 of normal chemical events at the level of the synapse. The monoamine hypothesis holds that several abnormalities may develop in NE, DA, or 5-HT neurons in the brain. The first is excessive reuptake (see figure 7-D). The effect of this abnormality is that significant amounts of neurotransmitter, that have already been released from the presynaptic cell, are rapidly reabsorbed. The result is decreased ability to stimulate postsynaptic receptors. The nerve cells, in a sense, are then unplugged. A second hypothesized malfunction involves decreased release of neurotransmitters into the synapse. This may be due to a reduction in the synthesis of the neurotransmitter and an inability to adequately store neurotransmitters in vesicles, and/or abnormalities in the process of vesicle migration and the creation of transmembrane pores.

A third way NE, DA, and 5-HT cells can shut down is when the naturally occurring enzyme monoamine oxidase (MAO) becomes too active, excessively degrading neurotransmitters. This results in major depression, but often a depression with its own unique symptomatic signature (see the previous section "Atypical depressions").

A fourth way cells can malfunction is by way of disruption of the synthesis of neuroprotective proteins, such as BDNF (brain-derived neurotropic factor). The production of this important protein is markedly reduced during episodes of severe depression. BDNF reduces the toxic effect of hypercortisolemia (an abnormal elevation in the stress hormone cortisol, seen to occur in 60 percent of people with major depression). One important mechanism of action of antidepressants is to increase the production of BDNF.

A final type of cellular dysfunction may be traced to abnormalities in receptors. This might involve a shift in the absolute numbers of receptors (or the ratio of inhibitory-to-excitatory receptors) and/or altered levels of receptor sensitivity, both of which can change the excitability levels of nerve cells. Such changes appear to be due to alterations in gene expression, which are likely to be secondary to the effects of second messengers.

Which of the cellular changes appear first and how they interact is not fully understood. However, as those conditions come to affect hundreds of thousands of NE, DA, or 5-HT cells throughout the limbic system and hypothalamus, biologic rhythms (such as sleep cycles) and drives (including hunger and sex) get off track; pleasure centers fail to respond (anhedonia); and emotional-control structures in the limbic system fail (resulting in lability or emotional dyscontrol). With time, the emergence

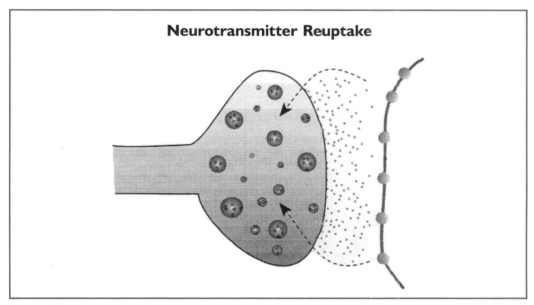

Neurotransmitter Reuptake

Figure 7-D

of neurovegetative symptoms is seen. Without treatment, this abnormal condition can persist for many months (on average six to eighteen months), and then it may begin to reestablish normal functioning; that is, the condition is often self-limiting, again, for reasons that are not well understood.

Biologic Consequences

Numerous physiological consequences can occur with severe depression (above and beyond the symptoms listed earlier). These are mentioned here, briefly:

- Extraordinarily high, sustained levels of cortisol (hypercortisolemia), seen in about 50 to 60 percent of those with major depression, have been associated with cell death in the hippocampus, atrophy of the anterior cingulate (a subcortical frontal-lobe brain structure) (Sapolsky 1996), and damage to the interior walls of arteries. The latter likely contributes to the higher incidence of coronary heart disease seen in people with chronic depression.

- Hypercortisolemia in depressed mothers during pregnancy may be harmful to the fetus (Sapolsky 1994).

- Abnormal brain metabolic states occur during depressive episodes, including:
  - Hypometabolism in the frontal lobes (especially the medial-orbital area; anterior cingulate; and lateral, dorsal prefrontal cortex).
  - Hypermetabolism in hypothalamus, amygdala, hippocampus, and infra-limbic cingulate (area 25) (Mayberg 1997).

- Reductions in secretion of growth hormone that may contribute to osteoporosis, and retarded growth and failure to thrive in children and elders.

- High cortisol levels leach out minerals from bone and contribute to osteoporosis.

- Immune-suppression (likely due to multiple factors, including chronic sleep deprivation and hypercortisolemia).

- Reduced synthesis of brain-derived neurotropic factor (BDNF), which is essential for neuronal maintenance, repair, and neurogenesis (Thoenen 1995).

This list is not all-inclusive. It is clear that beyond the tremendous emotional suffering, depressive disorders often take a significant toll on physical health.

Treatment

Treatment with antidepressant mediations is described in detail in chapter 16. However, discussion of some issues regarding treatment is warranted at this point.

Large-scale empirical treatment algorithm studies are beginning to provide guidelines for medication choices based on the clinical presentation. However, there is not an absolute way to determine which underlying neurotransmitter system (i.e., DA, 5-HT, or NE) may be the culprit in any particular depressed patient. Antidepressants fall into five broad classes: those that target NE, DA, 5-HT (the SSRIs), dual-action drugs (such as Effexor, which targets 5-HT and NE), and MAO inhibitors (see figure 7-E). Chapter 16, which covers antidepressants, will present some general guidelines for medication choices.

When the appropriate medication is found, generally after two to four weeks of treatment, the person begins to notice a reduction in symptoms (especially vegetative symptoms). Under ideal circumstances, the depression may be largely resolved within six to eight weeks (although it often takes longer). The clinical improvement is believed to correspond with a normalization of neuronal functioning. At such time, despite the improved clinical picture, medication discontinuation is not advised. Stopping medication at the point of symptomatic improvement has been associated with a very high acute relapse rate, at least 50 percent relapse within one month. Although the medication has returned the nerve cells to a more normal state, the cells are unstable and easily can regress if medication is not onboard. Thus, continued treatment with the antidepressants is necessary for at least six months. Then, cautious discontinuation generally results in stable functioning (the acute relapse rate drops to below 10 percent). Recurrence can occur months to years in the future, however, owing to the episodic/recurrent nature of depression.

Many millions of depressed patients have been helped with antidepressant medication. Clearly, these drugs often work when they are properly prescribed. Also, other approaches have been shown both to reduce depression and alter neurobiology, including the following:

- Electroconvulsive therapy (ECT)

- High-intensity light therapy

- Repetitive Transcranial Magnetic Stimulation (rTMS)

- Vagus nerve stimulation

- Exercise

- Psychotherapy

- Psychosurgery (rarely used)

It is important to underscore the fact that a number of the personal, emotional, and existential issues that make up the experience of a major depression are not magically resolved by antidepressants. Even under ideal circumstances when medications work well, most patients must engage in a good deal of soul-searching, mourning, and working through. The combined approaches of pharmacotherapy and psychotherapy offer the best chance of successful recovery from depression. This has been documented in studies investigating the combined use of antidepressants and three forms of psychotherapy especially designed for treating depression: cognitive-behavioral (Beck 1976; March et al. 2004), cognitive-behavioral analysis (McCullough 2000), and interpersonal psychotherapy (Klerman et al. 1984).

Selective Action of Antidepressant Medication

Generic Name	Brand Name	Norepinephrine Effects	Serotonin Effects	Monoamine Oxidase Effects	Dopamine Effects
imipramine	Tofranil	++	+++	0	0
desipramine	Norpramin	+++++	0	0	0
amitriptyline	Elavil	+	++++	0	0
nortriptyline	Aventyl, Pamelor	+++	++	0	0
protriptyline[a]	Vivactil	++++	+	0	0
trimipramine[a]	Surmontil	++	++	0	0
doxepin[a]	Sinequan, Adapin, Silenor	+++	++	0	0
maprotiline	Ludiomil	+++++	0	0	0
amoxapine	Asendin	++++	+	0	0
duloxetine	Cymbalta	++++	++++	0	0
venlafaxine	Effexor	++	+++	0	+
trazodone	Desyrel, Oleptro	0	+++++	0	0
fluoxetine	Prozac	0	+++++	0	0
paroxetine	Paxil, Pexeva	+	+++++	0	0
sertraline	Zoloft	0	+++++	0	+
bupropion[b]	Wellbutrin	+++	0	0	++
nefazodone	Serzone	+	+++	0	0
fluvoxamine	Luvox	0	+++++	0	0
clomipramine	Anafranil	+++	+++++	0	0
mirtazapine	Remeron	+++	+++	0	0
citalopram	Celexa	0	+++++	0	0
escitalopram	Lexapro	0	+++++	0	0
atomoxetine	Strattera	+++++	0	0	0
desvenlafaxine	Pristiq	++	+++	0	+
vilazodone	Viibryd	0	+++++	0	0
isocarboxazid	Marplan	+++	+++	+++++	+++
phenelzine	Nardil	+++	+++	+++++	+++
tranylcypromine	Parnate	+++	+++	+++++	+++
selegiline transdermal	Emsam	+++	+++	+++++	+++

a Uncertain but likely effects
b Atypical antidepressant; uncertain effects but likely to be a dopamine and norepinephrine agonist

Figure 7-E

QUICK REFERENCE
When to Refer for Medication Treatment

Event	Symptoms
Grief becomes clinical depression	Early morning awakening Serious weight loss Anhedonia Agitation
Major depression has vegetative symptoms	Sleep disturbance Appetite disturbance Fatigue Decreased sex drive Agitation or psychomotor retardation Anhedonia
Major depression has atypical symptoms	Pronounced fatigue Hypersomnia Increased appetite and weight gain Rejection sensitivity Reactive dysphoria
Dysthymia presents with sustained symptoms	Low energy Anhedonia
Daily functioning is markedly impaired	
Presence of severe suicidal impulses or psychotic symptoms	
Major depression or dysthymia fails to respond to psychotherapy	

8

Bipolar Disorders

The bipolar disorders (historically referred to as manic-depressive illness) are mood disorders characterized by the essential diagnostic feature of mania or hypomania. In general, these disorders follow cyclic patterns of mood, behavior, and thought alterations, alternating between mania or hypomania and depression. These episodic changes are only core features of a variable, heterogeneous group of illnesses. *DSM-IV-TR* classification distinguishes between bipolar I, bipolar II, cyclothymia, and bipolar disorder unspecified. Further diagnostic distinctions are made depending on severity of symptoms and time-course patterns. Pharmacologic treatment of the bipolar disorders is rapidly evolving, with the bulk of useful data having been generated in the last decade.

Differential Diagnosis

Mania rarely occurs as a primary psychiatric condition by itself, so the presence of a manic episode usually leads to a diagnosis of bipolar disorder, even in the absence of a clear depressive history. The manic episode as defined by *DSM-IV-TR* is "a distinct period of abnormally and persistently elevated, expansive, or irritable mood lasting at least one week (or any duration if hospitalization is necessary)" (p. 362). Additionally, manic episodes are defined as mild, moderate, or severe. If severe, psychotic features may be present, but this is not always the case. Associated with this mood disturbance are combinations of racing thoughts, pressured speech, grandiosity, increased activity, engaging in pleasurable activities, distractibility, and decreased need for sleep. If the above patterns are severe enough to impair occupational or social functioning, or to cause hospitalization, a diagnosis of mania is assigned.

A hypomanic episode, defined as lasting at least throughout a four-day period, is marked by an observable change in functioning and disturbance in mood that is uncharacteristic of the individual's usual nondepressed mood and level of functioning.

Hypomania is distinguished from mania by the absence of the significant impairment, or hospitalization, described previously.

The onset of mania can follow an abrupt or a gradual course. A useful stage-model categorization of acute mania has been described by Carlson and Goodwin (1973), as follows:

Stages of Acute Mania

Stage 1 (corresponds with hypomania):

- Increased psychomotor activity
- Emotional lability
- Euphoria or grandiosity
- Coherent but tangential thinking

Stage 2 (frank mania):

- Increased psychomotor activity
- Heightened emotional lability
- Hostility, anger
- Assaultive or explosive behavior
- Flight of ideas, cognitive disorganization
- Possible grandiose or paranoid delusions

Stage 3 (exhibited by some patients):

- Frenzied psychomotor activity
- Incoherent thought processes
- Ideas of reference, disorientation, delirium
- Florid psychosis (indistinguishable from other psychotic disorders, although usually mood congruent)

Case 13

George M. is a thirty-two-year-old man you saw briefly a number of years ago for several intensive therapy sessions following the death of his mother. You know of no other psychiatric history. His family history is significant because his mother was hospitalized twice with "some sort of mental problem." George was in law school at the time and was not informed of the specifics of his mother's illness. His paternal uncle committed suicide when George was fourteen.

He is, by his report, in a stable marriage of ten years and has two children. He has just been made a partner in a small, successful law firm. He prides himself on being skilled in various areas, including athletics and music.

George called your office yesterday requesting an appointment to discuss recent feelings of "anxiety and stress." When George arrives at your office, he is loud and demands to see you immediately because his "time is so valuable." The receptionist is able to escort him to your office fairly quickly, but not before he has attempted to pass out his business cards to other patients in the waiting room. He appears slightly disheveled, is unshaven, and states that he is "afraid to go to my office today," although he will not elaborate further.

During the interview he is unable to remain seated for very long and paces in front of the window. He states the reason for the appointment is for you to "help me straighten a few things out." He specifies that he has been working until 2:00 A.M. every day for the past week because of an upcoming case. He describes this as the "biggest case in recent history" for which he "will become famous." His speech is pressured, and his thought processes are tangential. When you comment that he smells of alcohol, he admits that he regularly needs "a couple of drinks" a day to bring himself "down." You recognize that George's symptoms may indicate a manic episode, and with some difficulty you persuade him to see one of your psychiatrist colleagues for further evaluation.

Mania may develop as a consequence of a general medical condition (see figure 8-A) or as a result of pharmacologic treatment (see figure 8-B).

Bipolar I Disorder

One or more manic or hypomanic episodes with one or more major depressive episodes generally constitute the diagnosis of bipolar I disorder. Depression in bipolar disorder meets diagnostic criteria for major depression, with the exceptions of shorter duration and increased frequency. A mixed episode is defined as at least a one-week period during which the criteria for both a manic episode and a depressive episode (except duration) are met. Mixed episodes are characterized by significant impairment in

Bipolar Disorder Facts

- Lifetime prevalence:
  Type I: 1 percent
  Type II: 4 percent
- Suicide rate: 15 to 20 percent
- Incidence of psychotic features: 47 to 75 percent
- Ratio of men to women:
  Type I: 1:1
  Type II: 1:2
- 60 to 65 percent of patients have positive family history
- Overrepresentation in higher socioeconomic and educational groups
- First episode is usually mania in males, depression in females
- Age of onset:
  Range: 20 to 40 years
  Average: 20 years
  Appearance of first symptoms in adolescence and childhood is not uncommon.
- Average episodes in a lifetime: 7 to 9
- Average recovery time for depressed state: 9 weeks
- Average recovery time for manic state: 5 weeks
- Average recovery time for mixed state: 14 weeks

Medical Conditions Associated with Mania

- Central nervous system trauma, for example, post-stroke
- Metabolic disorders such as hyperthyroidism
- Infectious diseases such as encephalitis
- Seizure disorders
- Central nervous system tumor

Figure 8-A

occupational or social functioning, hospitalization, or psychotic features. Depending on the current presentation, bipolar disorder is subclassified as one of the following (*DSM-IV-TR*):

Bipolar I Subclasses

A. Single manic episode—only one manic episode, no previous major depressive episodes

B. Most recent episode hypomanic—current (or most recent) episode hypomanic with at least one previous manic episode or mixed episode

C. Most recent episode manic—current (or most recent) episode manic with at least one previous depressive episode, manic episode, or mixed episode

D. Most recent episode mixed—current (or most recent) episode mixed with at least one previous depressive episode, manic episode, or mixed episode

E. Most recent episode depressed—current (or most recent) episode depressed with at least one previous manic episode, or mixed episode

F. Most recent episode unspecified—except for duration, current (or most recent) episode manic, hypomanic, mixed or depressive, with at least one manic episode or mixed episode

Between episodes, most bipolar patients are relatively asymptomatic, although many will continue to experience functional impairment after symptom resolution. With increasing age, episodes become more frequent and prolonged. As more recent outcome studies are published, evidence mounts that for many patients, the course of their disease will be particularly difficult, resulting in significant psychosocial morbidity. Unfavorable outcomes may be especially common in rapid cycling, secondary mania, and mixed mania (Keller et al. 1993; American Psychiatric Association 2000; Solomon et al. 1995; Goldberg, Harrow, and Grossman 1995; Evans, Byerly, and Greer 1995; Calabrese et al. 1996; Keck and McElroy 1996).

Beginning with Kraepelin's (1921) systematic classification of dysphoric mania, considerable attention has been paid to mixed states. His model was based on variable symptom patterns expressed in three areas: mood, thought, and motor activity. A factor analytic study of manic subtypes by Sato et al. (2002) provided support for Kraepelin's hypothesis. Mixed mania was once considered uncommon, and debate existed regarding whether it should be considered a subtype of mania or be designated as a distinct affective state. The mixed episode is now recognized in *DSM-IV-TR* as a discrete clinical entity. Earlier prevalence estimates by McElroy et al. (1992) of 30 percent, have not been disproven. Much of the early research provided evidence that mixed episodes can be more severe, chronic, and difficult to treat than pure manic or depressive episodes (Clothier, Swann, and Freeman 1992; McElroy et al. 1992; Dilsaver et al. 1993; Bowden et al. 1994; Swann 1995; Sachs 1996).

DSM-IV-TR associated features for a mixed episode are dysphoria and disorganized thinking or behavior. Demographically, mixed episodes may occur more frequently in younger patients or those over age sixty with bipolar disorder, and may be more common in males than females. A mixed episode can evolve from a manic or depressed episode, or may occur without a preceding mood disorder or episode. A mixed episode can evolve into a depressed episode or a manic episode, although the former is more common than the latter.

Recent attention has focused on developing more precise diagnostic indicators and treatment regimens for bipolar depression, mixed episodes, and rapid cycling. It is speculated that continued research may lead to the identification of separate and distinct bipolar I processes (Soares 2000; Goldberg 2000). For the treating therapist, it is important to point out that there is ongoing controversy regarding the role of antidepressants in bipolar depression. The potential for antidepressants to induce mania is well documented. Concerns about this effect have led, by extension, to the suggestion that antidepressant treatment may play a role in the development of rapid cycling. Correspondingly, the literature and expert guidelines are not in concordance regarding the use of antidepressants in bipolar I depression, especially for sequential courses of therapy. Likewise, there is disagreement regarding recommendations for the length of antidepressant treatment. Chapter 17 addresses medication treatment issues in more detail.

Bipolar II Disorder

Bipolar II disorder is defined as one or more depressive episodes and at least one episode of hypomania. It has been postulated that bipolar II is difficult to differentiate from major depression, for several reasons. First, many patients subjectively do not recognize periods of elevated mood as dysfunctional—or may even deny the existence of such periods because of the predominate depressive element. Second, the patient may primarily manifest irritability rather than classic mood and behavior symptoms of hypomania. Finally, there is considerable variation between individual clinicians' ability to reliably assess for hypomania. Note that while *DSM-IV-TR* criteria require a four-day duration for hypomania, in bipolar II disorder, there is substantial evidence that indicates the average length may be as short as two to three days (Akiskal et al. 2000).

Drugs That Can Induce Mania

- Stimulants (amphetamines)
- Antidepressants (especially tricyclic antidepressants)
- SAM-e
- Antihypertensives
- Corticosteroids (prednisone) in higher doses
- Anticholinergics (benztropine, trihexyphenidyl)
- Thyroid hormones (levothyroxine)

Figure 8-B

Case 14

Cheryl R. is a twenty-eight-year-old married woman with two children under three years of age. She has been referred by her family doctor, who has been treating her depression for nine months with fluoxetine, 20 mg daily. Her physician states that medication adjustment is not indicated and thinks "talking therapy" will be beneficial. Her psychiatric history is negative for hospitalizations, and she has never been in therapy. She describes a "lifetime of sadness" with periodic episodes of suicidal ideation during late adolescence.

Cheryl reports moderate improvement in her depression since starting the medication and wants to continue taking it. However, she says that some of her initial symptoms of irritability, tearfulness, and tiredness have never really improved. She reports continued initial insomnia and describes lying awake worrying about things.

Her major concern is that she is not the "best mother" she can be. On particularly "bad days," she places the children in front of the television and retreats to her room. She wishes she had more "good days," which occur about every three months and last about a week. During these periods she begins sewing and craft projects for the house, socializes with neighbors, exercises, and "feels on top of the world."

She appears slightly nervous and describes her mood as "pretty bad." She describes her marriage as "average" and her children as the "center of her life." She is moderately impatient with the interview questions relative to history taking, since she wants to "get on with things."

You are encouraged by Cheryl's motivation for treatment. However, you internally question whether she may fit the profile for bipolar II. In the process of the diagnostic interview, you elicit enough information indicative of hypomanic periods that predated the initiation of fluoxetine to warrant further consultation with her original prescriber or a psychiatrist.

Cyclothymia

The features of cyclothymia include periods of alternating depression and elation, of at least two years' duration, that do not meet criteria for either major depression or mania (see figure 8-C). During this two-year period, symptoms are never absent for more than two months. Social and occupational impairment may occur during the depressive phase but, typically, not during the hypomanic period. However, for many individuals, the pervasive, irregular pattern of mood lability eventually affects personal and work relationships. Because "mood swings" are a frequent complaint of individuals with certain personality disorders, it is important to identify the presence of the associated behavioral criteria for hypomania or depression before establishing a diagnosis of cyclothymia.

This is a chronic disorder, with approximately one-third of individuals later developing a major affective disorder (Akiskal et al., cited by Hirschfeld and Goodwin 1988). Cyclothymia is so strikingly consistent with bipolar disorder with regard to

---

Cyclothymia Criteria

- History of numerous hypomanic and depressive episodes
- The intensity of episodes does not warrant a diagnosis of major depression or full-blown mania
- Not due to any established organic factors or substance abuse

---

Figure 8-C

symptoms, family history, course, and treatment response that some clinicians argue for its categorization as a variant of bipolar disorder.

Although the "classic" manic is readily diagnosed, differentiating between diagnostic subtypes may be more difficult, especially when a seasonal pattern exists. Further disorders to rule out in the differential diagnosis include attention-deficit/hyperactivity disorder, schizophrenia, and schizoaffective disorder.

Bipolar Disorder Unspecified

Disorders with bipolar features that do not meet any specific bipolar disorder criteria fall into this category. *DSM-IV-TR* provides the following examples:

- Very rapid alterations in manic and depressive symptoms that meet symptom criteria, but not duration criteria

- Recurring hypomania without major depression symptomology

- Mania superimposed on certain delusional or psychotic disorders

- Hypomania with chronic depressive symptoms that does not meet the frequency criteria for cyclothymia

- Situations in which bipolar disorder cannot be determined as primary or secondary to medical conditions or substances

Episode Specifiers

Episode specifiers that apply to bipolar I disorder are listed below. Not all specifiers apply to all bipolar I disorders. The reader is referred to the *DSM-IV-TR* for full explanation:

- Severity/psychotic/remission

- Chronicity

- With catatonic features

- With melancholic features

- With atypical features

- With postpartum onset

The above episode specifiers also apply to bipolar II disorder, depressed.

Course Specifiers

DSM-IV-TR course specifiers that apply to bipolar I and bipolar II disorder include:

- With/without interepisode recovery

- Seasonal pattern

- Rapid cycling

Rapid-cycling bipolar disorder warrants special attention, due to the diagnostic and treatment challenges it presents. Rapid cycling is defined as at least four episodes of either mania, hypomania, or major depression in the previous twelve months. The characteristics of rapid cycling are these:

Rapid Cycling Bipolar Disorder

- Estimated incidence: 10 to 20 percent of bipolar patients.
- Of rapid cyclers, 70 to 90 percent are women (no link to menstrual cycle or menopausal status).
- May be associated with hypothyroidism, neurological conditions, head injury, mental retardation, and/or substance abuse.
- Poor lithium response.
- Cycle acceleration may be associated with antidepressant use.
- Poor long-term prognosis.
- Most cases of rapid cycling represent a time-limited complication of bipolar illness that lasts from a few months to one and one-half years. Less than 5 percent of patients with rapid cycling experience chronic rapid cycling (Gitlin 2002; Bowden 2003).

Suggested Model for Expanded Spectrum of Bipolar Disorders

In addition to the theoretical questions raised relative to dysphoric mania, other symptom patterns have been discussed as possible variants of bipolar disorder. Akiskal (1996); Akiskal and Bowden (2000); and Pies (2002) have presented an extensive case in support of defining bipolar disorders across a broader spectrum. Key points in their theory address softer expressions of bipolar I and bipolar II disorders, temperamental dysregulation, and the overlap between cycling affective states and personality disorders. Akiskal acknowledges that his ideas are controversial and await formal research examination. His arguments are included in this book, not as a criticism of established *DSM-IV-TR* criteria, but as a means of acknowledging that these ideas may be evident in clinical practice. Therapists may be faced with situations in which physician colleagues ascribe to this wider-spectrum nosology and elect to utilize mood stabilizing agents, or combinations, in the absence of the classic target symptoms of bipolar disorder. There are obvious challenges presented to the therapist in these scenarios, especially regarding assessment, treatment planning, therapeutic approach, and patient education.

Etiology

Even though bipolar disorder, formerly called *manic-depressive illness,* was first described by Kraeplin in 1898, causational and treatment questions persist. The introduction of lithium as an effective treatment in the 1970s sparked renewed research interest. Since that time, numerous theories have been investigated, most of which focused more on neurobiology and genetic transmission than on environmental influences, although the latter is not without importance. The complexity and expense of studying this disorder place limits on achieving consistent and replicable data. Throughout the 1970s, 1980s, and into the mid-1990s the theories focused on a variety of neurologic processes: neurotransmitters, synaptic activity, cell membrane function, and second messenger systems.

- **Dysregulation Theory.** J. Rosenthal et al.'s (1986) dysregulation theory includes (but by definition is not specific to) bipolar disorder. In this model, mood is regulated by several homeostatic mechanisms. The failure of a component part leads to the expression of mood outside of set limits, which are identified as the "symptoms" of mania and depression. R. Post, S. Weiss, and O. Chuang (1992) offer a similar explanation: that overactivity in either of the mediating "circuits" of mania or depression leads to the appearance of associated behavioral manifestations.

- **Chaotic Attractor Theory.** The chaotic attractor theory of J. P. Crutchfield et al. (1986) is intriguing and may help explain the unpredictable course of bipolar disorder. This model is predicated on a biochemical defect leading to dysregulation of neurotransmitter synthesis. The type of dysregulation is consistent, but the symptom presentation (either mania or depression) depends on the physiological or environmental conditions at the moment. Building on chaos theory, Gottschalk, Bauer, and Whybrow (1995) obtained results confirming a low-dimensional chaotic process in bipolar disorder.

- **Kindling Theory.** J. C. Ballenger and R. M. Post's (1980) kindling model of mood disorder is not completely adequate, but it has provided some valuable contributions to the reconceptualization of several psychiatric disorders. This hypothesis states that some psychiatric symptoms are the result of cumulative subclinical biochemical changes in the limbic system. This progressive buildup causes neurons to become more excitable until, eventually, clinically observable symptoms appear. The kindling model has been offered as an explanation for the progression and changes in bipolar disorder over time, especially the increasing frequency and severity of episodes that often occurs with aging.

In the late 1990s, research expanded to include a greater focus on molecular and cellular processes, signaling networks, and neuroplasticity. In the models summarized below, the evolution of this research is apparent. Due to the complex nature of this research we have outlined and clarified the major theoretical models, especially those that present new and thought-provoking ideas. Manji (2001), and Manji and Lennox (2000) have recently published very complete review articles that are referenced below, along with many secondary references.

- **Catecholamine Theory.** Although conclusions vary regarding the results obtained, in general, there is evidence suggesting that the catecholamine hypothesis of mood disorders extends to bipolar disorder, but probably not in a primary causative capacity (Goodwin and Jamison 1990; Schatzberg and Schildkraut 1995; Manji and Potter 1997, as cited in Manji 2001). Noradrenergic abnormalities predominate and are measured by concentrations of norepinephrine and its major metabolite, MHPG. Overall, urinary MHPG levels are lower in bipolar depressed patients and are higher during manic episodes. Urinary MHPG levels are lower in bipolar depression than in unipolar depression. In mania, CSF concentrations of NE and MHPG are elevated. There is less clear evidence for the role of other catecholamines in bipolar disorder. Serotonergic abnormalities have not been substantiated. However, areas that are being researched include reduced serotonin levels and alterations in the serotonin transporter. Preliminary research regarding the dopaminergic system implicates a decreased CSF concentration of HVA, the major dopamine metabolite (Willner 1995).

Although there are studies that have investigated the role of the cholinergic system in bipolar disorder, at this time there is no strong clinical evidence that implicates cholinergic abnormalities.

- **The HPA Axis Theory.** The HPA axis has been studied widely in mood disorders (see chapter 3). The strongest association between overactivation of the HPA axis and bipolar disorder appears to be in mixed states and in bipolar depression, with less convincing evidence in classic mania (Goodwin and Jamison 1990; Garlow, Musselman, and Nemeroff 1999).

- **Protein Signaling Network Theory.** At least two signaling pathways are thought to be implicated in bipolar disorder, the G protein pathway, discussed in chapter 3, and the protein kinase C (PKC) pathway. There is more evidence to support the proposed role of G proteins than of PKC, but research involving the latter is expanding. These systems have been likened to "cellular cogwheels" (Manji 2001) in that they function to integrate complex biochemical input and output and to regulate feedback mechanisms. In addition, these systems may play a role in maintaining cellular memory and plasticity (Bhalla and Iyengar 1999; Weng, Bhalla, and Iyengar 1999).

- **Calcium Signaling Theory.** Abnormalities in calcium signaling have long been postulated to play a role in bipolar disorder, extrapolated from evidence of higher-than-normal intracellular calcium levels in bipolar patients. However, the exact nature of what gives rise to these increases and how that might affect bipolarity has yet to be elucidated. There is mixed evidence that calcium channel blocking drugs are effective in treating bipolar disorder, which complicates conclusive interpretations. Research continues, with potential promising findings with nimodipine.

- **Neuroanatomical Theories: Cellular Resiliency.** As in schizophrenia research, efforts have been made to explore neuroanatomical abnormalities in mood disorders from a causational approach, as well as from a disease-consequence approach. To date, neuro-imaging and postmortem studies have shown enough positive results that research in this area is likely to expand greatly (Soares and Mann 1997; Manji et al. 2000). Key initial findings point to a decrease in CNS volume and cell numbers, neurons, and/or glia in mood disorders. Some results apply to major depression and some to bipolar disorder. An unexpected finding of these studies is the identification of a cytoprotective protein in the frontal cortex. This finding has sparked interest in defining the mechanism by which lithium and other mood stabilizers increase levels of this protein (see chapter 17 for further discussion). The existence of neuroprotective proteins holds great promise for furthering the understanding of mood disorders and for developing effective treatments.

- **Genetic and Familial Theories.** Familial, twin, and adoption studies support the theory that bipolar disorder is heritable. Bertelsen's early Danish twin studies have been supported in the intervening years, and it is generally accepted that the concordance rate for monozygotic twins is 50 to 60 percent for bipolar disorder (Tsuang and Faraone 1990). Even though the risk factor association in first-degree relatives is four to six times higher than in the general population, the exact mode of transmission has yet to be identified. Genetic linkage studies are complex and difficult to replicate. However, multiple chromosomes have been identified in various studies conducted over the last decade. Chromosome 22 has been implicated in both bipolar disorder and schizophrenia, raising questions as to how distinct the two conditions really are (Nurnberger and Foroud 2000; Potash and DePaulo 2000; Kelsoe et al. 2001).

In summary, the neurobiology of bipolar disorders is thought to encompass both functional and structural abnormalities at multiple levels of the CNS. Molecular and cellular alterations, systems and pathway disruptions, and compensatory processes are all areas of interest, either as independent factors or as elements of a cascade effect. Some of the most convincing evidence in favor of a biological etiology remains the relatively good response to pharmacotherapy and the extremely poor response to purely psychological interventions.

Unlike the biological theories discussed in chapter 7 and chapters 9 through 12 of this book, at this time the precise neurochemical dysfunctions in bipolar disorder have not been clearly established. Our intent is to provide you, as the therapist, with the fundamental knowledge necessary to address your patients' questions about their disorder and the medications prescribed.

Treatment

The evidence is so strongly compelling that bipolar is largely a biologic-based disorder that pharmacologic intervention is the mainstay of treatment. The details of treatment with various pharmacologic agents are discussed in chapter 17.

Although medications are the primary treatment modality for bipolar disorder, it is important to consider the impact of medications in conjunction with other forms of treatment. For instance, milieu therapy, when inpatient care is necessary, will be most effective after initial medication response has reestablished some degree of cooperation and insight. Psychotherapy, especially cognitive, behavioral, and psychoeducational approaches, is effective with the medication-stabilized patient. Group therapy, which can include families, will often revolve around acceptance of the disease as well as of the need for long-term medication treatment, and include a consideration of the side effects and the implications of noncompliance. In instances of medication-resistance or contraindications, ECT should be considered.

QUICK REFERENCE
When to Refer for Medication Treatment

Event	Symptoms
Mood indicates mania or hypomania	Expansiveness, overconfidence, euphoria, irritability, labile mood
Mood indicates depression	Criteria for major depression are met (see chapter 7)
Mood indicates mixed state	Manic and depressive symptoms
Thought process and judgment become impaired	Lack of insight, flight of ideas, grandiosity, tangentiality, paranoia, delusions, hallucinations
Behavior becomes inappropriate	Pressured speech, psychomotor hyperactivity, decreased need for sleep, hypersexual or promiscuous, increased spending, gambling
Grief becomes clinical depression	Early morning awakening, serious weight loss, anhedonia, agitation
Major depression has vegetative symptoms	Sleep disturbance, appetite disturbance, fatigue, decreased sex drive, agitation or psychomotor retardation, anhedonia
Major depression has atypical symptoms	Pronounced fatigue, hypersomnia, increased appetite and weight gain, rejection sensitivity, panic symptoms, reactive dysphoria
Dysthymia presents with sustained symptoms	Low energy, anhedonia
Daily functioning is markedly impaired	
Severe suicidal impulses or psychotic symptoms are present	
Major depression or dysthymia fails to respond to psychotherapy	

9

Anxiety Disorders

Anxiety disorders encompass a broad, heterogeneous group of psychiatric problems. Like depression, anxiety disorders have multiple etiologies. Some appear to be clearly related to biochemical abnormalities, while others are psychogenic in origin. And treatments vary considerably depending on the diagnosis and presumed underlying pathophysiology. Anxiety disorders have often been erroneously seen as mild or benign disorders. However, recent clinical and epidemiological studies indicate that anxiety disorders are quite common—more common even than depression—and exact a heavy toll on individuals and society alike. The current view sees anxiety disorders as often serious, chronic mental illnesses. Especially in severe cases, such as panic disorder, suicide rates are high, alcohol abuse rates reach 30 percent or more, medical services are inappropriately overutilized, and the cardiac-death rate is higher than average.

Differential Diagnosis

Before outlining the main features of each anxiety disorder, it is necessary to define two terms: *panic attacks* and *anxiety symptoms*. Panic attacks are very brief but extremely intense surges of anxiety. The major differences between a panic attack and more generalized anxiety symptoms are differences in the onset, duration, and intensity (see figure 9-A). Panic attacks often "come out of the blue"; that is, they are not necessarily provoked by stress. They come on suddenly, reach full intensity in ten minutes or less, are *extremely* intense, and last anywhere from one to thirty minutes and then subside. The patient feels as if he or she will actually die or go crazy, as we are not talking about uneasiness but full-blown panic.

The person may continue to feel nervous or upset for several hours, but the attack itself lasts only a matter of minutes. If a patient says, "I've had a continuous panic attack for the past three days," he or she may be having intense anxiety symptoms but not a true panic attack. In anxiety disorders without panic attacks, the anxiety symptoms can be very unpleasant but are much less intense; they also can be prolonged or generalized—that is, present most of the day and lasting from days to years. The distinction between anxiety and panic is very important when it comes to making an accurate diagnosis and choosing appropriate treatments. The symptoms of anxiety are as follows:

Symptoms of Anxiety

- Trembling, feeling shaky, restlessness, muscle tension
- Shortness of breath, smothering sensation
- Tachycardia (rapid heartbeat)
- Sweating and cold hands and feet
- Light-headedness and dizziness
- Paresthesias (tingling of the skin)
- Diarrhea, frequent urination, or both
- Feelings of unreality (derealization)
- Initial insomnia (difficulty falling asleep)
- Impaired attention and concentration
- Nervousness, edginess, or tension

Although *DSM-IV-TR* includes twelve types of anxiety disorders, the list of disorders in this chapter is somewhat more brief. Patients suffering from post-traumatic stress disorder (PTSD) and a related disorder, acute stress disorder, often do present with a host of anxiety symptoms; however, anxiety is but one aspect of PTSD. This syndrome also often includes symptoms of depression, transient psychosis, and dissociation. Thus, we have chosen not to address it here, but in a separate chapter (see chapter 12). Additionally, although obsessive-compulsive disorder (OCD) is considered to be an anxiety disorder, its pathophysiology and treatment vary enough from other anxiety disorders to warrant a separate chapter (see chapter 10).

Anxiety Symptoms Versus Panic Attacks

	Anxiety	Panic
Onset	Can be gradual	Very sudden
Duration	Prolonged	One to thirty minutes
Intensity	Mild to moderate	Severe
Precipitated by stressors	Generally	Often not

Figure 9-A

Ten anxiety syndromes can be distinguished, as follows:

1. Generalized anxiety disorder (GAD)

2. Anxiety associated with psychological stress (adjustment disorder with anxiety)

3. Specific phobias

4. Social phobias/social anxiety disorder

5. Agoraphobia without panic

6. Anxiety symptoms due to a general medical condition

7. Substance-induced anxiety disorder

8. Anxiety symptoms secondary to a primary mental disorder

9. "Neurotic" anxiety

10. Panic disorder

Anxiety Facts

- Lifetime prevalence rates for anxiety disorders: 25 percent.

- Thirty-seven million people per year suffer from anxiety disorders in the United States.

- Panic disorder patients are eighteen times more likely to make suicide attempts than normal controls.

- Incidence of anxiety disorders, women to men: 2:1.

- It is estimated that only 30 percent of patients with panic disorder receive treatment. Yet treatment is effective in 70 to 90 percent of those so afflicted.

Generalized anxiety disorder

Generalized anxiety disorder is characterized by chronic, low-level anxiety (without panic attacks). Patients with this disorder may have no specific current stressors. Life in general is stressful for them. Such people are often high-strung and are chronic worriers.

Anxiety associated with acute psychological stressors

In such disorders, anxiety symptoms are not evident prior to the onslaught of stressors; preclinically the person functioned well. Symptoms emerge in the wake of acute life stress.

Specific phobias

These phobias involve fears of specific objects, such as dogs, places, or heights. Anxiety is seen only in the phobic situation.

Social phobias/social anxiety disorder

Social phobias involve serious anxiety symptoms experienced only when the person is in social or interpersonal settings, such as speaking before a group, participating in a social gathering, or asking someone for a date.

Agoraphobia without panic

This disorder is characterized by intense fears of being in situations or places from which escape might be difficult or embarrassing. As in other phobias, the anxiety is accompanied by a strong tendency to avoid being in such feared places. Agoraphobia commonly develops in the course of panic disorder, but in agoraphobia without panic, there is no history of full-blown *spontaneous* panic attacks (see "Panic disorder," below). Experiences of anxiety are always associated either with entry into a feared place or situation, such as entering a crowded store, or with anticipation of such an event.

Anxiety symptoms due to general medical conditions, substance use or abuse, or another primary psychiatric disorder

In these disorders, the anxiety symptoms are secondary to another etiology.

Neurotic anxiety

Neurotic anxiety arises when an individual is beset by significant emotional issues or conflicts but maintains tight defenses against awareness of these inner issues. In other words, the conflicts are unconscious, and what one sees overtly are anxiety symptoms—often "generalized" and *sometimes* in the form of occasional panic attacks. Another version of neurotic anxiety is seen in individuals who are plagued by more conscious conflicts. Often such conflicts take the form of approach-avoidance, such as the person very much wanting to do something but worrying about offending others or violating certain internalized rules or "shoulds." The person feels inwardly torn and will often experience feelings of generalized anxiety.

Panic disorder

Panic disorder is characterized by recurring, intense panic attacks. Many times these attacks appear to be spontaneous, not provoked by identifiable stressors. As the disorder progresses, most patients begin to develop considerable anticipatory anxiety (a rather continuous, mild-to-moderate generalized anxiety as they come to worry when the next attack will occur) and phobias (agoraphobia is especially common). With time, alcohol abuse and depression commonly develop.

Since the etiology and treatment of these anxiety syndromes vary significantly, each is discussed separately below, with greater detail provided for the disorders that are felt to be more strongly biologically based.

Etiology

For decades, the psychoanalytic theory of neurosis rested on Freud's fundamental notions of the psychogenic origin of anxiety (Freud's second, or revised, theory of anxiety, 1923). Most neurotic disorders were felt to arise from the unconscious perception of danger: realistic anxiety (danger from the environment), moral anxiety (danger from the superego), and id anxiety (danger from the id). Such unconscious judgments involving potential danger provoked "signal anxiety" and ignited defensive operations. When defenses failed, patients experienced manifest anxiety symptoms.

Other dominant psychological views of anxiety have been proposed by cognitive theorists such as Beck (1976). The cognitive model suggests that anxiety is generated when people overevaluate the danger in certain situations or underestimate their coping ability. The perception of danger and loss of control can provoke fight-or-flight responses even in nondangerous circumstances. With anxious people, their perceptions of reality are skewed such that there are many misperceptions and "false alarms."

These psychological theories are not at all incompatible with biologic ones, though they were developed before the physiology of anxiety was well understood.

Biologic Theories

Let's now explore theories of biologic etiology. "Hardwired" into the nervous system of humans and many animals is a complex network of nerve pathways, brain structures, and glands that are responsible for eliciting the fight-or-flight response. This response triggers a multilevel neurochemical and hormonal reaction designed to mobilize the body and mind during times of potential danger. Nonessential physiological processes shut down (such as digestion and reproduction), and energy is channeled into a host of bodily functions preparing the organism for rapid action. The nervous system also shifts into a state of hyperarousal and vigilance. All of these changes, which occur rapidly and automatically, have evolved to assure survival when a person or animal confronts actual danger situations. Thus, fundamentally, the biologic mechanisms and processes underlying the fight-or-flight response are necessary and adaptive.

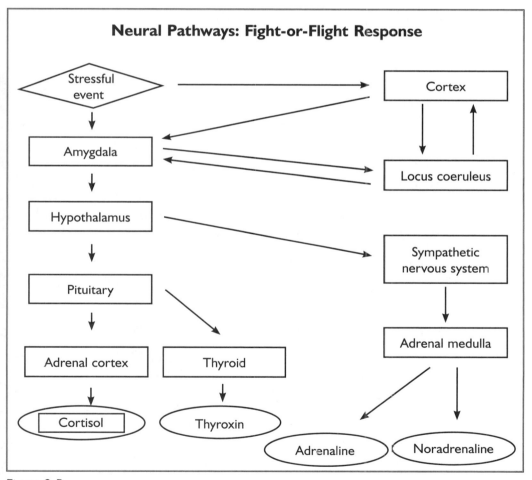

Figure 9-B

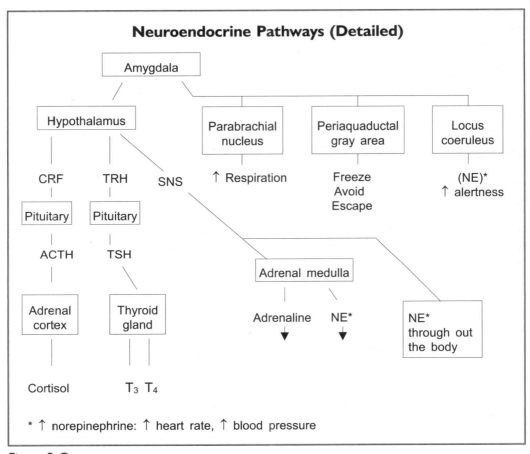

Neuroendocrine Pathways (Detailed)

Amygdala

Hypothalamus — Parabrachial nucleus — Periaquaductal gray area — Locus coeruleus

CRF   TRH   SNS   ↑ Respiration   Freeze Avoid Escape   (NE)* ↑ alertness

Pituitary   Pituitary

ACTH   TSH   Adrenal medulla

Adrenal cortex   Thyroid gland   Adrenaline   NE*   NE* through out the body

Cortisol   T₃ T₄

* ↑ norepinephrine: ↑ heart rate, ↑ blood pressure

Figure 9-C

The basic components of the fight-or-flight mechanism are depicted schematically in figures 9-B and 9-C. As stressful events are perceived at the level of the cortex and also processed in a crude way on the subcortical level (the amygdala), lower brain areas become activated. In a sense, the limbic system is put on alert. Should ongoing perception result in a conclusion that there is imminent danger, a burst of excitation emanates from a cluster of nerve cell bodies in the brain stem called the locus coeruleus (LC). The LC has sometimes been called the adrenal gland of the brain. The LC nerve cells, which project to the limbic system, are mediated by the neurotransmitter norepinephrine.

The limbic system and adjacent hypothalamus shift into high gear, and by way of the pituitary gland (and other downstream endocrine glands) and the sympathetic nervous system, a multitude of stress hormones are released into the system. The brain and body alike are then ready for action.

It is also important to discuss yet another feature of the nervous system that plays a role in anxiety. On the surface of the majority of nerve cells in the brain (including cells in the LC) are tiny gateways referred to as chloride ion channels (see figure 9-D). Chloride ions, which carry a slight negative charge, are in abundance in the fluid surrounding nerve cells. The ion channel can be activated (opened) when stimulated by the naturally occurring neurochemical gamma-aminobutyric acid, GABA for short (see figure 9-D, 2).

As the gate opens, the chloride ions are drawn in. When the nerve cell is infused with negative ions, its electrical characteristics are altered, resulting in decreased excitability (it is hyperpolarized). This operates as a sort of biological braking mechanism, serving to dampen "limbic alert" and calm overall brain excitation. Benzodiazepine molecules (the substances found in antianxiety medications) also bind to the chloride ion channels, further enhancing the in-flow of negative ions and thus producing a widespread calming in many areas of the brain (see figure 9-D, 3).

This model provides an understanding of the mechanism of action of anti-anxiety medications. It also has led to a theory that may explain some anxiety disorders. Since there is a receptor on the chloride ion channel that responds to benzodiazepine molecules, there is speculation that an endogenous benzodiazepine-like chemical may exist in the CNS. To date, however, such a chemical has yet to be identified (although some researchers believe that adenosine may be the chemical). However, should this theory hold true, it may provide an explanation for why some individuals are temperamentally more high-strung and less able to stay calm during stressful times, and why others experience chronic, generalized anxiety. Such individuals *may* suffer from a deficiency of this yet-to-be-identified endogenous neurochemical.

Excitability in the locus coeruleus (LC) is also mediated by serotonin (in this area of the brain, serotonin receptors are inhibitory). Thus any number of factors that lead to a global decrease in serotonin may affect the LC (i.e., it can become disinhibited and thus more sensitive to activation).

Acquired fears appear to be mediated primarily by the amygdala. After exposure to very frightening events, the amygdala encodes certain stimulus elements of the experience. Such memories have been shown to be quite indelible and highly resistant to extinction. Once etched into the memory circuits of the amygdala, this brain structure develops a sort of persistent hypersensitivity to activation by similar stimuli. One result is that reexposure to a similar anxiety-provoking event can result

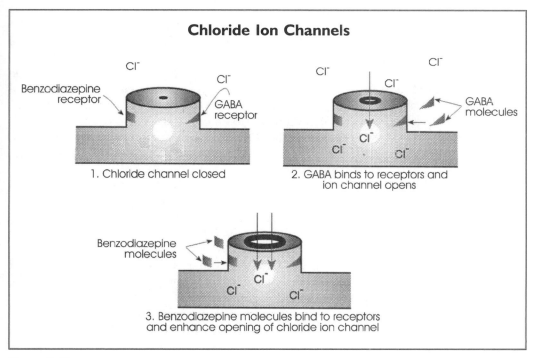

Figure 9-D

in significant or extreme reactivity. Also, generalization often occurs such that non-dangerous stimuli that somewhat resemble the original stressful event may readily provoke intense anxiety reactions; for example, the traumatized combat veteran who now experiences strong surges of anxiety when hearing the backfire from an automobile. There is speculation that serotonin also plays a role in inhibiting cellular reactivity in the amygdala (and serotonergic antidepressants are now considered to be first-line treatments for many anxiety disorders).

Neurobiologic structure and functioning underlying normal separation anxiety in young mammals also play a role in intense anxiety states in adult life; this is especially so with panic disorder. Often, in the six to twelve months prior to the emergence of panic disorder, people with the disorder experienced a significant interpersonal loss. This raises the speculation that such experiences may resensitize those neural circuits that once played a role in normal separation anxiety.

Finally, research on the impact of early child abuse and neglect suggests that such experiences may permanently alter the HPA axis and thus set the stage for chronic vulnerability to anxiety (Nemeroff 1997).

Please note: Biologic theories regarding obsessive-compulsive and post-traumatic stress disorder are dealt with in separate chapters (10 and 12, respectively), which deal specifically with these disorders.

With these biological models in mind, let's begin to look at specific anxiety disorders, many of which represent some type of malfunction in this otherwise adaptive physiological system.

Generalized anxiety disorder (GAD) and anxiety associated with acute stress

In GAD the individual is almost continuously predicting, anticipating, or imagining "dangerous" (unpleasant) events. The limbic system is kept in a perpetual state of alert—on guard for a multitude of "what-ifs." Since daily life rarely presents GAD patients with severely traumatic or life-threatening events, the level of activation does not reach the intensity of threshold of full-blown fight or flight. The result is a low-grade, but chronic, state of anxiety.

GAD is primarily believed to be a psychogenic disorder. However, there is some speculation that at least some GAD patients may suffer from a biologically mediated disorder. One hypothesis is that mentioned above: a deficiency of neurochemicals. Another model has emerged more recently. Treatment with serotonin agonists such as buspirone and 5-HT antidepressants (SSRIs and SNRIs) has been shown to reduce "what-ifing" (worry) in GAD patients. However, the mechanism of action and underlying pathophysiology are not well understood.

In stress-induced anxiety disorders, actual psychological stressors have evoked another version of ongoing limbic alert. And in the wake of severe stress, such patients often may have *occasional* full-blown panic attacks. These disorders emerge in response to life-threatening stressors (natural disasters, combat, assaults, automobile accidents) and in response to a host of emotional stressors (loss of a job, serious illness in a relative, marital separation). In many cases, the anxiety symptoms can be seen as normal responses; that is, they are not pathological. However, the symptoms can be severe enough to warrant treatment.

With GAD and stress-related anxiety, in all likelihood the basic neurobiology is not grossly abnormal. Rather, real or imagined stresses are provoking psychological reactions—which, of course, ultimately are biologically mediated.

Specific phobias

Phobias such as the fear of snakes, closed-in spaces, heights, and so on, are generally considered to be associated either with age-appropriate fears (fears that subside with maturation) or conditioned responses. There is little evidence that these disorders are due to biological dysfunction, and medication treatment is generally not warranted.

Social phobias

Social phobias are certainly influenced by developmental and other life experiences (such as the quality of early attachments, the development of appropriate social skills, and adequate experience interacting with others). At the same time, there is rather compelling evidence suggesting that social phobics (and their more pervasively impaired cousins—avoidant personalities) may have a biologically based disorder.

Animal studies have shown that when baby animals are separated from their parents, they typically enter a state of high arousal and agitation—frequently producing some form of vocal distress signal. This is obviously the case with human infants as well. Separation stresses appear to elicit extremely high levels of neuronal activity in the locus coeruleus (LC). One hypothesis holds that this brain area, in addition to its role in evoking fight-or-flight responses, may be a key brain structure designed to trigger arousal and distress behavior in infants separated from caregivers. Presumably, with psychological development and neurologic maturation, the threshold of LC activity gradually raises. Behaviorally, we see an increased capacity to tolerate separation as children and young animals mature.

What does this have to do with social phobias? One view is that the underlying fear in many social phobias is that the person will be embarrassed, humiliated, and ultimately rejected, which is equivalent to separation. This fear of rejection is also seen in avoidant personalities, so-called hysteroid-dysphorics, and many people suffering from borderline personality disorders. Animals treated with antidepressants or MAO inhibitors (drugs shown to reduce excitation in the LC) exhibit markedly decreased distress in the face of separation stresses. And during the past decade, clinical trials with antidepressants and MAO inhibitors have shown improvement in broad groups of patients with social phobias and rejection sensitivity. The theory contends that such patients may be chronically experiencing very low thresholds of arousal at the level of the LC— accounting for their exquisite sensitivity to humiliation, separation, and rejection.

Agoraphobia without panic

The anxiety experienced with this disorder occurs only when the patient must go into feared situations (such as a store) or in the moments before entering the phobic situation (anticipating anxiety). Although such experiences of anxiety ultimately do involve an activation of the limbic system, the primary disorder is felt to be largely psychogenic, a conditioned fear response. Medications are sometimes used to treat agoraphobia without panic; however, this disorder is not believed to be primarily biologically based.

Anxiety symptoms due to general medical conditions

Certain systemic medical illnesses and primary neurologic disorders can dysregulate CNS neurotransmitters and cause or contribute to anxiety symptoms (see figure 9-E). Note that most anxiety symptoms associated with these medical conditions present in the form of generalized anxiety, although panic attacks can also occur.

Medical Disorders Associated with Anxiety

- Adrenal tumor
- Alcoholism
- Angina pectoris
- Cardiac arrhythmia
- CNS degenerative disease
- Cushing's disease
- Coronary insufficiency
- Delirium[a]
- Hypoglycemia

- Hyperthyroidism
- Ménière's disease (early stages)
- Mitral valve prolapse[b]
- Parathyroid disease
- Partial-complex seizures
- Postconcussion syndrome
- Premenstrual syndrome
- Pulmonary embolism

a Delirium can occur as a result of many toxic and metabolic conditions and often produces anxiety and agitation.

b The mitral valve prolapse probably does not cause anxiety, but it has been found that MVP and anxiety disorders often coexist. This may be due to some common underlying genetic factor.

Figure 9-E

Substance-induced anxiety disorders

A common cause of anxiety symptoms can be traced to drug use or abuse (see figure 9-F).

Anxiety symptoms secondary to primary psychiatric disorders

Certainly, anxiety symptoms are seen in a very wide range of psychiatric disorders, including schizophrenia, mania, PTSD, agitated depressions, and severe personality disorders. It is important to keep in mind that anxiety symptoms do not necessarily signal a diagnosis of anxiety *disorder*. Almost without exception, however, when anxiety is associated with a more primary mental disorder, psychotropic medication treatment is aimed at the primary disorder. (Refer to appropriate chapters for descriptions of etiology and treatment.)

Drugs That Can Cause Anxiety

- Amphetamines
- Appetite suppressants
- Asthma medications
- Caffeine

- CNS depressants (withdrawal from)
- Cocaine
- Nasal decongestants
- Steroids

Figure 9-F

Neurotic anxiety

Although the term *neurosis* has fallen out of favor in some professional circles, the concept still has merit. As conceived of here, neurotic anxiety is a condition in which manifest symptoms of anxiety are evident but the underlying problem can ultimately be traced to unconscious conflicts or unrecognized inner emotional issues. A common example of this is illustrated in case 15.

Case 15

Rob S. is forty-two and recently lost his wife to breast cancer. Emotionally, he grits his teeth and blocks his inner grief. But the overcontainment of his inner feelings of loss has resulted in a tense, brittle adaptation. Rob feels little sadness, but his heart races, he experiences tension headaches, and he has initial insomnia. The problem does not lie in disordered neurons, but in overdefensiveness; and the solution is not to be found in a pill but, rather, in the process of working through and mourning (possibly in the context of psychotherapy). To assume a biological etiology and attempt to medicate away anxiety symptoms with this man would only create more distance between his conscious awareness and his inner, painful emotional concerns.

As mentioned earlier, some neurotic conflicts that generate anxiety may also be experienced on a conscious level. But, again, these are best seen as psychogenic rather than as biologically rooted problems.

Panic disorder

The biological factors that set the stage for the emergence of panic disorder may arise spontaneously (be truly endogenous) or can be set in motion by major life stressors as noted earlier. Biochemical factors likely operate to alter cellular functions in the LC, lowering the excitation threshold for those neurons.

Panic disorder begins with the eruption of full-blown panic attacks—many of which (as mentioned earlier) occur "out of the blue" in low- or no-stress situations. Some individuals with panic disorder suffer from relatively infrequent attacks (a few per month); in more severe cases, attacks can occur several times a day and oftentimes even during sleep. The *noradrenergic hypothesis* holds that the intense, recurring attacks are caused by hypersensitive neurons in the LC or a dysfunction in the natural braking mechanism in the LC nerve cells or both (see figure 9-G).

The nerve axon in figure 9-G impinges back on itself and releases its neurotransmitter norepinephrine (also called noradrenaline, hence the term *noradrenergic hypothesis*). The neurotransmitter typically stimulates inhibitory receptors on the cell body, acting to reduce excitability. However, in panic disorder, the inhibitory-alpha-2 receptors ("brakes") are believed to be dysfunctional (in a state of subsensitivity). Once stimulated, the LC cell continues to fire alerting signals to the limbic system, uninhibited by the normal braking mechanism. Antipanic medications (especially antidepressants) are hypothesized to have their effect by normalizing the operation of LC inhibitory receptors (see chapters 16 and 18). Other molecules that also have been found to exert inhibitory effects on LC neurons include: serotonin, GABA, and opiates. This helps to explain how SSRIs are often useful in treating panic disorder, and how certain minor tranquilizers may reduce panic symptoms (e.g., alprazolam, lorazepam, and clonazepam along with GABA activate chloride ion channels). Although opiates

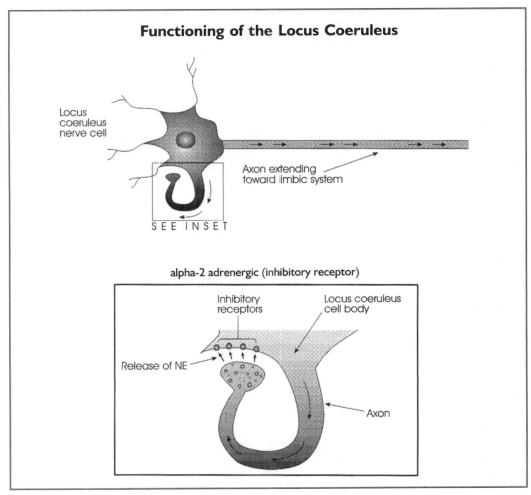

Functioning of the Locus Coeruleus

Locus coeruleus nerve cell

Axon extending toward limbic system

SEE INSET

alpha-2 adrenergic (inhibitory receptor)

Inhibitory receptors

Locus coeruleus cell body

Release of NE

Axon

Figure 9-G

are not approved or indicated for use in treating anxiety disorders, many narcotic addicts may be self-medicating with opiates to reduce anxiety symptoms.

Treatment

Generalized anxiety disorder

For many patients, psychological approaches are the treatment of choice. These techniques include stress management, cognitive-behavioral treatment,[1] relaxation training, meditation, and psychotherapy. Also, for GAD patients in good health who do not experience coexisting panic attacks, a program of regular, aerobic-level exercise can be very beneficial.

---

1. For a review of cognitive-behavioral treatments for anxiety disorders, the reader is referred to *Depression and Anxiety Management*, an audiotape by John Preston, New Harbinger Publications, 2000.

When medication is indicated, the clinician has four choices:

- Benzodiazepines (the class of drugs often termed *minor tranquilizers* or *anti-anxiety medications*) can be used in severe cases of GAD. However, the use of benzodiazepines to treat GAD has been the subject of considerable controversy. Great concern has arisen regarding potential benzodiazepine abuse and dependence. Certainly, people who chronically use benzodiazepines do develop a physiological dependence on these medications. Nonetheless, concern in the media and medical profession alike may have been overstated. The vast majority of chronically anxious patients do not abuse or become addicted to these medications and rarely require progressive increases in doses. The individuals who do, in fact, present a significant risk of abuse are people with a personal or family history of alcohol or other substance abuse. With such individuals, benzodiazepines are not appropriate. (Guidelines and cautions regarding treatment appear in chapters 14 and 18.)

- The atypical antianxiety medication buspirone has been used with some success with GAD patients. This medication offers the benefits of reduced rumination and worry, but without the problems of sedation and potential drug dependence seen with benzodiazepines. Buspirone is not addictive and thus provides a treatment option for GAD patients with substance abuse risk.

- Both tricyclic and serotonergic antidepressants (SSRIs and SNRIs) are being used increasingly to treat chronically anxious patients. (See chapter 16 for information regarding treatment with SSRI and SNRI antidepressants.)

- The antiseizure medication, gabapentin, is a non-habit-forming drug that can reduce anxiety.

Anxiety associated with acute stress

Again, for most individuals, psychological approaches are best suited for treating acute stress reactions. However, antianxiety medications can be an important adjunct to treatment, especially when the patient is experiencing considerable amounts of agitation or insomnia. The classic form of anxiety-related insomnia is initial insomnia (difficulty falling asleep). Middle insomnia or early morning awakening should alert the clinician to a diagnosis of depression. Medications used to treat daytime anxiety include the whole range of benzodiazepines, and for sleep, the so-called sedative-hypnotics (see chapter 18). Typically, drug treatment for acute stress is short-term (one to four weeks), in combination with crisis intervention and other psychological treatments.

Specific and social phobias

Specific phobias generally are not treated with psychotropic medications. Social phobias often respond well to cognitive-behavioral treatment. When medications are used, the clinician has two main alternatives: For occasional use—for example, to reduce anxiety associated with theatrical performances or public speaking—the beta blocker propranolol has been shown to be quite effective. This drug does little to alter the cognitive aspects of anxiety (worry) but effectively reduces many physiological symptoms, such as rapid heart rate. Anxious patients treated with propranolol take the medication only prior to the stressful event, ingesting 20 to 80 mg about one hour before.

More pervasive forms of social anxiety (and avoidant personality disorder) may be treated with MAO inhibitors, SSRIs, or SNRIs (see chapter 16), in addition to psychotherapy and social-skills training.

Agoraphobia without panic

The treatment of choice for this disorder includes psychotherapy, relaxation training, and behavioral treatment (graded exposure to feared situations). Such approaches have a solid track record of effectiveness, and medication treatment as a sole therapy generally is not effective. However, patients are often treated with psychotropic medications in the early phase of graded exposure therapy. Minor tranquilizers (benzodiazepines) and beta blockers (such as propranolol) can be used to somewhat reduce the level of anxiety as the patient begins gradually to reenter anxiety-provoking situations. As the patient starts to experience success and a sense of mastery, the medications can be gradually phased out.

Anxiety symptoms due to general medical conditions, substance abuse, or primary psychiatric disorder

These symptoms usually are not directly treated with psychotropic medications. Rather the primary medical disorder is treated, or the patient is referred for treatment of a chemical dependency problem (see chapter 14). When psychotropics are employed, they generally are used for short periods of time. Medications of choice are the benzodiazepines (although they should be used with extreme caution in patients with a substance abuse disorder).

As noted earlier, when a primary psychiatric disorder is diagnosed, generally medication treatment targets the primary illness, such as antipsychotics for schizophrenia or antidepressants for agitated depression.

Neurotic anxiety

In neurotic anxiety, medication treatment is generally contraindicated, since the reduction of overt anxiety symptoms can serve to further block awareness of core emotional conflicts. The exceptions are these:

- If the patient has inadequate ego strength to tolerate a more "uncovering" psychological approach.

- If the patient is not psychologically minded or has a low level of cognitive functioning.

- If the clinician must work with a highly symptomatic client in *very brief* therapy.

- If manifest anxiety symptoms are severe. In such cases, short-term treatment with benzodiazepines may help reduce suffering, restore functioning in daily life, and help the patient stabilize. This can then be followed by medication reduction and psychotherapy.

Panic disorder

Panic disorder is the anxiety disorder for which medication treatment plays its most important role. This often-devastating illness is quite responsive to combined medication and psychological treatment. It is helpful to focus on four somewhat discrete aspects of this disorder, each of which requires targeted treatments:

- Panic attacks

- Anticipatory anxiety

- Phobias

- Associated features—alcohol abuse, depression

Panic attacks must be either eliminated or greatly reduced in the initial phase of treatment. Some behavioral and cognitive techniques have been developed to reduce panic attacks, although antipanic medications take effect more rapidly and have a solid track record as safe and highly effective drugs. Antipanic medications fall into three groups:

- High-potency benzodiazepines, such as alprazolam, clonazepam, and lorazepam

- Antidepressants (tricyclics and SSRIs)[2]

- MAO inhibitors

See chapters 16 and 18 for more on these types of medications.

The first goal of treatment is to stop or reduce attacks. However, even when this is successful, anticipatory anxiety and phobias can, and often do, continue unabated. Thus, the second step is to reduce anticipatory anxiety and phobic avoidance using behavioral techniques, especially graded exposure and desensitization. These techniques are highly effective but only after there is good containment of panic symptoms.

Often, especially in more chronic cases, major depression and alcohol abuse/dependency, or both develop along with primary panic symptoms. In that event, appropriate antidepressant medication treatment and/or involvement in Alcoholics Anonymous or a chemical-dependency treatment program becomes necessary.

Finally, when primary anxiety or panic symptoms are resolved, many panic disorder patients often choose to pursue more traditional psychotherapy. As mentioned earlier, a number of panic patients have encountered major losses and must begin the journey of working through these major life changes. In our experience, however, insight-oriented treatment typically must await the resolution of primary panic symptoms.

Unfortunately, a large percentage of patients relapse when medications are discontinued: as many as 70 percent have a return of panic symptoms if medications are withdrawn a year after treatment is initiated. Panic disorder thus appears to be an often chronic condition. A nine-year follow-up study found that about half did not achieve remission (Svanborg, Wistedt, and Svanborg 2008). Thus the clinician should anticipate that medication treatment will last longer than one year. Then a trial discontinuation or medication reduction can be implemented to determine if continued treatment is necessary.

---

2. To date, all antidepressants have been shown to reduce panic symptoms, with one exception: bupropion. This antidepressant can at times exacerbate panic attacks and thus should be used with caution.

QUICK REFERENCE
When to Refer for Medication Treatment

The following anxiety disorders generally are not treated with psychotropic medications; a referral should be made only if the patient's symptoms are severe or fail to respond to psychological treatments:

- Generalized anxiety disorder
- Specific phobias
- Social phobias
- Agoraphobia without panic

If anxiety symptoms occur in the context of:

- A general medical condition
- Substance use or abuse
- Another primary psychiatric disorder

Then treat the primary disorder.

Psychotherapy is the treatment of choice for:

- Anxiety associated with acute stress
- Neurotic anxiety

Treat the following symptoms with medications only if symptoms are severe and fail to respond to psychological treatment:

- Initial insomnia
- Daytime agitation or restlessness
- Impaired concentration

Treatment with medication should be short term (I to 4 weeks).

A combination of medication and psychological therapy is the treatment of choice for panic disorder, as demonstrated by the following:

Event	Symptom
Recurring panic attacks	Sudden onset Intense anxiety Short duration (I to 30 minutes) Some attacks are spontaneous
Patient has had four or more attacks in past month	
Patient has developed significant anticipatory anxiety, phobias, avoidance	
Patient has developed secondary symptoms	Clinical depression Alcohol abuse

10

Obsessive-Compulsive Disorder

Until recently obsessive-compulsive disorder (OCD) was considered to be a very rare disorder. However, newer epidemiological studies show OCD to be just as common as panic disorder, and two to three times as common as schizophrenia.

OCD is a chronic psychiatric condition, often first emerging in childhood and potentially lasting a lifetime. It results in considerable emotional suffering. Yet until recent times, few of those afflicted sought treatment. This is probably due to the common tendency for OCD patients to experience humiliation and shame over symptoms that they generally consider to be "crazy" or "irrational" and thus not to seek out professional help.

Differential Diagnosis

The major features of this disorder are recurring obsessions (persistent intrusive, troublesome thoughts or urges that are recognized by the patient as senseless) and compulsions (repetitive behaviors or rituals enacted in response to an obsession, such as repeatedly checking to see if doors are locked, excessive hand washing, and counting). In order to meet the criteria for obsessive-compulsive disorder, the obsessions and compulsions must create significant distress and be time-consuming enough or otherwise interfere with normal routines, work, activities, or relationships (*DSM-IV-TR*).

Two-thirds of OCD patients are plagued by obsessions regarding dirtiness, contamination, and germs, with corresponding compulsions such as cleaning and hand washing. Another 20 percent primarily are worried about safety issues and engage in repetitive checking rituals (checking to see if doors are locked, if the stove is turned off, retracing their routes when driving to make sure they have not accidentally hit a pedestrian). The remaining patients are concerned with a sense of incompleteness, or lack of order or symmetry, and engage in rituals designed to make their environments "just right." At the heart of most obsessions and compulsions are two key elements:

Obsessive-Compulsive Disorder Facts
■ Lifetime prevalence: 2.5 percent.
■ Ratio of men to women: 1:1.
■ Age of onset: Although many cases of OCD begin in adolescence or early adulthood, about one-third begin in childhood. The incidence of OCD in children is 1 percent.
■ Course: Although some milder cases of OCD can be transient, most moderate-to-severe cases last for many years if untreated.

excessive self-doubt and intense worry regarding the safety of oneself and others. In addition to OCD symptoms, which are a tremendous source of suffering in their own right, two-thirds of OCD patients also experience episodes of major depression.

Many people will experience occasional obsessions and compulsions, especially when under stress or when they sense some loss of control over the environment or inner emotions. These more minor, transient obsessions and compulsions do not constitute OCD, which in contrast is a chronic and often incapacitating disorder.

Some similarities exist between OCD and obsessive-compulsive personality disorder (OCP); however, there are notable differences. For treatment purposes, it is important to distinguish between OCD and OCP. With OCD the person feels "under attack" by the obsessions and compulsive rituals; the symptoms are quite painful and ego-dystonic. In contrast, OCP traits (perfectionism, stinginess, emotional rigidity, overdevotion to work) are experienced as a part of oneself, or ego-syntonic.

Some patients are described as suffering from impulse-control disorders (ICD): gambling, overeating, and so on. Although OCD patients subjectively feel "seized" by an impulse to carry out rituals, notable differences exist between OCD and true ICDs. Those experiencing impulse-control problems find the actions, such as overeating, to be pleasurable. In contrast, OCD patients never enjoy carrying out rituals (beyond some reduction in anxiety). Also, impulse-control patients rarely are riddled with self-doubt or worries about harming others—again in sharp contrast to OCD. Finally, the medication treatments successful in OCD (described below) have been shown to be only modestly effective in most forms of impulse-control disorder.

Anorectics often exhibit a host of obsessions and compulsions (regarding eating—sizes and portions, times for meals, body weight)—yet two notable differences exist between anorectics and OCD patients. Obsessive-compulsive disorder patients almost always admit that the worries and rituals are irrational, whereas most anorectics don't appreciate the irrationality of their acts. Also, medications found to be effective for OCD generally are not effective in the treatment of anorexia nervosa.

Etiology

Traditional psychoanalytic theories posited psychogenic theories for what was once called obsessive-compulsive neurosis. These primarily involved early developmental experiences with perfectionistic, overly strict, and rigid parents who imposed unrealistic standards and stifled the child's emerging autonomy. These theories likely do apply to the development of OCP, but not necessarily OCD. In recent years a number of findings from clinical practice and neurobiology have convincingly argued a biological basis for OCD. Let's take a look at some of this evidence.

The disorder emerges early, often in late childhood, and maintains remarkable symptomatic stability throughout life. The incidence in the general population is 2.5

percent, yet it is 7 percent in first-degree relatives, suggesting a possible genetic loading for the disorder. Also, diseases such as certain types of encephalitis, that selectively damage areas of the basal ganglia (subcortical brain structures), have been shown to result in OCD-symptoms.

Probably most convincing are the findings from pharmacological and neuro-imaging studies. A very large number of clinical studies have shown that OCD patients can be helped by treatment with SSRI antidepressants. And this holds true even in OCD patients without coexisting depression. In addition, antidepressants that do not affect serotonin are not effective in alleviating OCD symptoms. The SSRI antidepressants selectively increase serotonin activity in the brain and probably more specifically in the basal ganglia, cingulate gyrus, and prefrontal cortex.

Finally, several studies of brain metabolic functioning reveal that in highly symptomatic OCD patients there is a significant increase in metabolic activity (thus increased activation) in the prefrontal cortex and basal ganglia. Furthermore, this abnormal metabolic activity becomes normalized when patients are treated with SSRI antidepressants (Baxter et al. 1992; Rapoport 1991; Schwartz and Begley 2003).

Two theories have emerged from these data. The first is that the frontal lobes normally act to inhibit or override the emergence of primitive instinctual urges. However, in OCD this inhibition fails, and we see the eruption of innate urges, or behavioral routines that resemble nest building, grooming, and the checking of territorial boundaries—instinctual behaviors associated with more primitive species. In this model, ordering, straightening, cleaning, hand washing, checking door locks, and so forth may reflect human versions of a breakthrough of these more primitive urges.

A second theory holds that there are naturally existing neural pathways that typically serve adaptive purposes, especially when people are exposed to potentially dangerous situations. The frontal cortex serves as the launching site for worry. When exposed to dangerous stimuli, the frontal lobes guide and direct sustained perceptual focus and attention. In essence, arousal is passed through a feedback circuit (see figure 10-A). In normal individuals this serves to maintain alertness and vigilance

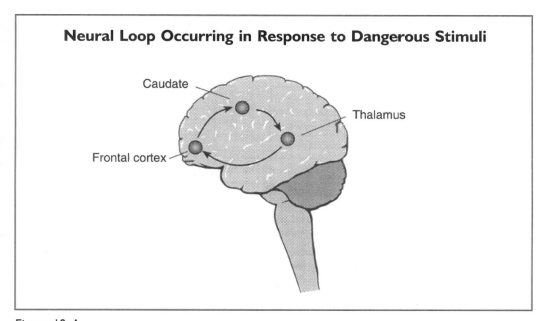

Neural Loop Occurring in Response to Dangerous Stimuli

Caudate

Thalamus

Frontal cortex

Figure 10-A

until it is determined that there is no danger; then the inner reverberating loop shuts down. Presumably, this neural loop fails to inhibit itself in OCD. The brain continues to sense danger (or to "worry" about danger) despite cognitive evidence to the contrary. The patient gets caught in an ongoing repetition of worry and engages in behavioral attempts to reduce the worry (the rituals). The caudate is richly innervated by 5-HT neurons. When these nerve cells are activated by 5-HT antidepressants, the inhibitory serotonergic cells reduce the excessive metabolic activity and shut down the maladaptive loop, and OCD symptoms diminish.

Treatment

Standard psychotherapy is notoriously ineffective with OCD. To date, two approaches to treatment are, however, proving to be helpful in reducing symptoms in this truly devastating mental illness.

The first are behavioral techniques: exposure and response prevention. Exposure amounts to systematic, gradual exposure to anxiety-provoking stimuli; for example, for a patient afraid of contamination by germs, the exposure trial might involve having the patient clean a toilet without using gloves. Response prevention amounts to helping the patient avoid rituals, such as avoiding excessive hand washing. The rituals, if carried out, usually reduce anxiety. With response prevention, the initial experience is that the patient will encounter considerable anxiety as he or she avoids the ritualistic behavior. Yet with repeated exposures or response prevention, gradually the anxiety diminishes. This is an emotionally difficult treatment to embark upon but one shown to be successful in up to 75 to 80 percent of patients—given an adequate number of trials, typically twenty to twenty-five sessions.

Medication treatment has become more successful with the advent of selective 5-HT antidepressants. These medications, as noted earlier, are given to OCD patients even if they are not clinically depressed. In addition to their antidepressant effects, these drugs reduce OCD symptoms directly. Treatment with medications for OCD generally requires doses higher than those used to treat clinical depression (see figure 10-B). Aside from higher doses, treatment guidelines are the same as for treating depression (see chapter 16).

Psychotropic medications are believed to be effective in 50 to 65 percent of OCD cases, generally showing a 50 to 60 percent reduction in symptoms. Complete remission is not common. Unfortunately, if patients stop medications, there is a 95 percent relapse rate; thus chronic treatment is necessary. In all likelihood, combined behavioral and pharmacologic treatment offers the best promise for successful outcome.

5-HT Antidepressants Useful in Treating OCD

Generic Name	Brand Name	Typical Depression Dose (mg/day)	Typical OCD Dose (mg/day)
Clomipramine	Anafranil	150–200	200–300
Fluoxetine	Prozac	20–40	20–80
Fluvoxamine	Luvox	100–300	100–500
Sertraline	Zoloft	50–150	50–200
Paroxetine	Paxil	20–30	20–50
Citalopram	Celexa	10–40	20–60
Escitalopram	Lexapro	5–20	10–30

Figure 10-B

QUICK REFERENCE
When to Refer for Medication Treatment

Event

Persistent symptoms that are ego-dystonic, create significant distress, and/or interfere with normal routines

Symptoms

Obsessions—intrusive, trouble-some thoughts or impulses

Compulsions—repetitive rituals enacted to reduce anxiety generated by obsessions

Comorbid clinical depression

11

Psychotic Disorders

This chapter deals with the group of disorders referred to as "psychotic disorders." The definition of the term *psychotic* has evolved over the course of previous *DSM* revisions. In the *DSM-IV-TR*, the meaning of psychotic refers to the presence of specific symptoms that vary depending on the condition. In general, though, these symptoms include false beliefs (delusions), seriously impaired perceptions (hallucinations) without awareness of their pathological nature, and disorganized thinking, as evidenced in speech and behavior. In addition to noting the presence of these symptoms, it is important to observe their content; for example, delusions may be paranoid ("I am being followed by the FBI"), and hallucinations may be self-deprecatory ("I hear a voice telling me I am bad").

Psychosis, per se, is not a diagnosis but a symptom. There are a number of types of psychotic disorders, which have traditionally been classified into two broad groups: functional psychoses and organic psychoses. The term *functional* refers to those psychoses with a presumed psychological etiology, and *organic* refers to those with a presumed biological etiology. Schizophrenia was traditionally classified as a functional psychosis; however, more recent research findings strongly suggest that schizophrenia has a biological basis; that is, it is an endogenous mental disorder. The distinction, however, is still important, but now different terminology is used. The functional disorders are referred to as "primary psychiatric disorders," and the organic disorders are referred to as "due to a general medical condition."

Differential Diagnosis

Psychotic Disorders Due to a General Medical Condition

The term "psychotic disorder due to a general medical condition" is used for those medical conditions that have psychotic symptoms. In the *DSM-IV-TR*, these conditions are divided into the following:

Psychotic Disorder Facts

■ 1 percent of the population has schizophrenia.

■ 1 to 4 percent of psychiatric admissions have delusional disorder.

■ 10 to 15 percent of medical-surgical patients in a general hospital have delirium.

■ 15 percent of patients diagnosed with dementia have a treatable condition.

■ Delirium is most common in the very young and the elderly.

■ Psychotic disorders due to a general medical condition, with delusions or hallucinations

■ Psychotic disorders due to a substance-induced disorder

Substance-related disorders that can be associated with psychotic symptoms can be produced by all classes of substances, that is, alcohol, hallucinogens, opioids, phencyclidine, sedative-hypnotics, and stimulants. Sometimes psychotic symptoms are more often associated with intoxication and, sometimes, more with withdrawal. Many medical conditions can produce psychotic symptoms, but the most common can be grouped into the following categories:

Medical Conditions That Can Cause Psychosis

■ Metabolic

Organ failure, such as renal failure

Hypoxia

Hypoglycemia

Vitamin deficiency

Endocrinopathy, such as hyperthyroidism

Fluid or electrolyte imbalance

Porphyria

■ Drug or alcohol intoxication or withdrawal

■ Infections

■ Epilepsy

■ Head injury

■ Vascular diseases, such as lupus

■ Intracranial tumor

■ Cerebral degenerative diseases

Dementia, such as Alzheimer's disease

Multiple sclerosis

Huntington's chorea

Parkinson's disease

Primary Psychoses

The primary psychoses can be divided into the following diagnoses:

- Brief psychotic disorder

- Delusional disorder

- Schizophrenia

- Schizophreniform disorder

- Schizoaffective disorder

- Shared psychotic disorder

- Psychotic disorder not otherwise specified (atypical)

- Major depression with psychotic features

- Bipolar disorder, manic

Brief psychotic disorder refers to a condition in which a person has psychotic symptoms lasting from one day to a month. There usually is some identifiable stressor that has precipitated the psychosis, and the person demonstrates significant emotional turmoil. The symptoms may be identical to those seen in schizophrenia, but they remit in a fairly brief period of time (less than one month).

Delusional disorder refers to a disorder with persistent nonbizarre delusions without bizarre behavior or prominent hallucinations. Thus, if someone has the delusion that he or she is under surveillance by the FBI, they may meet the criteria. But if delusions are bizarre—for example, if a patient thinks she is under surveillance by Martians—she does not meet the criteria. The disorder is classified by type of delusion: erotomanic, grandiose, jealous, persecutory, or somatic.

Schizophrenia refers to a disorder of longer than six months' duration with prominent psychotic symptoms. This disorder is discussed in detail below. *Schizophreniform disorder* has the same criteria as schizophrenia but is of less than six months' duration.

Schizoaffective disorder refers to a condition in which the person has not only schizophrenia but also significant episodes of mood disorder, either manic or depressive.

In *shared psychotic disorder*, the person develops psychosis as a result of an intense relationship and identification with someone who is already psychotic, for example, in folie à deux. Here the person typically has poorly defined self–other boundaries and will begin to mimic psychotic symptoms seen in the other individual. (Psychotic symptoms seen in severe affective disorders and mania and depressive psychoses are covered in chapters 7 and 8.)

Now let's discuss schizophrenia in more detail, using it as the prototype of primary psychosis.

Schizophrenia

Schizophrenia as a syndrome has been recognized for thousands of years. As long ago as the Hippocratic school, a syndrome called dementia (with behaviors and symptoms akin to schizophrenia) was recognized as distinct from mania and melancholia. Kraepelin (1921) described a syndrome he called "dementia praecox." This referred to

Schneiderian First-Rank Symptoms

- *Thought broadcasting*—belief that one's thoughts are escaping aloud into the external world

- *Experiences of alienation*—belief that one's thoughts, feelings, and actions are not one's own

- *Experiences of influence*—belief that one's thoughts, feelings, and actions are being controlled by some external agent

- *Complete auditory hallucinations*—hallucinations of voices coming from outside one's head

- *Delusional perceptions*—a real, normal perception to which one attaches a private meaning

a psychotic disorder with progressive debilitation leading to severe impairment of social and intellectual functioning. In his view, this syndrome was invariably progressive, with a very poor prognosis, although more recent research questions the progressive nature of all schizophrenic disorders.

The clinical picture of schizophrenia varies depending on the particular phase of the disorder. *DSM-IV-TR* divides the course of schizophrenia into three phases: prodromal, active, and residual. During the prodromal phase, patients show a deterioration in their level of functioning, without being actively psychotic. In this phase, the patient may show mostly "negative" symptoms (discussed below), such as isolativeness, blunted or flat affect, and lack of initiative. There may also be a disruption of sleep patterns. Often there is a deterioration of performance (at work or school), and sometimes in personal hygiene. There may be an abrupt change in behavior or lifestyle, such as a career change. In the active phase, the person is floridly psychotic, with disorganized thinking, delusions, and hallucinations. In the following residual phase, the patient continues to be impaired but without severe psychotic symptoms. Social isolation and peculiar affect and thinking may persist, to a degree.

For a diagnosis of schizophrenia, these three phases must last longer than six months and must not be due to a mood disorder. Three types of schizophrenia are delineated: catatonic (prominent movement disorder), disorganized (severe thought disorganization), and paranoid (prominent paranoid delusions with mild disorganization of thinking). Undifferentiated and residual types are categories for those who do not fit the above three types but have a mix of features.

Case 16

George A. was a nineteen-year-old college student who was brought to the student health clinic by his roommate. It was difficult to get a clear history from George because he kept changing the subject and making odd and disconnected statements. His roommate reported that George had been progressively more isolative the past four months. For the past month he had been staying up late at night and had become somewhat secretive. He wrote notes to himself in a special notebook and made odd comments about God and Christ and about something "coming soon." His personal hygiene had deteriorated, and he sometimes went several days without bathing or changing clothes.

George reported that he felt he was on a special mission to prepare for the second coming of Christ and that he sometimes heard God or the devil speaking to him. He thought it was necessary that he die or suffer in order to atone for his sins and the sins of the world. He admitted he was doing poorly in school, but explained that doing God's work was more important. His roommate, who had known him in high school, described him as quiet, shy, and somewhat of a loner. He had never dated.

George was treated with antipsychotic medication, and the delusions and hallucinations resolved. But he continued to have difficulty in college and eventually dropped out of school and returned home to stay with his family.

This case illustrates the prodromal, active, and residual phases. George A. is described as having a somewhat schizoid premorbid personality, as is classically described (although some studies have shown that this is present in only about 50 percent of those diagnosed with schizophrenia). This case also illustrates what are called positive and negative symptoms. For practical purposes, it is helpful to group schizophrenic symptoms into four categories, as outlined below. (Note that characterological features are not psychotic symptoms per se, but do often accompany the more core positive or negative symptoms.)

The distinction between positive and negative symptoms appears to be significant because of both their differential responses to medication and their differing clinical course and probable differing etiology. Recently, a third symptom cluster has been identified, the disorganized cluster (Arndt, Alliger, and Andreasen 1991; Liddle et al. 1989). This symptom cluster, like negative symptoms, correlates with cognitive impairment and frontal lobe dysfunction but has different behavioral manifestations.

There are now several theoretical models of the neurophysiological basis for these different types of symptoms and the course they follow in schizophrenia. They are discussed below:

Schizophrenia Symptoms

- Positive symptoms:
  Hallucinations
  Delusions
  Agitation
  Floridly bizarre behavior
  First-rank symptoms (see sidebar on the opposite page)

- Negative symptoms:
  Anhedonia
  Apathy
  Blunted affect
  Poverty of thought
  Feelings of emptiness
  Amotivational states

- Disorganization
  Behavioral disorganization
  Distractibility
  Thought disorder

- "Characterological" symptoms:
  Social isolation or alienation
  Marked feelings of inadequacy
  Poorly developed social skills

Etiology

Over the centuries, there have been a multitude of theories about the etiology of schizophrenia. These have ranged from religious, social, and psychological theories to more recent biological theories.

Early evidence of biological factors came from genetic studies. Twin studies showed that the rate of concordance was much higher for monozygotic (identical) than for dizygotic (fraternal) twins. Adoptive studies done by Kety et al. (1971) have shown that schizophrenia is much more prevalent in the biological relatives than in the adoptive families of those adopted at birth who are later diagnosed as schizophrenic. Since that study, many others have shown biological differences between schizophrenic subjects and controls:

- CT and MRI scans have demonstrated enlargement of the lateral ventricles and widened cortical sulci. This finding suggests that either there is brain atrophy or (more likely) that in some types of schizophrenia there has been abnormal brain development (Weinberger 1996). These abnormalities may increase over time.

- MRI scans have shown the presence of smaller anterior hippocampi (Weinberger et al. 1992) in schizophrenic subjects, which correlates with cognitive impairment (Nester et al. 1993).

- PET scan studies have shown decreased metabolic activity in the prefrontal cortex, which correlates with the severity of negative symptoms.

- Studies have found a positive correlation between levels of HVA (a dopamine metabolite) in plasma and clinical severity. Also, many studies have found an increase in the number of D2 receptors in the striatum and nucleus acumbens of schizophrenics (Bochus and Kleinman 1996; Lieberman et al. 1996; Gur et al. 1998; Knoll et al. 1998).

The Dopamine Model

The dopamine model was the predominant theory of biological causation for the past two decades. This theory hypothesized that schizophrenia is caused by abnormal dopaminergic activity in the brain. Dopamine neurons are located in a number of different brain regions. In the basal ganglia, these nerve cells help to regulate motor functioning. In areas of the limbic and reticular systems, dopamine neurons appear to play an important role in emotional control and the screening of stimuli.

The dopamine model holds that the basic physiological pathology involves primarily overactive or hyper-reactive dopamine neurons. The excessive dopamine activity can lead to behavioral agitation, a failure to adequately screen stimuli, and disorganization of perception and thought. This theory is supported by two observations: The first is that the potency of antipsychotic drugs has correlated closely with their ability to bind to and block the postsynaptic dopamine (D2) receptors in the mesolimbic system (see figure 11-A).

The second observation is that drugs that increase dopamine activity (such as amphetamines) can produce a paranoid psychosis similar to paranoid schizophrenia and, if given to schizophrenic patients, amphetamines may exacerbate psychotic symptoms.

Although the dopamine model has merit, the basic theory has been modified to help explain some clinical data (Davis et al. 1991). One of the strongest stimuli has

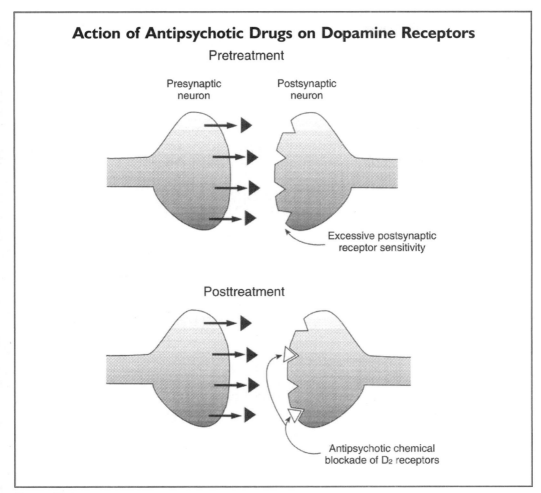

Action of Antipsychotic Drugs on Dopamine Receptors

Pretreatment

Presynaptic
neuron

Postsynaptic
neuron

Excessive postsynaptic
receptor sensitivity

Posttreatment

Antipsychotic chemical
blockade of D_2 receptors

Figure 11-A

been the finding that clozapine, although effective in the treatment of schizophrenia, is only a weak D2 blocker, because it is a reversible blocker. On the other hand, it is a fairly potent 5-HT2A and 5-HT2C antagonist. The 5-HT blocking ability appears to correlate with its effectiveness against negative symptoms. This has also been the case with second-generation antipsychotics (discussed in detail in chapter 19). (Note that second-generation antipsychotics were formerly called atypical antipsychotics.) Also, it has been shown that clozapine *does* significantly decrease dopaminergic activity in the mesolimbic area (despite the lack of D2 blockade) but not in the nigrostriatal tracts (thus the lack of extrapyramidal effects). What emerges is the following picture: In schizophrenia, there is hyperdopaminergic activity in the mesolimbic tracts that is associated with positive symptoms. In addition, there is decreased activity in the prefrontal cortex associated with negative symptoms. The exact relationship between these phenomena is not fully understood at this time. It has been suggested (Bochus and Kleinman 1996) that hypofunction of the glutamate neurons, which interconnect the four main areas shown to be abnormal in schizophrenia (prefrontal cortex, mesolimbic, striatum/ nucleus acumbens, and medial temporal lobe), may be the underlying pathophysiology. The different neurochemical basis dictates alternative treatment approaches: the use of second-generation antipsychotics (discussed in detail in chapter 19).

The Glutamate Model

Another theory was proposed over fifty years ago (Luby et al. 1962) as the phency-clidine (PCP) model of schizophrenia. This was based on the discovery that PCP exerts its effect by blocking the action of glutamate at the N-methyl-D-aspartate (NMDA) receptor in the brain. The advantage of this model is that PCP, unlike amphetamines, induces negativism and apathy in addition to disorganized thinking. It is hypoth-esized that in schizophrenia there is a primary dysregulation of the glutamate system resulting in cognitive deficits and that the dopaminergic hyperactivity, and resultant positive symptoms, are secondary phenomena (Goff and Coyle 2001).

The Neurodevelopmental/Neurodegenerative Model

The neurodevelopmental model proposes that in schizophrenia there is a defect, possibly genetically determined or from an event (e.g., a viral infection) during intra-uterine or early infantile development, that leads to abnormal development later in life, especially during the synaptic "pruning" during adolescence (Hoffman and McGlashan 1997). This model suggests that the pathophysiological processes of schizo-phrenia develop over time until they produce overt symptomatology. Treatment would then be directed, not just at the final psychotic symptoms, but toward correcting the abnormal development.

Some evidence suggests that schizophrenia is a neurodegenerative disorder leading to poorer functioning and progressively diminished cognitive functioning after each psychotic episode (Lieberman 1999; Tsuang, Stone, and Faraone 2000). A number of studies using MRI imaging to measure brain and ventricular volume have shown progressive enlargement of the lateral ventricles, and corresponding loss of brain tissue. Furthermore, these changes correlate with deterioration in condition, and precede the first psychotic episode. Other studies have shown elevation of both dopamine and glutamate. Taken together, this evidence suggests that *in some cases* schizophrenia is a progressive neurodegenerative disorder with progressive loss of neurons and cognitive function. Newer evidence (Harvey and Keefe 2001) suggests that the second-generation antipsychotics may greatly reduce, or possibly eliminate, this deterioration. The evidence suggests that early intervention and treatment may lead to marked improvement in the overall course of the illness. On the other hand, older studies (Bleuler 1968) have suggested that almost half of schizophrenic patients substantially improved or recovered.

Whatever the precise neurophysiological pathogenesis of schizophrenia may turn out to be, several things are clear:

- There is not just one type of schizophrenia. Different people with schizo-phrenia may have very differing courses, for example, good-prognosis versus poor-prognosis schizophrenia. These have differing neuroanatomical find-ings and, presumably, differing pathogeneses.

- The etiology of schizophrenia is complex. A simple theory like the dopamine model cannot fully explain the disorder. A full understanding will take into account factors at the intracellular, synaptic, and neural network levels.

- The genetic factors are complex. They are certainly polygenic and seem to overlap with other disorders.

Treatment

We can consider the positive and negative symptoms listed earlier as target symptoms for antipsychotic medication treatment. Antipsychotic medications are now considered an important, if not essential, component in the treatment of schizophrenia. The focus of treatment is not only the resolution of psychotic symptoms but also relapse prevention. Unfortunately, schizophrenia is a disorder in which relapse is extremely common. It is estimated that following a psychotic episode and subsequent recovery, 70 percent of patients will relapse within a year if treated with either placebo or no medication at all. With continued antipsychotic treatment the relapse rate can drop to 30 to 40 percent. Studies have shown that low-dose and intermittent treatment are associated with poorer outcome, as measured by number of hospitalizations (Carpenter et al. 1990; Kane 1990).

In addition, there is now evidence to support the notion that being psychotic is damaging to the brain (Loebel et al. 1992). It is as if the more the dopamine circuits are used, the more the psychotic pathways become etched into the brain. Loebel and associates studied the relationship between duration of illness and clinical outcome in a group of untreated, first-episode schizophrenic patients. The study showed that patients who had been psychotic longer prior to treatment tended to have a poorer treatment response. This is consistent with the observation that prolonged hallucinogen or stimulant abuse is associated with incomplete clearing of mental status. It also suggests some type of kindling phenomena or toxic effect of psychosis and supports the need for prompt treatment with antipsychotic medications. As is said, "neurons that fire together, wire together."

Besides antipsychotic medications, both typical and atypical, other medications may be useful in the treatment of schizophrenia. These include lithium, carbamazepine, benzodiazepines, reserpine, propranolol, antidepressants, and antiparkinsonian drugs. Most of these are used to treat associated features of schizophrenia and are used in addition to, not instead of, antipsychotic medication. Lithium may be helpful to reduce psychotic and affective symptoms. It was once thought that lithium would benefit only those patients who were actually bipolar or schizoaffective, but even some patients without apparent affective symptoms can benefit from lithium. Benzodiazepines (minor tranquilizers) may be helpful in relieving some of the negative symptoms, in addition to anxiety and agitation. Antiparkinsonian medications are usually effective for the extrapyramidal side effects of antipsychotic medications. Antidepressants may be helpful when there are significant comorbid depressive symptoms. Propranolol (a beta blocker) is often helpful for akathisia (a common side effect of antipsychotic medications) and can sometimes reduce agitation.

The goal of medication treatment is to reduce symptoms so that the person can function better and benefit more from other forms of treatment, such as individual, group, or family therapy, and social or vocational rehabilitation. An important part of such therapy involves educating the patient about prodromal symptoms and effects and side effects of medications. It is also important to address patients' beliefs that taking medications means they are sick (and conversely, that not taking medications means they aren't). Especially with paranoid patients, the belief that medications are a means of being controlled by others must be worked through.

Sometimes people with schizophrenia feel better when not taking antipsychotic medications because they are able to entertain more grandiose notions about themselves and thereby lift their moods. Even more commonly, premature discontinuation occurs because patients are plagued by very unpleasant medication side effects.

Appropriate education of patients regarding side effects and medical intervention (many side effects can be controlled with other medications) can improve the quality of life and greatly enhance compliance. It may be helpful to present medications as a tool for people to use to help them control their illness, as a diabetic uses insulin.

Any of the psychotic disorders, regardless of etiology, may respond to antipsychotic medications. Where there is an underlying medical illness causing the psychosis, it is crucial to treat the underlying disorder. However, even in that case, antipsychotic medication may help reduce symptomatology. In the case of drug-induced and brief reactive psychosis, it may be appropriate not to use antipsychotic medications initially and instead to await the resolution of the psychotic symptoms using only supportive treatments. In the cases of the other psychoses, it is usually best to treat with antipsychotic medications for at least six months.

QUICK REFERENCE
When to Refer for Medication Treatment

Event	Symptoms
Psychosis due to a general medical condition	Delusions Hallucinations
Depression with psychotic features	Delusions Hallucinations Catatonic features
Schizophrenia	Positive symptoms
Other psychotic disorders	Delusions Hallucinations
Drug-induced state (including intoxication)	Severe paranoid delusions Hallucinations
Severe personality disorder	Disorganized thinking Prominent paranoia Poor impulse control
Manic episode	Prominent delusions Severe agitation

12

Post-Traumatic Stress Disorder

Natural disasters, catastrophic illnesses, combat exposure, incest, rape, and assault are but a few life experiences that can unleash a wave of intense emotional stress. Acute stress reactions or "traumatic neuroses" were first addressed in the clinical literature during World War I, as thousands of soldiers returned from the front suffering from severe anxiety, insomnia, and nightmares attributed to "shell shock." The understanding of acute stress reactions was furthered by the pioneering work of Eric Lindeman.

In 1942, during an after-football celebration at the Coconut Grove nightclub in Boston, a disastrous fire claimed the lives of 499 people and stunned the community. Lindeman and his colleagues quickly rushed in and provided free counseling services for a large group of people, including survivors of the fire and relatives of the victims. At the same time they provided crisis intervention, the mental health team was able to carefully study this group of people. Lindeman discovered tremendous regularity in the symptoms that people reported: vacillation between overwhelming painful emotions and periods of numbness, a strong need or impulse to repeat the tragic events in their minds over and over again, nightmares, and a host of psychosomatic symptoms.

In 1976, psychiatrist Mardi Horowitz published a book entitled *Stress Response Syndromes*. In this landmark publication, Dr. Horowitz carved out a very useful model for understanding what appears to be a common pattern of human emotional response to significant stress and shed new light on the various aspects of PTSD symptomatology. Horowitz developed this model based on his review of numerous field studies (including Lindeman's), a good deal of clinical work treating mentally healthy people who had experienced major stresses, and even some experimental studies. Horowitz concluded that across a broad spectrum of stressful events (deaths of loved ones, physical assault, natural disaster, even viewing upsetting movies), most people exhibit a typical pattern of response. The various phases of the stress response syndrome helped to explain the differing and often dramatically shifting symptoms seen in PTSD.

Let's take a look at the stress response syndrome (see figure 12-A). The full stress response syndrome is seen most clearly in situations where the stressful event is sudden and intense, although a host of events may trigger this reaction. Each of the boxes in the figure represents a state of mind or emotion. The stress response reaction begins with awareness of some painful event.

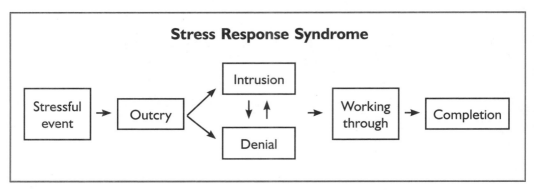

Stress Response Syndrome

Figure 12-A

The first phase is outcry. In a sense, a state of outcry is simultaneously an eruption of intense, unpleasant emotion (sadness, fear, and so on) *and* denial ("I can't believe it. It can't be true"). The person is in a state of shock and may be engulfed by very strong emotions. This phase of the reaction can last for a few minutes, a few hours, or a few days. Rather quickly, the person moves into phase two, which may be either a state of intrusion or a state of denial.

Intrusion occurs when a person experiences waves of intense emotion and a strong impulse to think about, imagine, remember, or mentally relive the stressful event. These experiences are deemed "intrusive" because generally the strong feelings and repetitive thoughts are not brought on willfully. During a state of intrusion, emotions feel very raw and people feel extremely vulnerable, easily overwhelmed, and close to tears. They startle easily, don't sleep well, and often have nightmares. When intrusive experiences are especially intense, the individual may transiently lose reality testing and manifest psychotic-like symptoms, such as auditory or visual hallucinations.

Phase two includes a stage of denial. Denial may occur directly following outcry or may come on the heels of a period of intrusion. As noted earlier, denial is a state of emotional numbness; people often feel nothing. Other symptoms during the stages of denial include dissociative experiences (feelings of detachment, estrangement, impaired concentration, forgetfulness), avoidance of situations that may be associated with the trauma, and marked general social withdrawal.

Although *DSM-IV-TR* includes post-traumatic stress disorder as an anxiety disorder, in some respects this may be a misnomer. Clearly, anxiety symptoms predominate in PTSD, but it is very common for PTSD patients to exhibit major depression, transient psychosis, and substance abuse as well. The symptoms of PTSD can be organized into six categories, as follows:

Symptoms of PTSD

- Persistent reexperiencing of the trauma
    - Distressing, intrusive recollections of the event (images, affects, cognitions)
    - Recurring nightmares regarding the trauma
    - "Flashbacks" or déjà vu (sensations as if the traumatic episode were happening in the present)
- Increased arousal
    - Sleep disturbances
    - Startle response
    - Irritability
    - Hypervigilance
- Transient psychotic symptoms
    - Derealization
    - Illusions
    - Hallucinations (visual or auditory)
- Avoidance
    - Avoiding discussion of the traumatic events
    - Avoiding activities or people and places that could provoke recollections of the trauma
    - General social withdrawal
- Numbing
    - Blunted affective responses
    - Feelings of emptiness
    - Feelings of estrangement or detachment
    - Clouding of consciousness
- Associated features
    - Major depression
    - Panic attacks
    - Substance abuse (often seen as an attempt to "self-medicate," to reduce anxiety or intrusive experiences)

Differential Diagnosis

It is important to note that traumatic life events often do not result in PTSD. Depression and substance abuse are actually more common than post-traumatic reactions. Having said that, let's discuss PTSD. PTSD is subdivided into the following clinical presentations: acute (duration of symptoms is less than three months) and chronic (duration of symptoms is more than three months). Also two versions of PTSD are seen clinically: acute onset (the traumatic event has just recently occurred) and delayed onset (the onset of severe symptoms occurs at least six months after the traumatic event). Beyond these distinctions, other variables are extremely important to consider both in terms of diagnosis and treatment.

PTSD Facts

Lifetime prevalence rate may be as high as 14 percent (Zisook et al. 1999). Each year a large number of people are exposed to overwhelmingly stressful events. Such encounters may be reflected by the following data. Each year it is estimated that:

- 1.5 to 2 million children are judged to be at risk for physical abuse by parents.

- 2.4 million children are *reported* to child protective services: 49 percent for neglect, 27 percent for physical abuse, 16 percent for sexual abuse, and 8 percent for emotional abuse.

- There are 1.9 million *reported cases* of violent crime: 25,000 murders, 107,000 rapes. Twenty-four percent of American households per year are victimized by crime.

- There are 36,000 infant deaths, 77,000 accidental deaths, 27,000 suicides, and many other sudden traumatic deaths.

- Countless thousands of people are exposed to natural disasters and traumatic medical crises, witness deaths or gruesome accidents, or are victims of some form of terrorism.

Most of those suffering from PTSD experience serious symptoms for many months or years, unless they are treated.

Lenore Terr (1991) aptly notes that *generally* single-blow traumas have a less devastating effect on psychologic functioning than recurring traumas. In the latter case are situations such as repeated child abuse and molestation, systematic terrorizing, and recurring spousal abuse. The age at which trauma occurs also plays a crucial role in our understanding of psychological sequelae. Very early, severe, recurring child abuse often not only results in primary symptoms of PTSD but may also interfere significantly with fundamental personality development. The outcome may be coexisting PTSD and borderline or other severe personality disorder.

Since PTSD can have a variety of symptomatic presentations (owing to the above-mentioned variables and whether the person is in the intrusion or denial stage of the stress response syndrome), it is wise first to formulate the overall diagnosis and then delineate particular target symptoms (see symptom list, on the previous page). In all forms of PTSD, ultimately the psychiatric symptoms can be traced to the patient's exposure to extremely overwhelming psychosocial stressors. And in almost all cases, a common element is the person's experience of extraordinary helplessness or powerlessness in the face of such stressors.

Etiology

Volumes have been written about the psychological origins and consequences of severe trauma, and it is beyond the scope of this book to attempt a review. Suffice it to say that the majority of PTSD symptoms can be understood as arising largely from psychogenic sources. However, some authors have proposed interesting theories regarding biological factors in PTSD, which we will review here. The primary work in this area has been done by Bessel A. van der Kolk (1987) and Charles Nemeroff (1997). In this chapter we will look at six models in which biology potentially can be altered by psychological stress.

Attachment and the repetition compulsion

PTSD due to early, severe child abuse or neglect may leave not only emotional scars, but also neurobiology may be altered. Severe stress during childhood and infancy in both humans and animals can result in an increased need for attachment and protection. Studies with birds, dogs, and monkeys show that infants will strongly seek out attachments even with abusive parents, especially under stress. This behavioral pattern, seen so strongly in other species, may provide some understanding of the common human tendency for abused individuals to cling to and gravitate toward abusive parents and spouses. Since it is seen across diverse species, this may reflect an underlying neurobiologically mediated reaction pattern.

The repetitive involvement in apparently aversive or abusive relationships (sometimes called the repetition compulsion) may be related to hypersensitivity of the separation-stress center in the brain (see the discussion in chapter 9), which has been shown to respond favorably to treatment with antidepressants, especially MAO inhibitors and SSRIs.

Attachment and impaired affect modulation

When the traumatic experience has occurred early in life, another consequence, conversely, may be inadequate attachment and bonding. This may be especially true if the nature of the trauma was profound neglect. One common consequence of inadequate or insecure attachment is poor affective regulation. Studies with monkeys have revealed that isolated, neglected infants often develop persistent aggressive and self-destructive behaviors (such as biting) and, in general, impaired abilities for emotional regulation. Clearly many PTSD patients also show chronic problems with emotional control and at times manifest symptoms of self-mutilation (Harlow and Harlow 1971; Sackett 1965). This may account for both chronic emotional arousal and an increased vulnerability to later traumatic life events (van der Kolk 1987).

Following early trauma, permanent alterations in the nervous system have also been documented, including persistent elevations in the neuropeptide CRF and atrophy of the hippocampus (Post and Weiss 1997; Sapolsky 1996; Nemeroff 1997). Also, see chapter 13.

Hyperarousal

When animals are exposed to inescapable shock, they exhibit consistent behavioral reactions—initially hypervigilance or arousal and ultimately a profound state of withdrawal and "depression." In addition, such animals eventually show a significant depletion of norepinephrine, likely accompanied by changes in NE receptor sensitivity in parts of the brain. Alterations of receptor sensitivity may leave the animals in a state of chronic hyperarousal. In essence, their nervous systems may be permanently altered such that traumatized animals and people alike are relatively unable to dampen or inhibit excessive emotional arousal. Antidepressants that affect norepinephrine appear to alter receptor sensitivity, both in humans and animals. Serotonergic antidepressants may also indirectly inhibit hypersensitive NE cells (Nagy et al. 1993) and, thus, can play a role in treating hyperarousal in PTSD patients. Hyperarousal may also be due to more or less permanent dysregulation of the hypothalamic-pituitary-adrenal axis damage to the hippocampus and anterior cingulated gyrus (Sapolsky 1996; Heim and Nemeroff 2002).

Intrusive symptoms

L. M. Nagy and colleagues (1993) reported that PTSD patients treated with high doses of fluoxetine (a serotonergic antidepressant) showed a significant reduction in flashbacks and other intrusive symptoms. Interestingly, as intrusive experiences decreased, so did symptoms of avoidance and numbing. (Again, the reductions were at levels that were statistically significant.) (Also see Tucker et al. 2003.) Furthermore, van der Kolk and other researchers have hypothesized that flashback experiences may be traced (neurobiologically) to "stress-induced reaction of LC—hippocampus/amygdala pathways." As we saw in chapter 9, the locus coeruleus is mediated by norepinephrine, and selective serotonin antidepressants also clearly have an inhibitory effect on LC activation.

Acute, toxic levels of glutamate and cortisol

In the immediate aftermath of severe trauma, marked increases in the neurotransmitter, glutamate, and the stress hormone, cortisol, may reach toxic levels and damage parts of the brain associated with affect regulation. This has been supported by both human and animal studies (Southwick et al. 1999; Heim et al. 2000; Heim and Nemeroff 2002). Experimental treatments with acute administration of alpha-2 agonists (e.g., clonidine), which dampen activation of noradrenergic cells in the locus coeruleus, are producing promising results. It may be possible to rapidly treat at-risk individuals following severely traumatic events and prevent brain damage due to excessive cortisol and glutamate activity, thus reducing the likelihood of chronic hyperarousal and other manifestations of affect dysregulation (Southwick et al. 1999; Shinba et al. 2001).

Kindling

Finally, it has been hypothesized that severely traumatic experiences may result in a sort of kindling effect, in which repeated episodes of trauma change brain functioning and even brain morphology. Severe trauma may *progressively* increase the likelihood that subsequent stresses are responded to with even more intense affective symptoms (see chapter 2). Animal models have suggested a kindling effect following emotional trauma (for instance, Kraemer, Ebert, and Lake 1984), although at present this theory remains mostly speculative. There are clinical and anecdotal reports that some PTSD patients benefit from treatment with lithium carbonate, divalproex, or carbamazepine, which have been shown to inhibit kindling effects.

Summary

Animal models strongly support the notion that severely traumatic experiences alter brain functioning and may more or less permanently change an organism's biologic capacity for response to stressful stimuli. It is likely that this occurs for human beings as well. Thus, although PTSD can be seen as *induced by* environmental-psychologic stressors, the *impact* is on both psyche and soma. The resulting disorder is best understood as a psychological and neurobiological problem.

Treatment

The treatment of choice for PTSD is psychotherapy (most effective is exposure-based cognitive therapy). It is essential that these patients gradually come to face the painful memories of traumatic experiences—come to terms with the realities of their lives. The process of "working through" is often quite prolonged and fraught with periodic emotional upheaval. Typically, PTSD patients must navigate through repeated periods of intrusion and denial on their way toward psychological resolution and symptomatic improvement. During this treatment, it is crucial that affective reexperiencing

PTSD Symptoms That Respond to Medication

Target Symptoms	Class of Medication
Intrusive experiences: "flashbacks,"[a] avoidance, and numbing[b]	SSRI antidepressants, buspirone augmentation of SSRI, second-generation antipsychotics
Hyperarousal[c]	Antidepressants, benzodiazepines, α-2 adrenergic agonists, anticonvulsants
Transient psychosis, marked derealization[d]	Low-dose antipsychotics
Nightmares	Prazosin (Minipress)
Treatment-resistant PTSD[e]	Second-generation antipsychotics, anticonvulsants
Depression[a]	Antidepressants
Panic attacks	Antidepressants, MAO inhibitors, high-potency benzodiazepines

a Nagy et al. (1993); Davidson, Roth, and Newman (1991); Hidalgo and Davidson (2000); Connor et al. (1999); Hidalgo et al. (1999); Stein et al. (2000); van der Kolk et al. (1994); Brady et al. (2000); Davidson et al. (1990); Hammer et al. (1997); Wells et al. (1991); Ahearn, Winston, et al. (2003); Davidson (2003)

b As intrusive symptoms are reduced and affective control improves, often numbing and avoidance diminish (Tucker et al. 2003).

c van der Kolk (1987); Forster et al. (1995); Berigan and Holzgang (1995); Fesler (1991); Tucker et al. (2003)

d Kapfhammer and Hippius (1998); Hori (1998); Joseph (1997); Krashin and Oates (1999); Ahearn, Krohn, et al. (2003); Ahearn, Winston, et al. (2003); Hamner et al. (2003)

e Antipsychotics: Stein, Kline, and Matloff (2002); Hamner et al. (2003)
Anticonvulsants: Otte et al. (2004); Petty et al. (2002)

Figure 12-B

of painful events be "dosed" (gradual, paced exposure) so as to not overwhelm or retraumatize the patient. Medications can be used in treating certain aspects of PTSD but are not the primary treatment. In all cases, psychotropic medications should target particular, serious symptoms *as they arise*. Figure 12-B summarizes common target symptoms and provides treatment implications drawn from the limited studies and clinical experience available.

Central to appropriate pharmacological treatment of PTSD is the restoration of some sense of control over turbulent emotions. When medications are appropriately used, in the context of a solid and safe patient-therapist relationship, the improved emotional control can serve as a sort of antidote for what is otherwise a feeling of powerlessness. Ultimately, the ability to face painful realities with a degree of mastery is at the heart of recovery from PTSD.

At times, excessively high doses of benzodiazepines or antipsychotics have been used (often inappropriately) in desperate attempts to snuff out eruptions of painful affect. This approach can backfire, as it results in a chemically induced state of "dissociation." The patient may then be unable to access inner emotions or memories, and the process of working through comes to a halt. Also, overly aggressive medication treatment can be experienced by the patient as an assault in its own right—another case of being controlled by a powerful other. In cases of extremely severe intrusive symptoms or psychosis, aggressive pharmacotherapy may be necessary, but it should be seen only as a short-term solution that continues only until the patient has regained a measure of stability. At that time the dosage of benzodiazepines or antipsychotics should be reduced or eliminated. Additionally, it should be noted that prolonged use of benzodiazepines has been associated with a poorer outcome (Gelpin et al. 1996).

When the PTSD patient develops a full-blown clinical depression or a severe, entrenched panic disorder, antidepressants can be quite helpful. When PTSD patients are treated with antidepressants, the course of treatment almost invariably must be lengthy (as in treating all panic disorders and major depression)—at least nine to twelve months (see chapters 7 and 16).

QUICK REFERENCE
When to Refer for Medication Treatment

Psychotherapy is the treatment of choice for most cases of PTSD. Psychotropic medications can be used when the patient presents with any of the following:

- Persistent ego weakness and an inability to tolerate exploratory psychotherapy or exposure-based treatment.

- Low level of cognitive functioning.

- When the following target symptoms become too intense and overwhelming or markedly interfere with functioning in daily life, *short-term* medication treatment is indicated:

   Intrusive experiences, flashbacks

   Transient psychosis

   Marked derealization

   Avoidance and numbing

- When these target symptoms become too intense and overwhelming or markedly interfere with functioning in daily life, *longer-term* medication treatment is indicated:

   Major depression

   Panic disorder

   Persistent psychotic symptoms

13

Borderline Personality Disorders

The concept of borderline disorders has slowly emerged from Hoch's early description of pseudoneurotic schizophrenia and Grinker's landmark study in 1968. Nosological and theoretical controversy has surrounded this very common diagnostic group. It has often been referred to as a "wastebasket" diagnosis—a depository for those clients who are severely impaired, hard to diagnose, or especially difficult to treat. All therapists encounter people with severe levels of character pathology. These folks are said to exhibit a very "loud" form of psychopathology; they suffer a lot and cause great suffering in others. According to Allan Frances (1989) borderline patients often seek out psychotherapy and psychotropic medication treatment—and often overdose on both!

Differential Diagnosis

Borderline disorders have been viewed both from a behavioral-symptomatic perspective (such as that of *DSM-IV-TR*) and a theoretical perspective (for example, borderline personality organization à la Kernberg and others). As Grinker and many subsequent researchers and clinicians agree, borderline patients are not all alike; they present in many different sizes and shapes. You can see borderline characteristics in the context of a number of different personality styles: schizoid-detached, obsessional, paranoid, narcissistic, and histrionic. However, all varieties share a few common characteristics as outlined in the box on the next page.

Beyond these commonalties are a considerable variety of symptomatic presentations. The particular behaviors observed are colored by the patient's style (obsessional, histrionic, and so on), the nature of his or her current social support network, and the presence or absence of comorbid Axis I disorders (see Preston 2006).

Borderline Personality
Disorders Facts

■ The incidence of severe
personality disorders in the
general population is difficult
to determine. However, in
some community mental
health clinics, up to 25 percent
of clients present with an
Axis II borderline personality
disorder.

■ Among borderline patients,
the lifetime mortality rate by
suicide may be as high as 10
percent.

■ Recent longitudinal studies
suggest that two-thirds of
borderline patients experience
a significant reduction in
emotional instability and
impulsivity after age forty-
five. Thus appropriate crisis
management and supportive
medication treatment can
play an important role in
sustaining functioning and
survival until patients reach
their fourth decade.

**Core Symptoms of Borderline
Personality Disorders**

■ Generalized ego impairment

■ Chronic emotional instability

■ Chaotic interpersonal relations

■ Feelings of emptiness

■ Impaired sense of self

■ Low frustration tolerance

■ Impulsivity

■ Primitive defenses, such as splitting,
acting out

■ Irritability and anger-control problems

The critical defining feature that can help the clinician be more certain of a borderline diagnosis is the history. As noted in chapter 6, many individuals may transiently experience borderline characteristics while in the throes of a major Axis I disorder (for example, a depression or PTSD), only to recompensate when the Axis I problem resolves. A more definitive diagnosis of borderline disorder emerges when there is a well-documented history of ego impairment dating back to adolescence or early adulthood— "stable instability."

DSM-IV-TR focuses largely on one version of borderline disorder (a type of histrionic-dependent borderline). Speaking more broadly in this book, we will refer to borderline disorders as including a host of personality "styles" that share the common core features listed above. In addition, it is helpful to delineate three subgroups of borderlines. These subgroups have been derived both by research methods (cluster and factor analysis) and by a method that psychopharmacologist Donald Klein calls "pharmacological behavioral dissection." This latter approach looks at how different groups of patients respond to psychotropic medications; based on their response patterns, subtypes can be identified.

Hysteroid-dysphoric

These borderline clients present with a significant degree of emotional lability and are exquisitely sensitive to interpersonal rejection, loss, and abandonment. As a consequence, they often cannot tolerate being alone and may engage in desperate attempts to maintain attachments, including clinging behavior and manipulative suicidal threats or gestures. These patients are at great risk for recurring depression.

Schizotypal

These borderline patients chronically display odd thinking—ideas of reference, magical thinking, vagueness, very idiosyncratic beliefs—and periodically experience marked episodes of depersonalization or derealization and transient psychoses. Such people likely represent a truer sort of borderline schizophrenia.

Angry-impulsive

These people are characterized by their pervasively hostile-aggressive way of interacting with others. They have very low frustration tolerance and can be quite volatile. As a result, their interpersonal relations are replete either with ongoing intense friction or multiple rejections.

In addition to these subtypes, it is important to keep in mind that many, if not most, borderline personalities have comorbid Axis I disorders—especially common are major depression and substance abuse. These coexisting disorders always complicate the picture and must be dealt with in any approach to treatment. In particular, longitudinal studies following the course and outcome of borderline personality disorders over the life span suggest very clearly that those patients who continue to do poorly are those who continue to abuse alcohol and other substances. Thus treatment of chemical dependency problems *must* be addressed.

Etiology

Most writings addressing the etiology of borderline disorders focus on psychological factors—especially traumatic events and serious developmental failures in the early family of origin (Mahler, Kernberg, Kohut, Masterson, and so on). Biological theories are, at this time, only speculative. They include the following:

- Inborn or constitutional factors in the CNS may leave certain children with defects in their ability to psychologically "metabolize" early interpersonal experiences adequately. Thus, even if raised in a "good enough" home, some kids simply may not acquire adequate emotional nurturance and sustenance from otherwise good parents.

- Inborn or constitutional factors may lead to the development of a difficult temperamental style, such as an irritable, restless infant. Some children cry excessively, seem extremely sensitive to mild stressors, or are unable to be soothed. There certainly are times when such children evoke ongoing negative reactions in otherwise good parents (frustration, withdrawal of affection, and so on). Thus the child is both biologically at risk (less capable of handling stress, more sensitive) and prone to behave in ways that may provoke less-than-optimal parental interactions or bonding. The secondary parental-child friction likely contributes to ongoing problems with psychological growth.

- Early, severely traumatic experiences (especially neglect) may alter brain development, resulting in chronic neurotransmitter abnormalities (see chapter 12) and structural changes in the nervous system.

In the theories above, the particular biological-based abnormalities or dysfunctions may become manifest in various symptom clusters, as noted earlier: hysteroid-dysphoria, schizotypal, and angry-impulsive. It may be hypothesized that these subtypes of borderline disorders have neurochemical abnormalities, as outlined in figure 13-A. It must be emphasized, however, that at present such theories are quite speculative and not yet verified by well-controlled studies. Many studies attempting to identify biological markers in borderline disorders have shown inconclusive results. These results are largely due to designs in which diagnostic subtypes are collapsed into an overly heterogeneous group of patients in which there is no control for comorbid Axis I disorders.

Hypothesized Neurochemical Dysfunctions of Borderline Disorder Subtypes

Subtype	Neurotransmitter	Location
Hysteroid-dysphoria	NE	Locus coeruleus
Schizotypal	DA	Mesolimbic, frontal cortex, and reticular formation
Angry-impulsive	5-HT	Prefrontal cortex

Figure 13-A

Treatment

No medication treatment can directly treat personality disorders, per se. Rather, psychotropic medications are used to ameliorate certain target symptoms. From results of the limited studies available, the medications of choice appear to be those listed in the Quick Reference (on the next page). The reduction in target symptoms can contribute significantly to improved coping ability and reduced levels of emotional despair. It is clear that no magic pill can cure deep characterological wounds, but targeted medication treatment of borderline patients can be an important adjunct to psychotherapy and crisis management.

Cautions

Three cautions are important to note:

- Treatment with antianxiety medications (benzodiazepines) is risky with borderline patients. These patients are certainly at risk for tranquilizer abuse. In addition, clinical experience, as well as research, shows that chronic use of benzodiazepines can contribute to emotional dyscontrol and increased suicidality with borderline patients (Cowdry and Gardner 1988; Hori 1998).

- Since some borderline patients are at risk for transient psychosis, the antidepressant bupropion (a dopamine agonist) should be used with caution. This drug, which is an effective antidepressant, may precipitate psychosis in prepsychotic individuals.

■ Because this group as a whole engages in frequent suicidal acting out, it is advisable to treat borderline patients with medications that have been found to have a low degree of toxicity when taken in overdose. These include antipsychotics and the following antidepressants: SSRIs, trazodone, venlafaxine, and bupropion (note the previous caution). Most other antidepressants are quite toxic when taken in overdose.

QUICK REFERENCE
Medications for Treating Borderline Subtypes[d]

Borderline Subtype	Class of Medication
Hysteroid-dysphoria[a]	SSRIs, anticonvulsants
Schizotypal[b]	Second-generation antipsychotics
Angry-impulsive, labile[c]	SSRI antidepressants, lithium, anticonvulsants, second-generation antipsychotics, omega-3 fatty acids
Comorbid major depression	Antidepressants
Comorbid panic disorder	Antidepressants

a Cowdry and Gardner (1988); Gardner and Cowdry (1986); Liebowitz and Klein (1981); Townsend, Cambre, and Barber (2001)

b Soloff et al. (1986); Frances and Soloff (1988); Goldberg et al. (1986); Gitlin (1993); Schulz et al. (1999); Coccaro (1998); Hori (1998); Hilger, Barnes, and Kasper (2003); Rocca et al. (2002)

c Norden (1989a); Cornelius et al. (1991); Salzman et al. (1995); Markovitz et al. (1991); Hori (1998); Stein et al. (2000); Moleman et al. (1999); Coccaro (1998); Bogenschutz and Nurnberg (2004); Rizvi (2002); Townsend, Cambre, and Barber (2001); Hilger, Barnes, and Kasper (2003); Rocca et al. (2002)

d General reviews: Kapfhammer and Hippius (1998); Hori (1998); Joseph (1997); Krashin and Oates (1999); Turner (1999); Turnbull (1998); Links, Boggild, and Sarin (2001)

14

Substance-Related Disorders

Substance abuse and related disorders represent a major problem area facing the clinician. Despite the "war on drugs," they continue to be a widespread problem: at least 5 percent of Americans are alcoholic, and stimulant abuse is a serious problem among teenagers and young adults. Any solution to these problems will undoubtedly involve social and political factors in addition to clinical programs. This chapter focuses on the differing types of clinical syndromes related to each commonly abused substance, and medications that may be useful as an adjunct to treatment.

Often the clinician will be confronted with a client who has substance-use problems in addition to a psychiatric disorder (comorbidity or dual diagnosis) or whose psychiatric disorder may be a direct result of substance use. In either case, treatment of the substance disorder will be crucial to the treatment of the psychiatric disorder. In the past, substance use was often seen as a form of self-medication—the person was using the drug to "treat" an emotional disorder, and psychotherapy was attempted in an effort to cure the person of the need for the substance—usually to no avail. In recent years, the evidence has shown that achieving abstinence is frequently a precondition for effectively dealing with psychological issues. In fact, the emotional problems may be significantly diminished by the person's achieving abstinence. For example, most (but not all) alcohol-related depression resolves within one to two weeks of abstinence. The interaction between substance-related disorders and other psychiatric disorders (like that between Axis I and Axis II disorders) is a complex one. We try here to clarify some of the more well-defined relationships.

Differential Diagnosis

Substance-related disorders are divided in *DSM-IV-TR* into dependence, abuse, intoxication, and withdrawal. In addition, each substance may have related disorders phenomenologically similar to other disorders: delirium, dementia, amnestic, psychotic, mood, anxiety, sex, and sleep disorders.

Substance-Abuse Facts

- Alcoholism affects 5 to 10 percent of the adult population.

- Alcoholism plays a major role in the following causes of death: accident, homicide, suicide, and alcoholic cirrhosis.

- One million Americans are reported to be addicted to cocaine, and over five million use cocaine regularly.

- Billions of dollars are spent annually on the treatment and prosecution of drug users.

- 30 to 50 percent of those in mental health treatment have a significant substance-abuse disorder.

Substance dependence is defined in *DSM-IV-TR* as a pattern of substance use leading to significant impairment or distress, demonstrated by at least three of the following:

- Tolerance—diminished effect from the same amount of the substance, often leading to use of increased amounts to achieve the same effect

- Withdrawal—onset of withdrawal syndrome if the substance is discontinued, often leading to continued use to avoid withdrawal symptoms

- Substance is taken more often than intended

- Persistent use despite efforts to cut down

- Great deal of effort is expended to obtain or continue use of the substance, or recover from its effects

- Other important activities are reduced in order to continue substance use

- Continued substance use despite knowledge that it is harmful

The *DSM-IV-TR* defines *substance abuse* as a pattern of substance use leading to significant impairment or distress, demonstrated by at least one of the following:

- Impairment of home, work, or school performance as a result of substance use

- Hazardous behavior resulting from substance use

- Legal problems resulting from substance use

- Continued substance use despite significant resultant problems

Intoxication refers to an acutely altered mental state due to ingestion of (or exposure to) a substance that is not caused by a medical condition or other mental disorder.

Withdrawal refers to an altered state produced by cessation or reduction of use of a substance that causes significant impairment in functioning in important areas and is not caused by a medical condition or other mental disorder. The disorder may be "persisting"—may continue even though substance use has stopped and the withdrawal syndrome has been resolved.

Figures 13-A and 13-B list substances and the clinical syndromes they can produce. Not all substances can cause every syndrome. For example, phencyclidine (PCP) can produce a very severe psychosis during intoxication but has no withdrawal syndrome, whereas sedative-hypnotics (such as benzodiazepines) can produce all of the substance diagnoses, as can alcohol. In the remainder of this chapter we review several of the major classes of substances associated with clinical disorders.

Major Substance Diagnoses

Substance	Dependence	Abuse	Intoxication	Withdrawal	Persisting
Alcohol	X	X	X	X	X
Hallucinogens	X	X	X		X
Opioids	X	X	X	X	
Phencyclidine	X	X	X		
Sedative-hypnotics	X	X	X	X	X
Stimulants	X	X	X	X	

Figure 14-A

Substance-Induced Disorders That Mimic Other Disorders

Substance	Delirium	Dementia	Amnestic	Psychotic	Mood	Anxiety
Alcohol	X	X	X	X	X	X
Hallucinogens	X			X	X	X
Opioids	X			X	X	
Phencyclidine	X			X	X	X
Sedative-hypnotics	X	X	X	X	X	X
Stimulants	X			X	X	X

Figure 14-B

Alcohol

Alcohol (ethanol) is a water-soluble substance that is rapidly absorbed and readily crosses the blood-brain barrier. It is a CNS depressant and is metabolized by the liver. It is also a gastric irritant and is toxic to liver cells and neurons. Alcohol is probably the most-studied substance of abuse (and the most abused substance). It is associated with dependence, abuse, withdrawal, intoxication, delirium, dementia, amnesia, delusions, hallucinations, mood disorder, anxiety disorder, sexual dysfunction, and sleep disorder.

There is much evidence demonstrating that alcoholism is familial, but the exact biological mechanism remains unclear. Several studies have tried to find a biological marker for alcoholism. Studies have shown a differential sensitivity to alcohol in alcoholics versus nonalcoholics (Pollock 1992). Schuckit, Gold, and Risch (1987) have shown that sons of alcoholics had significantly lower prolactin levels in response to ethanol challenge. Smith and colleagues (1992) showed that alcoholics were more likely to show *Taq* 1 A1 restriction, fragment-length polymorphism of the D2 dopamine receptor gene, a genetic abnormality (and dopamine controls prolactin release). The significance of these findings, however, remains speculative, and the search continues for the biological basis of alcoholism.

Psychiatric symptoms are very common in alcohol intoxication and withdrawal, but studies by Schuckit show that most of these symptoms improve greatly within one to four weeks of abstinence and are likely to abate over several months (Brown and Schuckit 1988; Schuckit, Irwin, and Brown 1990). The three diagnoses associated with increased risk of alcoholism are schizophrenia, mania, and antisocial personality disorder. As a depressant, alcohol tends to produce depressive symptoms during intoxication and anxiety symptoms during withdrawal and abstinence. These syndromes often mimic major depression or an anxiety disorder, but they will usually resolve within two weeks of abstinence and do not require prolonged treatment.

Medications can play an important role in the treatment of alcohol-related disorders. Figure 12-C lists medications that can be used in the treatment of alcohol-related disorders. Most of those medications are covered in part three of this book. The exception is disulfiram (Antabuse), a medication used to assist in the maintenance of abstinence. Disulfiram causes an accumulation of acetaldehyde if a person drinks alcohol while taking it, which leads to an unpleasant and potentially dangerous reaction involving flushing, throbbing headache, nausea, and vomiting. Only certain people are appropriate for disulfiram treatment. Some are able to remain abstinent without it; some will drink in spite of it. In between are those who will be able to reinforce their desire for abstinence by taking 250 to 500 mg of disulfiram once daily. Naltrexone, an opiate antagonist, has also shown some promise in helping maintain abstinence by reducing craving for alcohol (Bender 1993). Acamprosate (Campral) is a medication recently approved for maintenance of abstinence from alcohol. It is thought to reduce craving by its action on the glutamate and GABA neurotransmitter systems. It is recommended that it be started immediately following detoxification. Acamprosate

---

Alcohol-Related Disorders and Medications for Treating Them

Disorder	Medication
Intoxication	Thiamine, folate, multivitamins
Withdrawal	Benzodiazepines
Abstinence maintenance	Antabuse, naltrexone, topiramate[a] acamprosate, lithium,[a] SSRIs[a]
Delirium	Benzodiazepines
Dementia	—
Amnesia	Thiamine
Delusional disorder	Benzodiazepines, antipsychotics
Hallucinosis	Benzodiazepines, antipsychotics
Mood disorder	Antidepressants[a]
Anxiety disorder	Benzodiazepines, buspirone

a Likely, but not proven

Figure 14-C

must be taken three times per day and has few side effects, mostly gastrointestinal. It can be taken in conjunction with naltrexone to provide additional craving-reduction.

Stimulants

Amphetamines ("crank," "speed," "bennies" "ecstasy" [XTC]) and cocaine ("crack," "freebase") have become common substances of abuse. They are CNS stimulants that act on the dopaminergic system. Research suggests that a dopamine-medicated endogenous reward system in the limbic system is activated by amphetamines and cocaine. Amphetamines produce increased release of dopamine and norepinephrine along with their attendant peptides, and decreased reuptake. This leads to increased dopaminergic and noradrenergic activity and symptoms of euphoria, paranoia, and hyperexcitability. The half-life of dextroamphetamine is about ten hours. Cocaine produces similar pharmacologic effects but has a shorter duration of action and in some forms, especially crack cocaine, produces more intense effects, thus making it more addictive.

To understand the pharmacologic treatment of stimulant dependency it is helpful to look at the different phases of use on a neuronal level (see figure 14-D). During acute intoxication there is increased release of catecholamines (dopamine and norepinephrine) and enkephalins, along with decreased reuptake, leading to increased catecholamine activity. In the acute withdrawal state there is a reduction of available neurotransmitters (due to depletion and reduced reuptake). This leaves a state of reduced catecholamine activity and feelings of craving, depression, and restlessness. With chronic use, there is development of tolerance, further reduced availability of neurotransmitters, and an increased number of receptors (supersensitivity) leading to lower occupancy and feelings of craving, depression, and anhedonia.

Pharmacological treatment of stimulant use is different for each phase of use. During acute intoxication, medications can be used to block the effects of dopamine and norepinephrine. During withdrawal, medications are used to reduce craving (and hopefully subsequent use). The medications used to treat amphetamine use (see figure 14-E) generally potentiate the effects of norepinephrine, dopamine, or both. Most of those medications are discussed in part three of this book. Bromocriptine is a D2 dopamine agonist. Amantadine increases dopamine activity. L-dopa is a dopamine precursor that leads to increased dopamine synthesis. All these medications increase

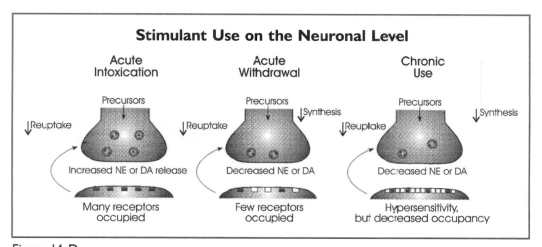

Stimulant Use on the Neuronal Level

Acute Intoxication — Acute Withdrawal — Chronic Use

Figure 14-D

Medications Used to Treat Phases of Stimulant Use

State	Medications
Intoxication	Beta blockers
	Clonidine
	Benzodiazepines
	Antipsychotics
Withdrawal/Abstinence	Buproprion
Maintenance	Antabuse
	Acamprosate
	Topiramate
	Modafanil

Figure 14-E

dopamine activity, thereby reducing the feelings of craving produced by dopamine depletion. It should be noted, however, that dopaminergic medications can produce psychotic symptoms, so the dose must be monitored closely. The effectiveness of these medications continues to be under investigation. They are not a panacea, but are often helpful in reducing symptoms of withdrawal and craving.

Opiates

Heroin was first synthesized from morphine over a century ago. Since then, it has become one of the most abused substances. Research into why it produces such powerful effects has led to the discovery of specific opiate receptors and endogenous opioids (enkephalins and endorphins). These peptides appear to be neurotransmitters involved with the sensation of pain and pleasure. A number of opiates and synthetic opioids are available and can lead to dependency, including morphine, heroin, propoxyphene (Darvon), methadone, meperidine (Demerol), pentazocine (Talwin), hydromorphone (Dilaudid), oxycodone (Percodan, Oxycontin), and hydrocodone (Vicodin, Damason-P), and codeine.

Different medications are used to treat different phases of opiate use (see figure 14-F). Acute opiate (opioid) intoxication leads to sedation, pupillary constriction, and respiratory depression and can be fatal. There are specific opiate antagonists that block the opiate receptors and rapidly reverse these effects: naloxone and naltrexone. Opiate withdrawal is characterized by anxiety, agitation, sweating, gastrointestinal upset, tremulousness, and running nose. It is treated by using an opiate such as propoxyphene (Darvon), methadone, or clonidine, or a combination of these drugs.

There are two strategies for treating dependence or abuse. One is to use methadone, a long-acting synthetic opiate that is well tolerated and reduces craving for other opiates such as heroin. Methadone is used for maintenance treatment because, with its long half-life, it produces less of a "high" and is less prone to abuse. It is now available only in certain federally approved treatment sites. The other is to have the client take an opiate antagonist (naloxone, naltrexone, or buprenorphine) so that the effect of the opiate will be blocked if it is used.

Medications Used to Treat Phases of Opiate Use	
State	**Medication**
Acute intoxication	Naloxone (injectable)
	Naltrexone (oral)
Acute withdrawal	Opiates, especially methadone and buprenorphine
	Clonidine
	Benzodiazepines
Abstinence maintainance	Methadone
	Naltrexone or buprenorphine
	LAAM (L-alpha-acetylmethadol)

Figure 14-F

Hallucinogens

Various substances can produce transient psychotic states, often accompanied by visual, auditory, or olfactory hallucinations. These include LSD (lysergic acid diethylamide), mescaline, psilocybin, and PCP. These drugs are not associated with dependence or withdrawal, but they can produce a florid psychosis during acute intoxication. This effect can usually be allowed to run its course (usually twelve to twenty-four hours), but sometimes medications (such as antianxiety or antipsychotic) need to be used to decrease agitation and stabilize blood pressure.

Sometimes patients will report a reexperiencing or "flashback" of hallucinations they had during a previous ingestion of hallucinogen. These reactions likewise usually do not require treatment with medication but, when severe, may benefit from antianxiety or antipsychotic medication. Severe overdoses of PCP can lead to convulsions and may require emergency medical treatment.

Other Drugs

Other substances of abuse—including caffeine, cannabis, inhalants, and nicotine—are not covered here since they are less important clinically. Caffeine intoxication can lead to anxiety or confusion. Inhalants can cause an organic psychosis and are very neurotoxic—leading to permanent neurological deficit. Nicotine dependence can be treated with a nicotine gum or patch, bupropion (Zyban) or vareniclike (Chantix) (in conjunction with cognitive-behavioral treatment). Sedative abuse and dependence is discussed in chapter 18, on antianxiety medications.

QUICK REFERENCE
Treatment of Substance-Related Disorders

Alcohol	Symptoms	Treatment
Intoxication	Confusion, slurred speech, ataxia, delirium	Supportive; thiamine, vitamins
Withdrawal	Anxiety, agitation, possible hallucinations, possible convulsions	Benzodiazepines
Abstinence maintenance	Craving, irritability	Naltrexone, acamprosate, Antabuse, Topiramate
Stimulants		
Intoxication	Anxiety, agitation	Supportive; benzodiazepines, beta blockers, clonidine
	Paranoid psychosis	Antipsychotics
Withdrawal	Anergia, irritabililty	Supportive; modafanil, acamprosate
	Depressed mood	Cyclic antidepressants, buproprion
Opiates		
Intoxication	Sedation, respiratory depression	Naloxone, naltrexone
Withdrawal	Anxiety, agitation, sweating, tremors	Clonidine, benzodiazepines, opiates (methadone or buprenorphine)
Abstinence maintenance	Craving, irritability	Methadone naltrexone, buprenorphine
Hallucinogens		
Intoxication	Agitation, prominent hallucinations	Benzodiazepines, antipsychotics
Withdrawal	No withdrawal syndrome	

15

Other Miscellaneous Disorders

There are several types of disorders that, although they are encountered less often in clinical practice, we have chosen to discuss in this chapter. Compared to disorders discussed in earlier chapters, their biological basis is less well understood at this time, and the role of medications may be less clear. These disorders are Tourette syndrome, eating disorders (anorexia and bulimia nervosa), attention-deficit disorder (ADHD), self-mutilation, sleep disorders, obesity, aggression, and chronic pain.

Tourette Syndrome

Tourette (or Gilles de la Tourette) syndrome is characterized by motor and vocal tics—sudden involuntary movements or vocalizations. It is most known for coprolalia (sudden yelling of obscenities), but this is seen only in 25 to 30 percent of cases. Motor tics typically involve the head and neck. Vocal tics may be guttural sounds, repeated coughing, or words. Tourette is now generally considered a neurological disorder, although symptoms may be exacerbated by anxiety or tension. It appears to involve dysfunction of dopaminergic pathways and is treated with dopamine D2 blockers—haloperidol or pimozide, in low to moderate doses. Persons with Tourette have a higher incidence of obsessive-compulsive disorder (OCD), attention-deficit/hyperactivity disorder (ADHD), and other learning disorders (Stern et al. 2000). This is probably because Tourette can involve multiple areas of the brain, some of which are also associated with OCD and ADHD. Theories regarding the etiology of Tourette include genetic (Robertson and Stern 1997) and autoimmune mechanisms related to strep infection (Bowes 2001).

Eating Disorders

Eating disorders are divided into two main types in *DSM-IV-TR*: anorexia nervosa and bulimia nervosa. Anorexia nervosa involves significant weight loss and maintenance of a very low body weight, by restriction of intake, purging, or both, often in combination with excessive exercising.

The *DSM-IV-TR* diagnostic criteria are:

■ Body weight less than 85 percent of that expected

■ Fear of gaining weight

■ Distorted perception of one's weight (thinking oneself fat when actually one is very thin)

■ Missing at least three consecutive menstrual cycles (where applicable)

Bulimia nervosa involves repeated episodes of binging and purging: eating large amounts of food (everything in the refrigerator) and then purging through self-induced vomiting or use of laxatives or diuretics. In addition, according to the *DSM-IV-TR*:

■ Both the binge eating and compensatory behaviors occur, on average, at least twice a week for three months.

■ Self-esteem is overly influenced by weight.

■ Disturbance does not occur only during periods of anorexia nervosa.

Much research has investigated personality characteristics, psychological issues, family dynamics, and the biological basis of anorexia and bulimia. Anorexia usually requires a multimodal, if not a multidisciplinary, treatment approach. The severe nutritional deficiency causes a multitude of problems that must be addressed medically and which make response to medication treatment alone poor. Indeed, no medication has shown significant consistent benefit in the treatment of anorexia. One theory holds that patients with anorexia become addicted to starvation; it is known that endorphins are released during prolonged fasting. This theory holds that anorectics have a biological vulnerability to becoming addicted to fasting. Studies have shown some benefit of naltrexone (an opiate antagonist) in the treatment of anorexia—the explanation being that it blocks the "high" of fasting and thereby removes the incentive (Luby, Marrazzi, and Kinzie 1987). Other medications are *sometimes* helpful; these include antidepressants, antipsychotics, cyproheptadine, and lithium (see figure 15-A). These drugs can be especially useful when there are coexisting features, for instance, antidepressants when depressive features are present or SSRIs when obsessional symptoms are prominent.

Bulimia, in contrast, often benefits from treatment with antidepressants (40 to 70 percent respond) and is considered by some to be a depressive variant. All types of antidepressants have proven useful, although it should be remembered that bupropion (Wellbutrin) is contraindicated in eating disorders because of increased incidence of convulsions. Selective serotonin reuptake inhibitors (SSRIs) have been quite effective and, because of their low side-effect profile, are often tried first. Topiramate (Topamax), an anticonvulsant, has also been shown to have efficacy but, because of its side effects, should be used only after other medications have proven ineffective.

Binge-eating disorder is not a separate disorder in the *DSM-IV-TR* and, thus, falls under "Eating Disorder Not Otherwise Specified." It has been receiving increasing attention and research. Binge-eating disorder is similar to bulimia, but without

Medications for Treating Eating Disorders	
Disorder	**Medication**
Anorexia	Naloxone
	antidepressants
	antipsychotics
	cyproheptadine
	lithium
Bulimia	Antidepressants (SSRIs, TCAs, or MAOIs), naltrexone, ondansetron, topiramate

Figure 15-A

the purging. It is usually associated with some degree of obesity. In addition to nonmedical treatments, such as diet and exercise, several medications can be helpful. Often antidepressants (SSRIs or bupropion) are used. Sibutramine, an anorectic agent (diet pill), can be helpful. Also, the anticonvulsants topiramate and zonisamide have shown some efficacy but, again, because of their side effects, are used only after other treatments have failed (Yager et al. 2006).

Residual Attention-Deficit/Hyperactivity Disorder (ADHD)

ADHD is a disorder that first appears in childhood, but at least half of those who develop ADHD will have residual symptoms that persist into adulthood. Often, these adults have been previously undiagnosed and present with depressive symptoms or problems with work or relationships. Adults with ADHD may report irritability, impulsivity, traffic accidents, forgetfulness, poor time management, and difficulty finishing tasks. A careful evaluation is essential to recognizing residual ADHD in adulthood. ADHD is discussed in detail in chapter 23.

Self-Mutilation

Self-mutilation refers to deliberate self-injury without the intent to die. It is most commonly encountered in three groups of patients: those with organic disorders (including mental retardation), psychotic disorders, and personality disorders. Self-mutilation is often a clinical issue in patients with severe personality disorders who, for example, repeatedly make lacerations (often fairly superficial) on their wrists or forearms. They may describe that, as they watch the blood flow from the cut, it feels as if some internal tension is flowing out of them.

Recently, there has been growing interest into the possible biological substrate of this type of behavior. Studies have involved the opiate, dopamine, and serotonin systems. It has been shown that endorphins (endogenous opiates) are released by painful stimulation. Opiate antagonists (such as naltrexone) have been helpful in reducing self-injurious behavior (Winchel and Stanley 1991). Self-injurious behavior in animals has been increased by dopamine agonists and decreased by dopamine blockers. Serotonin has also been implicated, partly by the similarity between self-mutilation and some behaviors seen in obsessive-compulsive disorder—irresistible urges to commit an act and the resulting relief from anxiety that follows commission. Selective serotonin reuptake inhibitors have been shown to be somewhat helpful in treating trichotillomania (hair pulling).

A wide variety of medications are sometimes helpful in self-injurious behavior. Those that sometimes have been found to help in self-injurious behavior in the context of a personality disorder include MAO inhibitors, SSRIs, carbamazepine, lithium, antipsychotics, and benzodiazepines. The choice of medication should be based on the associated features present. Thus, when depressive features are present, try an SSRI; when there are symptoms of atypical depression and rejection sensitivity, an MAOI; and when psychotic features are present, an antipsychotic. This is an area where there are no clear guidelines for medication use and no guarantee of effectiveness. However, using trial and error, one can often find a drug that has significant benefit.

Insomnia and Sleep Disorders

In this section we cover normal sleep and sleep disorders, with a focus on two primary sleep disorders: sleep apnea and restless legs syndrome (also called periodic limb movements of sleep). Disrupted sleep both exacerbates and is exacerbated by psychiatric disorders. Thus restful sleep plays a key role in emotional well-being.

Sleep

Although we do not yet understand the precise way in which sleep is restorative, we do know that it is very important to our health and functioning. Sleep helps consolidate memory and it processes emotionally charged experience. Many studies have shown that inadequate sleep leads to impaired functioning. In fact, it is estimated that over 50,000 highway accidents per year can be traced to driver fatigue (Knipling and Wang 1994). Research by Dr. William Dement, the former director of the Stanford Sleep Clinic, found that the average person needs eight to nine hours of sleep to be fully rested. Dr. Dement concluded that most people are in a chronically sleep-deprived state (personal communication). Sleep deprivation leads to:

- Fatigue (of course).

- Reduced ability to think clearly, maintain attention, and retrieve information from memory.

- Reduced emotional control, which leads to increased irritability and reactivity.

- Paradoxically, it sometimes leads to increased insomnia.

There are different patterns of sleep disturbance:

- Difficulty falling asleep (initial insomnia)

- Restless sleep: tossing and turning all night, with frequent awakenings

- Early morning awakening: waking several hours before morning, such as 3:00 to 4:00 A.M., and having difficulty falling back to sleep

- Hypersomnia: sleeping excessively

Normal Sleep

During normal sleep, we cycle through multiple stages of sleep. These stages are divided into REM (rapid eye movement) sleep and NREM (nonrapid eye movement) sleep. As we fall asleep, we slip into stage 1 of NREM sleep. Then we gradually go deeper into sleep: into stage 2 and stage 3 of NREM sleep, and then back up into REM sleep. After REM sleep (also known as dream sleep) we go back into stage 1 of NREM sleep and begin the cycle again. Each cycle takes 75 to 90 minutes, so we have four to six cycles per night.

As the night progresses, we spend more time in REM sleep. We may not reach stage 3 of NREM sleep in every cycle. The degree of restfulness derived from sleep seems to depend on the amount of time spent in deep sleep; that is, on the amount of time spent in stages 2 and 3 of NREM sleep. It's normal to awaken one or two times per night. This usually happens as we come out of REM sleep and start a new sleep cycle. As long as the time awake is brief, it should not interfere with getting a good night's rest.

As we age, our sleep "efficiency" decreases; that is, we become less able to sleep soundly through the night, and have more awakenings and less deep sleep. This is why older people often sleep less at night, often only five hours, and compensate by taking a nap in the afternoon.

Causes of Insomnia

All types of sleep disturbance can be caused by stress, tension, anxiety, depression, or other psychiatric disorders. In this case, the sleep disorder is called a secondary insomnia because it is due to another condition. There are also primary insomnias, such as sleep apnea and restless legs syndrome, in which the sleep disturbance is the main symptom of the disorder. These are described below. The main causes of secondary insomnia are:

- Situational stress and worry

- Anxiety, depression, and other emotional disorders

- Medications, drugs, and alcohol

- Medical illness

Situational stress and worry are very common causes of sleep disturbance. Probably everyone has experienced them at one time or another. They usually cause difficulty falling asleep or restless sleep. Fortunately, the insomnia usually resolves within a few days, or when the stress is reduced. Sometimes stress leads to disturbing dreams or nightmares that interfere with sleep. Improved sleep hygiene often helps this issue.

Most psychiatric disorders can affect sleep. When this is the case, the best approach is to treat the primary disorder, for example, treat the depression. Unfortunately, sometimes sleep does not improve, even when the symptoms of the disorder are greatly improved. For instance, sometimes treatment with an antidepressant will lead to significant improvement in mood, but the person may still have difficulty falling asleep. In this case, sleeping pills or other sedative medications are often used.

Many medications and other drugs adversely affect sleep. The most common offenders are:

- Caffeine
- Decongestants (e.g., pseudoephedrine, often found in cold medications)
- Alcohol
- Tranquilizers (e.g., Xanax, Ativan, Valium)
- Sleeping pills
- Steroids
- Bronchodilators (used to treat asthma)

It may be surprising to see alcohol, tranquilizers, and sleeping pills on this list. Indeed, they are often effective in helping people fall asleep. But then two things happen: First, there is often a rebound when the drug or alcohol wears off, so the person awakens in the middle of the night and has difficulty falling back to sleep. In addition, some sleeping pills (but not all) and most tranquilizers disturb the quality of sleep by reducing the amount of time spent in deep sleep. Thus sedatives can interfere with sleep even though the person may be sedated or asleep for more than eight hours.

Many, if not most, medical illnesses can also cause sleep disturbance. Medical conditions that commonly cause insomnia include:

- Chronic pain conditions
- Congestive heart failure
- Respiratory diseases, including chronic lung disease
- Acid reflux (GERD)
- Hot flashes associated with perimenopause or menopause
- Hyperthyroidism

Sleep Hygiene

Sleep hygiene refers to the steps that one can take to prepare the body and mind for sleep and, thereby, improve the quality of sleep. This is done by starting to shift toward quieter, more peaceful activities at least three hours prior to bedtime. The mind has a difficult time falling asleep when it is excited and activated. Gradually slowing down several hours before going to bed helps the mind ease into sleep. A routine of going to bed and getting up at (fairly) consistent times is also helpful. Moreover, it is helpful to use the bed mainly for sleeping (and intimacy), and not for watching TV, eating, sorting mail, and so forth. Specific things to avoid in the evening include:

- Bright light
- Intense exercise (although regular exercise earlier in the day improves sleep)
- Loud music and emotionally charged entertainment

- Intense discussions or arguments

In addition, engaging in one or more of the following activities can help to quiet the body and mind:

- Meditating or practicing progressive relaxation quiet both the body and the mind. There are several commercially available audio CDs that describe these activities.

- Watching a peaceful (or boring) TV show or reading a boring book may help. (Do not read the news.)

- Taking a warm bath.

- Eating carbohydrate-rich food (e.g., fruits and vegetables but not sweets) or tryptophan-rich foods (such as milk) can aid sleep.

- Listening to peaceful music.

- Sleeping cool (heavy covers or electric blankets may feel cozy but can interfere with entering into deep and slow wave sleep). The ideal temperature for sleep is 68 degrees.

Sleep Disorders

The primary sleep disorders include sleep apnea and restless legs syndrome (also referred to as periodic limb movements in sleep, or PLMS). These are disorders whose main symptom is fatigue caused by disturbed sleep.

Sleep Apnea

Sleep apnea is characterized by transient periods of the cessation of breathing, or apnea, during sleep. These periods last only a few seconds, but they are enough to cause a partial awakening, and thus disturb sleep. They may occur several hundred times each night. Diagnosis can be made by a polysomnogram, taken during a sleep study in which breathing, EEG (electroencephalogram), and other vital signs are monitored during sleep. The main symptom of sleep apnea is daytime fatigue, but it is also often associated with loud snoring, or awakening gasping for breath during the night. Often the person is unaware of the apneic episodes and is aware only of being tired all the time.

Sleep apnea can be caused either by the collapse of the muscles of the throat during sleep (obstructive type) or by the failure of the respiratory center in the brain to instruct the lungs to breathe during sleep (central type). Generally, sleep apnea is treated with a CPAP (breathing) machine or surgery. These treatments are fairly effective for treating obstructive apnea, but they are of little benefit in central apnea.

Restless Legs Syndrome

Restless legs syndrome (RLS) involves, as the name suggests, a sensation of restlessness of the legs. Most people with RLS also have periodic limb movements in sleep (PLMS), meaning they move their arms and legs frequently during sleep. RLS, like PLMS, also results in fatigue. It is usually diagnosed by taking a case history, but the diagnosis can be confirmed by polysomnography. RLS and PLMS are usually treated with a medication that increases the activity of dopamine, such as pramipexole (Mirapex) or ropinirole (Requip). Other medications sometimes used include tranquilizers (e.g., clonazepam), opiates, or anticonvulsants, (e.g, gabapentin). RLS is worsened by some antidepressants and caffeine. For that reason treatment often involves reducing offending medications and caffeine.

Medications for Restless Legs Syndrome (and PLMS)		
Generic	Brand	Dosage
pramipexole	Mirapex	0.125–2 mg
ropinirole	Requip	0.25–4 mg

Sleeping Medications

Sleep medications, referred to as *hypnotics*, are used to treat insomnia, regardless of the cause. Because of this and because they are very effective and have few side effects, they have become immensely popular. As reported by the *New York Times*, IMS America found that Americans received over 49 million prescriptions for hypnotics in 2006 (Mooallem 2007). The National Sleep Foundation survey (2005) found that 25 percent of all Americans take a hypnotic every year. Insomnia is a very common problem and Americans spend millions of dollars every year on sleeping pills. But despite their effectiveness and relative safety, there are several important considerations about their use to take into account:

- When poor sleep is due to another medical condition, such as depression, sleep apnea, or congestive heart failure, the most important thing is to treat the primary condition.

- Most sleep medications, except zolpidem (Ambien), zaleplon (Sonata), eszopiclone (Lunesta), and ramelteon (Rozerem), reduce the amount of deep sleep and, therefore, may contribute to daytime fatigue.

- Sometimes sleeping pills cause sedation, especially in the morning.

- Sometimes sleeping pills cause amnesia. This means that people sometimes do not remember things they have done. A classic example is the person who wakes up in the morning to find cracker crumbs in his or her bed, and does not remember having eaten crackers during the night. Of greater concern are those who drive their cars in this condition. This has been most reported with triazolam (Halcion) and zolpidem (Ambien) and appears to be associated with a short drug half-life.

- Most sleeping pills are habit-forming. Usually, this means they should be used only for a short time. With continued use, tolerance often develops, requiring an increase in dose, and then dependence results. Pretty soon, instead of taking the medication to sleep, you can no longer sleep without it. If the medication is to be used for more than several weeks, it's best not to take it more than three nights per week. Ramelteon (rozerem) is the only sleeping pill that is not habit-forming. This may be because it works at the melatonin receptor, which does not release dopamine and, therefore, may not lead to being habit-forming. Other medications that produce sedation, but are not sleeping pills, are often used for sleep because they are not habit-forming. These include trazodone (Desyrel), quetiapine (Seroquel), mirtazepine (Remeron), and diphenhydramine (Benadryl). Because these medications have more serious side effects (except for diphenhydramine), generally they are reserved for more severe or chronic forms of insomnia. The benzodiazepine anti-anxiety medications (such as Ativan or Xanax) are sometimes also used for sleep and have the same problems as the benzodiazepine hypnotics, such as Valium; that is, they are habit-forming and suppress deep sleep.

Hypnotics		
Generic	**Brand**	**Daily Doses**[1]
flurazepam	Dalmane	15–60 mg
temazepam	Restoril	15–30 mg
triazolam	Halcion	0.25–0.5 mg
estazolam	Prosom	1–2 mg
quazepam	Doral	7.5–15 mg
zolpidem	Ambien, Ambien CR	5–12.5 mg
	Intermezzo	1.75 mg
zaleplon	Sonata	5–10 mg
eszopiclone	Lunesta	1–3 mg
ramelteon[1]	Rozerem	4–16 mg
Other:		
diphenhydramine	Benadryl	25–100 mg
melatonin	Melatonin	1–3 mg
trazodone	Desyrel	25–100 mg
doxepin	Silenor	3–6 mg

[1] To treat initial insomnia

Obesity

New pharmacological treatments have been developed for the treatment of obesity. They should not be used as the sole treatment for obesity, but can be helpful adjuncts to other forms of treatment, such as exercise, dietary restriction, and behavioral modification. Obesity is usually defined as a body mass index (calculated by dividing weight in kilograms by height in meters squared) greater than 30. Phentermine (Fastin, Ionamin) is a stimulant that can cause anxiety and insomnia, and must be used with caution if taken with antidepressants, especially the SSRIs. Sibutramine (Meridia) is a serotonin and norepinephrine reuptake inhibitor with some demonstrated efficacy (Hanotin et al. 1998). It can cause elevations of heart rate and blood pressure. Orlistat is another new medication for obesity that works by inhibiting the digestion and absorption of fat. It inhibits the enzyme lipase so that about one-third of dietary fat is not absorbed (Drent and van der Veen 1993).

Aggression

Aggression, including irritability, hostility, or violent behavior, is usually a symptom of a psychiatric or neurological disorder. Below is a list of some examples of such disorders:

- ADHD
- Antisocial personality disorder
- Borderline personality disorder
- Conduct disorder
- Delirium
- Dementias
- Depression
- Explosive disorder
- Medication-induced aggression
- Mania
- Mental retardation
- Paranoid disorder
- Postconcussion syndrome
- Schizophrenia
- Substance-use disorders
- Temporal lobe epilepsy

In these cases, the preferred strategy is to treat the primary disorder. There have been indications (Fava, Anderson, and Rusenbaum 1993) that some angry outbursts may be similar to panic attacks, but instead of flight, or fear, there is fight, or anger. Aggression has been shown to be responsive to antidepressant medications. In addition, there are a number of medications listed next that have a somewhat nonspecific antiaggression effect. In choosing a medication it is helpful to choose on the basis of associated features.

Medication Type	Associated Features
■ Anticonvulsants (e.g., carbamazepine)	Labile mood, poor impulse control, organicity
■ Antipsychotics	Disorganized behavior
■ Beta blockers (e.g., propranolol)	Organicity (e.g., dementia)
■ Buspirone	Organicity
■ Clonidine	Anxiety, agitation
■ Lithium	Labile mood, impulsivity
■ SSRIs	Anger "attacks"

Chronic Pain

Antidepressant medications have been shown to often be helpful in chronic pain syndromes. These medications are effective only for chronic pain and not for acute pain. They help reduce pain and, when combined with narcotic analgesics, potentiate the effects of the narcotic. The cyclic antidepressants (e.g., amitriptyline, doxepin, nortriptyline, and duloxetine [Cymbalta] are the best studied and have the most supporting evidence. When there is not an accompanying depression, lower than the usual antidepressant doses may be effective. Venlafaxine and duloxetine are also effective because they affect both serotonin and norepinephrine, like the cyclic antidepressants. There are a few studies showing the effectiveness of the SSRIs but some studies that do not.

Part Three

Medications

Part three deals with the different classes of psychopharmaceuticals, including dosage and choice of medication, side effects, and mechanism of action (where and insofar as it has been established). Also covered are precautions for monitoring medication effects and serum levels, and guidelines for educating patients and their families about the effects and side effects of these drugs.

16

Antidepressant Medications

The term *antidepressants* refers to a large, important group of medications used to treat depression. In recent years, they have grown enormously in frequency of prescription and popularity as well as notoriety. This growth is due to increased awareness of depression and decreased troublesome side effects from the newer agents.

Antidepressants were developed in the 1950s. Iproniazid, an agent used to treat tuberculosis, was inadvertently found to produce an improvement in mood. Ultimately, it was discovered to be an inhibitor of monoamine oxidase (MAO)—an enzyme used to break down catecholamines (dopamine, norepinephrine, and serotonin) in neurons. This led to the development of an entire class of antidepressants: the monoamine oxidase inhibitors, or MAOIs.

At about the same time, the drug imipramine was first produced. It was originally developed as a phenothiazine (antipsychotic) but was found to have antidepressant properties. Soon came amitriptyline, followed later by other "tricyclic" and "heterocyclic" antidepressants.

We now have at least six major groups of antidepressants: cyclic antidepressants, selective serotonin reuptake inhibitors (SSRIs), serotonin and norepinephrine reuptake inhibitors (SNRIs), norepinephrine reuptake inhibitors (NRIs), monoamine oxidase inhibitors (MAOIs), and the atypicals. In addition, sometimes stimulants (such as Ritalin or Dexedrine) are used to treat depression, and there are some reports of the use of buspirone (Buspar).

Despite our knowledge of some of the important mechanisms of action of these medications, we still do not really know how they relieve depression. It is theorized that they start a process that leads to neuro-endocrine effects, for example, decreased CRF (corticotropin releasing factor) and/or, through intracellular second messengers, to increased BDNF (brain-derived neurotropic factor), leading to improvement (Musselman et al. 1998).

Types of Antidepressant Drugs

Tricyclics

For many years, tricyclic antidepressants (TCAs) and heterocyclics were the mainstay of the treatment of severe depression. The following is a list with their brand names:

Cyclic Antidepressants	
Generic Name	**Brand Name**
Amitriptyline	Elavil
Amoxapine	Asendin
Clomipramine	Anafranil
Desipramine	Norpramin
Doxepin	Sinequan, Adapin, Silenor
Imipramine	Tofranil
Maprotiline	Ludiomil
Nortriptyline	Pamelor, Aventyl
Protriptyline	Vivactil
Trazodone	Desyrel, Oleptro
Trimipramine	Surmontil

No antidepressant has been proven consistently superior to another, but they do differ significantly in terms of side effects. All of the tricyclics have the same side effects, but in varying degrees. These side effects can be grouped as follows:

- Anticholinergic

- Adrenergic

- Antihistaminic

- Miscellaneous

The tricyclics are considered "dirty" drugs in that they react with a number of receptors besides the one responsible for the therapeutic effect, resulting in a host of side effects (see figure 16-A). Anticholinergic side effects range from unpleasant (dry mouth, dry skin, blurred vision, and constipation) to serious (paralytic ileus, cessation of movement of the intestine, which can lead to intestinal rupture and death; and urinary retention, inability to urinate, which in serious cases can lead to rupture of the bladder). Adrenergic side effects include sweating, sexual dysfunction, and orthostatic hypotension—sudden drop in the blood pressure upon rising and a sensation of light-headedness. This condition can lead to a fall and, in turn, to fractures, which can have serious medical consequences, especially in the elderly. Antihistaminic effects include sedation and weight gain. Miscellaneous side effects include lowered seizure threshold, cardiac arrhythmia, hepatitis, agranulocytosis, rashes, sweating,

Side Effects of Cyclic Antidepressants

	Anticholinergic	Sedation	Orthostatic
Amitriptyline	++++	++++	+++
Amoxapine	++	+	++
Clomipramine	+++	+++	++
Desipramine	+	+/0	+
Doxepin	++++	++++	+++
Imipramine	++	++	++
Maprotiline	++	++	+++
Nortriptyline	++	++	+
Protriptyline	++	++	++
Trazodone	0	+	++
Trimipramine	++	++++	+++

Figure 16-A

anxiety, and elevated heart rate. Tricyclics are quite toxic and even a small overdose can be lethal.

Selective Serotonin Reuptake Inhibitors

The SSRIs are a newer class of antidepressants. They have been used widely because they are generally as effective as the tricyclics but have significantly fewer side effects and are safer in overdosage. The first SSRI on the market was fluoxetine (Prozac). Five newer agents are citalopram (Celexa), escitalopram (Lexapro), fluvoxamine (Luvox), paroxetine (Paxil), and sertraline (Zoloft). They share the same side effects but in varying degrees (see figure 16-B). Unlike the tricyclics, they are relatively "clean," and interact very little with other receptors besides the serotonin 5-HT reuptake receptor. Their side effects tend to be related to increased serotonin activity: nausea, gastrointestinal upset, sweating, anxiety, insomnia, headache, restlessness, and sexual dysfunction. They can have very mild anticholinergic side effects and can cause dry mouth, sedation, and blurred vision (Paxil has modest anticholinergic effects). Such side effects generally are considerably less intense than those seen with cyclic antidepressants. After several months of treatment, patients taking SSRIs can develop a syndrome including loss of energy, passivity, decreased pleasure, and decreased libido, which resembles, but is not the same as, the depression for which they are being treated. This may, with close patient monitoring, respond to the addition of buproprion or a stimulant such as methylphenidate or modafinil.

Sexual dysfunction, delayed or absent ejaculation in men, and anorgasmia in men and women, are common SSRI side effects. Decreased libido may also be caused by the SSRIs. These side effects often may be diminished by dose reduction, drug holidays, or the use of other medications as antidotes, such as Viagra, cyproheptadine, or buproprion.

Another difference between the antidepressants is their half-lives. Paroxetine has a half-life of approximately one day, sertraline one to two days, and fluoxetine seven to ten days. A long half-life is an advantage in maintaining a stable blood level but may be a disadvantage when stopping the medication. It takes six weeks to reach a steady state with fluoxetine and six weeks to eliminate it from the body after discontinuation.

Serotonin and Norepinephrine Reuptake Inhibitors

The serotonin and norepinephrine reuptake inhibitors (SNRIs) are dual-action antidepressants, affecting both serotonin and norepinephrine. The SNRIs include venlafaxine (Effexor), desvenlafaxine (Pristiq), duloxetine (Cymbalta), and mirtazapine (Remeron). Venlafaxine and duloxetine are blockers of the reuptake of both serotonin and norepinephrine, and mirtazapine is an alpha-2-adrenoreceptor blocker, producing increased serotonin and norepinephrine activity. Some of the older cyclic antidepressants are also dual-action, but they are not included here because they have many other effects. There is evidence that duloxetine, venlafaxine, and mirtazapine are somewhat more effective than the SSRIs in the treatment of severe depression (Clerc, Ruimy, and Verdeau-Palles 1994; Wheatley et al. 1998). However, duloxetine, venlafaxine, and mirtazapine have additional side effects relative to the SSRIs.

Side Effects of SSRIs and Atypical Antidepressants

	Anxiety	Sedation	Insomnia	Nausea	Sexual Dysfunction
SSRIs					
Citalopram	+	0	+	+	++
Escitalopram	+	0	+	+	+
Fluoxetine	++	±	++	+	++
Fluvoxamine	±	++	±	++	++
Paroxetine	±	++	±	+	++
Sertraline	+	+	+	++	++
SNRIs					
Desvenlafaxine	+	+	+	++	+
Duloxetine	+	+	+	+	+
Mirtazapine	±	++	±	+	++
Venlafaxine	+	+	+	++	+
NRI					
Atomoxetine	+	++	±	+	0
Atypical					
Bupropion	++	±	+	+	0
Nefazodone	±	±	+	+	±
Vilazodone	±	±	+	+	±

Figure 16-B

Norepinephrine Reuptake Inhibitors (NRIs)

Atomoxetine (Strattera) is a relatively new medication FDA-approved for the treatment of ADHD. It is a selective blocker of norepinephrine reuptake. It is not FDA approved for the treatment of depression, but its pharmacological action is that of an antidepressant, and it has been shown to have antidepressant effects. Reboxetine (Vestra) is an NRI antidepressant available in Europe but not currently in the United States. As a class, the NRIs tend to be especially effective at improving energy and cognition, and they have little or no effect on sexual function. On the negative side, they may tend to cause anxiety, loss of appetite, and, paradoxically, sedation.

Atypical Antidepressants

Bupropion (Wellbutrin) is an antidepressant with unique properties. Along with mirtazapine (see above), it is one of the antidepressants whose mechanism of action is *not* reuptake inhibition. It appears to work in a complex way to increase noradrenergic activity. In addition, it has weak dopaminergic activity, resulting in some stimulant effect. It has side effects of anxiety and insomnia. It had received much attention because of its tendency to lower the seizure thresholds in patients with eating disorders. However, the newer sustained-release formulations (Wellbutrin SR and Wellbutrin XL) do not present this problem any more than other antidepressants, if given in doses of 300 mg or less per day. (Note: All antidepressants lower seizure thresholds to a degree.) Bupropion is also one of the most common agents used to augment SSRIs and has an additional positive feature in that it has fewer sexual side effects.

Nefazodone (Serzone), like venlafaxine, is an antidepressant that affects multiple neurotransmitter systems. Like trazodone, nefazodone is a potent 5-HT2A receptor blocker. In addition, it is both a serotonin and norepinephrine reuptake inhibitor. The most common side effects are nausea, headache, anxiety, sedation, and dizziness. It has been associated with drug interactions, and there is a warning regarding its use with Xanax. Serzone has been associated with liver toxicity, and in rare cases this has led to hepatic failure. It is currently only available in generic form.

Buspirone (BuSpar) is a medication used mainly for the treatment of anxiety. However, there are several reports of its effectiveness as an antidepressant in higher doses (40 to 60 mg per day and up). In the recently completed STAR-D study (supported by NIMH) buspirone was shown to be an effective augmenting agent. It has the side effects of anxiety (paradoxically), nausea, headache, and dizziness.

Vilazodone (Viibryd) is an SSRI and a 5-HT1A partial agonist. These pharmacodynamics suggest that in addition to antidepressant effects, vilazodone is likely to be effective in treating anxiety.

Monoamine Oxidase Inhibitors

The MAO inhibitors represent a group of antidepressants now used mainly when other antidepressants have failed in the treatment of major depression and panic disorder. This is partly because of the risk of a hypertensive reaction. The MAOIs

---

1. In a study by Bieck and Antonin (1988) 50 percent of patients taking tranylcypromine (Parnate) showed a significant hypertensive reaction from taking 8 mg of tyramine.

Tyramine Contents in Food Products

Food	Tyramine Content per Serving
Fish	
Lumpfish roe	0.2 mg/50 g
Sliced schmaltz herring in oil	0.2 mg/50 g
Pickled herring[a]	negligible
Smoked salmon	negligible
Salmon mousse	0.7 mg/30 g
Meat and sausage	
Salami	5.6 mg/30 g
Mortadella	5.5 mg/30 g
Air-dried sausage	3.8 mg/30 g
Chicken liver	1.5 mg/30 g
Bologna	1.0 mg/30 g
Aged sausage	0.9 mg/30 g
Smoked meat	0.5 mg/30 g
Corned beef	0.3 mg/30 g
Kielbasa sausage	0.2 mg/30 g
Fruit	
Avocado[a]	negligible
Banana[a]	negligible
Banana peel	1.424 mg/banana
Raisins[a]	negligible
Figs[a]	negligible
Other	
Marmite concentrated yeast extract	6.45 mg/10 g
Sauerkraut	13.87 mg
Beef bouillon mix	231.25 mg/package
Beef bouillon	102 mg/cube
Soy sauce	0.2 mg/10 ml
Yogurt[a]	negligible
Fava beans[a]	negligible
Beer[b]	0.3–1.5 mg
Wine	0–0.5 mg

a Previously thought to be higher in tyramine

b Some types of beer have been recently identified as having dangerously high tyramine content. See Tailor et al. (1994).

Source: Shulman et al. (1989).

Figure 16-C

can cause a severe and sudden rise in blood pressure, potentially leading to cerebral hemorrhage or death. Such a reaction can be caused by eating foods high in tyramine content (see figure 16-C) or taking sympathomimetic drugs, such as decongestants or other antidepressants.[1] Thus, it is recommended that people taking MAOIs wear a medic alert bracelet and seek medical attention immediately at the first sign of a hypertensive reaction (severe, pounding occipital headache). In one study of 182 people taking MAOIs, 12 hypertensive reactions occurred, with no fatalities, giving a rate of about 7 percent (Rabkin et al. 1985). In addition to the hypertensive reactions, which are fortunately uncommon, there are a number of other side effects that can be troublesome. These include sedation, insomnia, agitation, confusion, orthostatic symptoms, and edema.

Phenelzine (Nardil) and tranylcypromine (Parnate) are the two most common MAOIs. Two newer MAOIs are being studied to evaluate their clinical use; both have a reduced risk of hypertensive reaction. Selegiline (Deprenyl and Ensam: transdermal patch) is an MAO-B inhibitor (inhibits type B MAO) that is used in the treatment of Parkinson's disease and may be especially useful for treating depression in patients with Parkinson's. Ensam is a transdermal patch that has been approved by the FDA for treating depression. Meclobemide, a reversible MAO-A inhibitor, is currently used in Europe and Canada and is not available in this country.

Stimulants

Stimulants have been used as antidepressants for many years, especially dextroamphetamine (Dexedrine) and methylphenidate (Ritalin). They have the side effects of anxiety, insomnia, agitation, and appetite suppression. They can be quite effective as augmenting agents for antidepressants.

Mechanism of Action

The antidepressants, generally, produce their therapeutic effects by blocking the reuptake of one or more neurotransmitters (norepinephrine, serotonin, and dopamine), which leads to a decrease (down-regulation) of the number of postsynaptic receptors—generally within seven to twenty-one days, coinciding with the onset of clinical effect (see chapter 3). It is thought that the down-regulation of postsynaptic receptors is part of a complex series of steps involving secondary messengers, which lead to the turning on and off of selected genes and transcription of mRNA. The MAOIs block monoamine oxidase, which metabolizes the NE, 5-HT, and DA stored at the nerve ending of the presynaptic neuron—thereby making more neurotransmitter available. Stimulants increase the release of catecholamines. Buspirone is a 5-HT IA receptor blocker.

Antidepressants generally produce effects within two to three weeks. Once therapeutic benefit has been obtained, it is important that the patient continue the medication for at least six months. Discontinuing in less than six months is likely to lead to relapse. In treating a patient's first depression, it is reasonable to gradually discontinue the medication after six to twelve months. If the patient has had two or more depressions, it is probably best to continue the medication because the likelihood of recurrence is significant (70 to 80 percent or more). Recent studies have also shown that subsequent depressive episodes may be less responsive to treatment. Therefore, in such cases the best treatment is to prevent relapse by continuation of medication.

Comparison of Antidepressants

Celexa (citalopram): Advantages: Minimal documented interaction with other drugs. Minimal sedation/weight gain.
Disadvantages: May cause anxiety initially: At doses above 40 mg a day, may cause cardiac problems.

Cymbalta (duloxetine): Advantages: Good for severe depression.
Disadvantages: May cause nausea, sedation.

Effexor (venlafaxine): Advantages: Good for severe depression, social anxiety and GAD, and possibly chronic pain.
Disadvantages: May cause hypertension. Increased gastrointestinal side effects.

Lexapro (escitalopram): Advantages: Minimal documented interaction with other medications and minimal sedation/weight gain.
Disadvantages: May cause anxiety initially.

MAO inhibitors: Advantages: Especially potent in treatment-resistant depressions.
Disadvantages: Drug-drug and drug-food interactions can be dangerous.

Paxil (paroxetine): Advantages: Good antianxiety benefit.
Disadvantages: More prone to discontinuation symptoms, weight gain, may interact with other medications. Contraindicated in pregnancy.

Prozac (fluoxetine): Advantages: Activating (energizing), long half-life.
Disadvantages: May cause initial activation (anxiety) that subsides in a week or two. May interact with other medications.

Remeron (mirtazapine): Advantages: Good for severe depression, insomnia. Less sexual dysfunction. Indicated in treating geriatric depressed patients who often show failure to thrive and marked weight loss.
Disadvantages: Significant weight gain and sedation.

Serzone (nefazodone): Advantages: Good at reducing anxiety. Fewer sexual side effects.
Disadvantages: Sedating. Prone to medication interactions. Rare reports of liver damage.

Strattera (atomoxetine): Advantages: Good for cognitive symptoms. Minimal sexual side effects.
Disadvantages: May cause sedation or anxiety.

Wellbutrin (buproprion): Advantages: Energizing, few sexual side effects, less weight gain.
Disadvantages: May increase anxiety and insomnia. Can cause seizures, especially at doses over 400 mg/day.

Zoloft (sertraline): Advantages: Neither too sedating, nor too prone to cause anxiety.
Disadvantages: More prone to gastrointestinal side effects.

Viibryd (vilazodone): Advantages: Can treat comorbid anxiety.
Disadvantages: At the time of this printing, none determined as yet, because the drug is new.

Figure 16-D

Another consideration in the treatment of depression after the initial phase is treating to remission, as opposed to improvement. Most studies showing antidepressant benefit use 50 percent improvement in symptoms (usually 50 percent reduction in the Ham-D score) as the criterion for treatment response. However, people with this level of response still may be significantly depressed. They may feel better, but still be impaired in their social or occupational functioning. Treating to remission (Ham-D score of 7 or less) may require raising the dose of the antidepressant or augmenting or switching to another antidepressant (see figure 16-D).

Dosages

In order for medications to be effective, they must be taken at an adequate dose (see figure 16-E) for an adequate period of time. There seems to be a threshold effect, with subtherapeutic doses producing little or no benefit. However, achieving an effective dose may be difficult due to side effects.

Initially, you will see only side effects. Over the course of one to two weeks, tolerance to side effects will develop and the dosage can be increased. It is always a good idea to start with a very low dose (5 to 10 mg of fluoxetine or 37.5 mg venlafaxine), in case the person is particularly sensitive to side effects. One severe reaction to medication can have very destructive consequences for the therapeutic relationship and the willingness to try further medications.

For the SSRIs, nausea can often be managed by taking the medication with a meal. Insomnia may require taking the medication only in the morning and sometimes by taking a sedating medication, like trazodone, at bedtime. Anxiety can be reduced by avoiding caffeine and oral decongestants and short term use of benzodiazepines. Sedation can be reduced by taking the medication at bedtime. Sexual dysfunction often can be improved by adjunctive medications like Viagra or Wellbutrin.

For the tricyclics, dry mouth is common and can be managed by drinking water, chewing gum, or using a synthetic saliva (available at a pharmacy). Constipation can be managed with a stool softener such as Metamucil or DSS. Orthostatic symptoms can be managed by avoiding dehydration, adding salt to the diet, standing up gradually, and holding onto something for a few seconds after standing.

Many more measures can be taken to manage other side effects, but they are beyond the scope of this book. When these measures do not work and the patient complains of troublesome or intolerable side effects, one can decrease the dosage (which may lead to a loss of benefit) or change to another medication, as is addressed in the next section.

Choice of Medication

Choosing an antidepressant involves considering a number of factors. One important consideration is the person's previous response to medication, if any, and his or her family history of response to medication. Another important consideration is the presence of associated symptoms and comorbidity; for example, does the person have panic attacks, OCD, or PTSD? Consideration should be given to whether the person may have a bipolar disorder, because antidepressant treatment can cause a manic episode in the absence of an antimanic agent (see chapter 17).

Antidepressant Doses*

Drug	Dose (mg/day)
Cyclics	
Amitriptyline	75–300
Doxepin	75–300
Imipramine	75–300
Trimipramine	75–300
Clomipramine	75–200
Amoxapine	150–400
Desipramine	75–300
Maprotiline	75–225
Nortriptyline	50–150
Protriptyline	15–60
Trazodone	150–400
SSRIs	
Fluoxetine	20–80
Sertraline	50–200
Paroxetine	20–60
Fluvoxamine	50–300
Citalopram	10–40
Escitalopram	5–20
Atypical, SNRIs, NRIs	
Atomoxetine	60–120
Bupropion SR and XL	150–400
Desvenlafaxine	50–400
Duloxetine	20–100
Mirtazapine	15–45
Nefazodone	100–600
Venlafaxine XR	75–350
Vilazodone	10-40
MAOIs	
Phenelzine	30–90
Tranylcypromine	20–60
Isocarboxazid	20–40
Selegiline transdermal	6–12

* Doses for children and adolescents: See appendix B.

Figure 16-E

Blood Levels of Antidepressants

Drug	Typical Plasma Concentration (mg/ml)
Amitriptyline	100–250
Doxepin	100–250
Imipramine	200–300
Trimipramine	250–300
Clomipramine	200–300
Amoxapine	150–500
Desipramine	100–250
Maprotiline	250–300
Nortriptyline	50–150
Protriptyline	100–250
Trazodone	800–1600
Fluoxetine	200–700
Bupropion	25–100
Sertraline	32–190

Figure 16-F

With the possible exception of severe and melancholic depression (for which dual-action antidepressants appear to be more effective), all antidepressants have similar efficacy. So, the next consideration is to minimize undesirable side effects.

Due probably to feelings of hopelessness and pessimism, depressed patients are especially prone to discontinuing medication prematurely. This is particularly the case when they encounter significant side effects. Thus, choosing an antidepressant with minimal side effects becomes a crucial part of ensuring an adequate medication trial. On the other hand, sometimes medication is chosen on the basis of its side effects. Thus, if a patient complains of anxiety and insomnia, you might use a sedating medication. Or, conversely, if the individual complains of lack of energy, you might choose a nonsedating or energizing antidepressant. Most professionals feel that because of their safety, efficacy, and lack of side effects, the SSRIs or one of the newer antidepressants are the first choice in the treatment of depression. TCAs are now reserved for use only when other, safer antidepressants have been ineffective. When they *are* used, the secondary amines (refers to chemical structure), amoxapine, desipramine, maprotiline, nortriptyline, and protriptyline, are preferred because they have reduced side effects.

Whichever antidepressant is chosen first, the question of what to try if the first one doesn't work may arise. But what is considered a nonresponse? Before you abandon one medication for another, it is important that the patient experience an "adequate" clinical trial. This means adequate time at an adequate dose—at least four weeks, and some studies suggest eight to twelve weeks because there is a small percentage of late responders. But then, what is an adequate dose—the usual dose, such as 20 mg of fluoxetine, or the maximum tolerated dose? (Again, blood levels sometimes help. See figure 16-F.) Medication compliance must also be considered.

The STAR-D (Sequenced Treatment Strategies for Reducing Depression) program has found some superiority to switching *classes* of antidepressants (i.e., if first treated with an SSRI, switch to a norepinephrine or dopamine reuptake inhibitor, such as bupropion) versus switching *within* class (i.e., from one SSRI to another SSRI). An even higher-yield strategy is augmentation (discussed under "Treatment-Resistant Depression" below).

Special considerations also apply to certain classes of patients when selecting an antidepressant—see figure 16-G.

Special Considerations in Choosing an Antidepressant

Patient Type	Medication Choices
Anxious	SSRIs, SNRIs
Anergic	Bupropion or NRIs
Atypical	SSRIs, MAOIs, or bupropion (watch for possible bipolar disorder)
Child	SSRIs
Choices to avoid	
Obesity	TCAs, mirtazapine
Seizure disorder	Bupropion (doses over 300mg/day)
Cardiac disease	TCAs
Elderly	TCAs
Comorbidity	
Marked irritability	SSRIs
OCD	SSRIs, clomipramine
Panic disorder	All antidepressants except bupropion
Chronic pain	TCAs, venlafaxine, duloxetine
Dysthymia	SSRIs
High suicide risk	Less toxic antidepressants (avoid TCAs and MAOIs)
Premenstrual dysphoria	SSRIs
Psychotic	Symbyax (olanzapine and fluoxetine combination), amoxepine, venlafaxine, TCAs
Severe, recurrent	SNRIs or SSRI/bupropion combination

Figure 16-G

Phases of Treatment

It is helpful to consider three phases in the treatment of major depression. These are outlined below:

Acute Treatment: Begins with the first dose and extends until the patient is asymptomatic (in good case scenarios, this may be from six to eight weeks).

Continuation Treatment: To avoid acute relapse, it is strongly suggested that patients continue treatment for a minimum of six months beyond the acute phase.

Also, recent studies indicate that the patient should be maintained on the same dose used during the acute phase. Remember to treat to remission, not just improvement.

Maintenance Treatment: Relapse prevention is an important aspect of treatment, especially in those patients judged to have recurrent episodes (or those at risk for recurrence). Continued (lifelong) treatment provides the best outcome for such individuals. The following guidelines are offered:

1. *First Episode:* At the end of the continuation phase, gradually reduce the dose (over a period of one to two months) and, assuming no return of depressive symptoms, discontinue. Educate the patient to be alert to any signs of recurrence (e.g., poor sleep, fatigue, and so on) and should this occur, as soon as possible reinstigate treatment.

2. *Second Episode:*

    a. *With "Risk Factors"* (which include family history of mood disorders, first episode occurring prior to the age of eighteen, and/or most recent episode has severe symptoms): Recommend lifelong medication treatment to prevent recurrence.

    b. *Without "Risk Factors":* Gradually discontinue medications.

3. *Third or Subsequent Episodes:* Recommend lifelong medication treatment.

Problematic Side Effects

Three side effects are often encountered that can lead to patient discontinuation. The first is *activation*. This is an acute onset side effect seen within the first few hours after starting an antidepressant or when doses are increased. It presents with nervousness and anxiety; activation may also cause initial insomnia. It is important to distinguish between activation and switching.

Switching occurs when a person being treated with an antidepressant is provoked into a manic state. One significant difference between activation and switching is that, generally, switching does not occur until after several weeks of antidepressant treatment (versus the rapid onset of activation).

It is also important to note that when a patient experiences activation, this side effect has nothing to do with bipolar disorder; that is, it is not diagnostic of an underlying bipolar disorder. Activation feels very uncomfortable and is a common reason for patient-initiated discontinuation. Generally, activation can be successfully addressed by co-administering a low dose of a tranquilizer (e.g., lorazepam, 0.25 to 0.5 mg twice a day) during the first three weeks of antidepressant treatment and then phased out. Activation, if it occurs, typically lasts only a week or two.

A second problematic side effect is sexual dysfunction. It is worth noting that rates of sexual dysfunction in the general (nondepressed) population are quite high. In addition, depression itself is often associated with decreased libido. In a very large study by Clayton et al. (2002), when careful histories were elicited from the patient and a significant other, many reported sexual problems predated to the onset of antidepressant treatment, and a good many sexual symptoms (especially reduced sex drive) appeared to be related to the depression (again, evident prior to starting medication treatments). When these preexisting problems were taken into account, Clayton and colleagues found rates of drug-related sexual side effects to range from 14 to 39 percent for the newer antidepressants (the one exception was Wellbutrin with a rate of 7 percent).

The primary sexual side effect was *inorgasmia* (difficulty achieving an orgasm despite adequate arousal). Impotency was rare. The best-supported treatments for such sexual side effects are the addition of Wellbutrin 150 to 300 mg per day, with improvement seen generally within a few weeks. Also, administration of Viagra is often helpful (both in men and women). This strategy requires a dose of 50 to 100 mg one hour before intimate relations. Interestingly, although Viagra was developed and approved for treating male erectile dysfunction, it appears to have other benefits, that is, increasing the ability to achieve orgasm in both genders.

Antidepressants can increase libido when it has been decreased by depression. On the other hand, antidepressants, especially SSRIs, can decrease libido over time.

There also have been case reports of *genital anesthesia* (decreased sensitivity) and what has come to be known as *ejaculatory anhedonia* (ejaculation but without pleasure). Prevalence rates for this problem are not clearly known nor are any particular treatments.

The final side effect is weight gain. This is most notable with the antidepressant Remeron. Generally, this is an undesirable side effect; however, when depression presents with anorexia and pronounced weight loss, this medication can be helpful. This is most frequently seen in the elderly who, when clinically depressed, often show "failure to thrive" accompanied by marked weight loss. Most other newer-generation antidepressants do not appear to cause weight gain, at least not during the first few months of treatment. Any weight gain seen during this time is most commonly a consequence of a reduction in depression and return to normal appetite. However, about 10 percent of patients on longer-term antidepressant treatment do report weight gain (this may not become readily apparent until after a number of months of treatment). Why this occurs is not clearly understood, but it does not appear to be associated with increased caloric intake. The speculation is that for this small group of patients, the drug has somehow affected metabolic rates, and they are simply not burning as many calories. Caloric restriction and exercise may be needed to combat this side effect.

Antidepressants and the Issue of Increased Suicidality

This important issue is covered in detail in chapter 23 (see the sidebar on page 261).

Treatment-Resistant Depression

Many people are inadequately treated for depression and have minimal positive response, usually due to poor compliance and inadequate trials. However, true *treatment-resistant depression* (TRD) refers to a depression that has failed to respond to adequate trials of two or more antidepressants. As many as 10 to 20 percent of people with depression may fall into this category.

A full discussion of the treatment of TRD is beyond the scope of this book, but it will be helpful for you to be familiar with some of the typical strategies used in such cases. The following list should be considered in the treatment of resistant depression, but it is by no means exhaustive:

- Check the diagnosis: Are depressive symptoms due to characterological disorder, medical illness, or psychotic disorder?

- Is it a type of depression that typically is not responsive to medication treatment (such as psychological-reactive depression) so that psychotherapy is instead the treatment of choice?

- Check the dose: Has the medication dose been too low? (It may help to check the blood level.) Has the patient taken the medication as prescribed and for a long enough period of time (at least four to six weeks at adequate dose)? Adequate trials require, if necessary, pushing the dose to upper limits and making sure that the patient has been compliant. High-dose strategies are often very successful if they can be tolerated. Frequently, a failure to fully respond may be due to inadequate compliance.

- Check for substance abuse, especially alcohol.

- Change the medication: Usually you will want to try another class of medication (NE, 5-HT, MAOI). (Figure 16-H lists particular neutotransmitters associated with antidepressant effects.) See the algorithm at the end of this chapter as a general guideline for a systematic progression of medication trials.

- Augmentation: The addition of a second medication (referred to as *augmentation*) often yields a positive response. The strategy is to add a medication with a different mechanism of action to try to get a synergistic effect. There is little scientific evidence to guide us in our choice of augmenting agent, but a survey of clinicians at Harvard (Mischoulon et al. 1999) revealed that the most common medication combination was an SSRI with Wellbutrin. The second most common was an SSRI with Buspar, followed by the addition of Ritalin to an antidepressant. Other augmenting agents include lithium, thyroid, the new stimulant medication modafinil (Provigil), and second-generation antipsychotics (e.g., olanzapine or risperidone).

- Consider electroconvulsive treatment (ECT) (see sidebar at end of chapter), transcranial magnetic stimulation (TMS),* vagal nerve stimulation (VNS), or RU 486 (mifepristone).*

- Never forget psychotherapy.

Patient Education

Education of patients about antidepressants has several facets. First, education about the biological aspects of depression is helpful, especially so that they do not view taking medication as a sign of moral weakness. Next, it is important to describe what to expect from the antidepressants: what typical side effects are, that the medication is not habit forming, that a clinical response typically takes two to four weeks to be achieved, that side effects diminish over time, and that other medications can be tried if the first one does not work. For people taking MAOIs, education about foods and medications to avoid is crucial.

---

* Currently undergoing clinical trials—considered experimental at this time.

Selective Action of Antidepressant Medications

Generic Name	Brand Name	Norepine- phrine Effects	Serotonin Effects	Monoamine Oxidase Effects	Dopamine Effects
Amitriptyline	Elavil	+	++++	0	0
Amoxapine	Asendin	++++	+	0	0
Atomoxetine	Strattera	+++++	0	0	0
Bupropion[b]	Wellbutrin	++	0	0	++
Citalopram	Celexa	0	+++++	0	0
Clomipramine	Anafranil	+++	+++++	0	0
Desipramine	Norpramin	+++++	0	0	0
Desvenlafaxine	Pristiq	++	++++	0	+
Doxepin[a]	Sinequan, Adapin Silenor	+++	++	0	0
Duloxetine	Cymbalta	++++	++++	0	0
Escitalopram	Lexapro	0	+++++	0	0
Fluoxetine	Prozac, Sarafem	0	+++++	0	0
Fluvoxamine	Luvox	0	+++++	0	0
Imipramine	Tofranil	++	+++	0	0
Isocarboxazid	Marplan	+++	+++	+++++	+++
Maprotiline	Ludiomil	+++++	0	0	0
Mirtazapine	Remeron	+++	+++	0	0
Nefazodone	Serzone	+	+++	0	0
Nortriptyline	Aventyl, Pamelor	+++	++	0	0
Paroxetine	Paxil, Pexeva	+	+++++	0	0
Phenelzine	Nardil	+++	+++	+++++	+++
Protriptyline[a]	Vivactil	++++	+	0	0
Selegiline transdermal	Emsam	+++	+++	+++++	+++
Sertraline	Zoloft	0	+++++	0	+
Tranylcypromine	Parnate	+++	+++	+++++	+++
Trazdone	Desyrel Oleptro	0	+++++	0	0
Trimipramine[a]	Surmontil	++	++	0	0
Venlafaxine	Effexor	++	++++	0	+
Vilazodone	Viibryd	0	+++++	0	0

a Uncertain, but likely, effects

b Atypical antidepressant; uncertain effects but likely to be a dopamine and norepineph- rine agonist

Figure 16-H

Handbook of Clinical Psychopharmacology for Therapists

The most common cause of medication failure is failure to take enough medication for long enough. Discussion about side effects can be very helpful in helping someone continue the medication long enough to benefit. This can be difficult, because initially there are only side effects and no benefits; only later are there benefits and diminished side effects. Through supportive therapy you can often help your depressed patient to overcome annoyance or distress over side effects (preoccupation with somatic symptoms), discouragement about delayed benefits, and pessimism about the outcome. In these ways, you can help your client to continue in treatment and achieve greater benefit.

Never discontinue abruptly or without medical monitoring. Acute discontinuation can cause nausea, general malaise, achiness, and return of depressive symptoms.

Over-the-Counter Options

Three over-the-counter (OTC) products have been shown to have efficacy in treating depression. The herb, *Saint-John's-wort*, has research support for effectiveness in treating mild-to-moderate depression. The dosing is 300 to 600 mg three times a day, and generally daily treatment for a minimum of six to eight weeks is required before the onset of symptomatic improvement. Two cautions are important to note. First, since the FDA does not regulate herbals, there is no guarantee that all products have adequate or standardized amounts of the psychoactive ingredient. Second, Saint-John's-wort has been shown to induce liver enzymes and thus presents with significant drug-drug interaction problems. Although this product has few side effects when taken alone, serious drug interactions have been reported when it is combined with other prescription drugs, including antidepressants. Should a patient be taking Saint-John's-wort and the decision is made to switch treatment to a prescription antidepressant, a one-week washout is strongly advised before initiating the new medication.

SAM-e (s-adenosyl-methionine) is another OTC product with some research support for effectiveness in treating mild-to-severe depression. The effective dosage range is from 400 to 1600 mg per day. Onset for symptomatic improvement appears to be similar to that seen with the use of prescription antidepressants. At the time of the publication of this book, serious drug-drug interactions have not been reported, therefore caution is warranted until this medication has been more fully evaluated. (Also see chapter 20.)

Omega-3 fatty acids (such as EPA and DHA, which can be purchased over the counter) have been shown to be an effective adjunct in the treatment of unipolar and bipolar depression (Stoll et al. 1999). Early studies evaluated the effectiveness of high doses (9 grams per day), but more recent clinical experience suggests that doses of 0.5 grams twice daily can be effective. Currently, this is considered to be an experimental treatment, but there are several positive studies, and the side effects are minimal: mild gastrointestinal symptoms and a fishy odor (Peet and Horrobin 2002).

ECT: Electroconvulsive Therapy

During the late 1930s it was observed that people suffering from both epilepsy and serious mental illnesses exhibited an interesting phenomenon in the aftermath of a seizure. Often, such individuals would experience a noticeable reduction in psychiatric symptoms after having seizures; the effect would last from a few days to a couple of weeks. Based on this observation, numerous attempts were made to intentionally induce seizures in psychiatric patients who did not otherwise have epilepsy. It was found that the safest way to accomplish this was by delivering an electrical shock to the head. The duration of the shock was a couple of seconds, resulting in a grand mal seizure. It was found that a series of "shock treatments" (generally nine to twelve, given at a rate of three per week) were required to produce a significant diminution in psychiatric symptoms. Especially since there were no other viable medical treatments for severe mental illness during the 1930s, this new procedure caught on and was used extensively for the next three decades.

Indiscriminate use of electroconvulsive therapy (ECT) was common in these early days. There were a number of serious complications that accompanied the treatment (e.g., spinal fractures). And the public's view of ECT, characterized in numerous movies, was of an inhumane, horrific, and frightening procedure. During the 1950s it also gradually became clear that ECT was not especially effective for some types of illnesses (e.g., schizophrenia).

Eventually, clinical experience showed that the best outcomes from ECT were with people with severe mood disorders (i.e., very severe depression with melancholic features; psychotic depressions; and severe, acute mania). In more recent times, techniques for administering ECT have changed dramatically. This currently includes the use of powerful muscle relaxers (to prevent severe motor contractions that had been previously encountered) and the use of a general anesthesia; prior to the treatment per se, the patient is fully anesthetized. Serious or persistent side effects now are considered to be rare. However, it is important to note that all patients receiving ECT do experience significant memory problems that continue throughout the treatments and generally for four to six weeks after treatments have ended. Cognitive problems persisting after this time are rare.

Although ECT can dramatically and quickly improve mood, ongoing medication treatments (antidepressants, antipsychotics in cases of psychotic depressions, and mood stabilizers in cases of mania) are crucial for the prevention of acute relapse.

ECT is often considered a treatment of last resort, but when used with appropriately diagnosed patients, it can be extremely effective and, at times, a life-saving procedure. And ECT remains the "gold standard" for severe depressions.

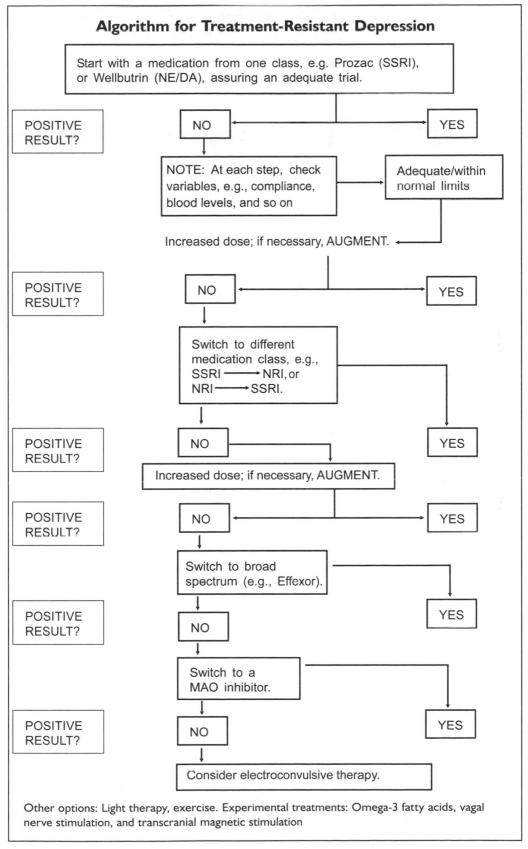

Algorithm for Treatment-Resistant Depression

Start with a medication from one class, e.g. Prozac (SSRI), or Wellbutrin (NE/DA), assuring an adequate trial.

POSITIVE RESULT? — NO ← YES

NOTE: At each step, check variables, e.g., compliance, blood levels, and so on → Adequate/within normal limits

Increased dose; if necessary, AUGMENT. ←

POSITIVE RESULT? — NO ← YES

Switch to different medication class, e.g., SSRI ⟶ NRI, or NRI ⟶ SSRI.

POSITIVE RESULT? — NO ← YES

Increased dose; if necessary, AUGMENT.

POSITIVE RESULT? — NO ← YES

Switch to broad spectrum (e.g., Effexor). — YES

POSITIVE RESULT? — NO

Switch to a MAO inhibitor. — YES

POSITIVE RESULT? — NO

Consider electroconvulsive therapy.

Other options: Light therapy, exercise. Experimental treatments: Omega-3 fatty acids, vagal nerve stimulation, and transcranial magnetic stimulation

Medications for Treating Depression (Cyclic Antidepressants)

Generic Name	Brand Name	Average Daily Dosage Range (mg/day)	Side Effects (usually diminish; may require attention if persist)	Side Effects Requiring Immediate Attention	Significant Drug Interactions* (not all-inclusive)
Amitriptyline	Elavil	75-300	■ Blurred vision	■ Changes in blood pressure	■ Amphetamines
Amoxapine	Asendin	150-400	■ Breast enlargement	■ Confusion	■ Anti-arrythmics
Clomipramine	Anafranil	75-200	■ Discharge from the breast	■ Excitation or mania	■ Anticoagulants (blood thinners)
Desipramine	Norpramin	75-300	■ Dizziness	■ Extreme constipation	■ Antipsychotics
Doxepin	Sinequan	75-300	■ Dry mouth	■ Extreme eye or skin sensitivity to sunlight	■ Bupropion
Imipramine	Tofranil	75-300	■ Increased appetite	■ Extreme sedation	■ Carbamazepine
Maprotiline	Ludiomil	75-225	■ Mild to moderate constipation	■ Irregular heart rate	■ Cimetidine
Nefazodone	Generic only	100-600	■ Persistent sore throat	■ Problems with urination (difficult or painful urination; unable to urinate)	■ Clonidine
Nortriptyline	Pamelor	50-150	■ Sexual problems		■ Drugs that depress the CNS (antihistamines, narcotics, muscle relaxants, and barbiturates)
Protriptyline	Vivactil	15-60	■ Tremor of the hands	■ Seizure	■ Drugs used during surgery
Trazodone	Desyrel	150-400	■ Weight gain	■ Shortness of breath	■ MAOI antidepressants (phenelzine, isocarboxazid, and tranylcypromine)
Trimipramine	Surmontil	75-300		■ Yellow skin or eyes	■ MAOI drugs (selegiline, isoniazid, linezolid)
					■ Quinolones
					■ SSRI antidepressants
					■ Thyroid hormones

Warnings/Precautions

■ Not indicated during pregnancy or while breastfeeding

■ Liver or kidney impairment may require dosage adjustment or discontinuation of treatment

■ Can trigger mania/hypomania

■ May increase the risk of suicidal thinking in young adults, adolescents, and children

■ Cardiac monitoring as indicated

■ Blood level monitoring required for some cyclic antidepressants

■ Increased intraocular pressure

■ Orthostatic hypotension

■ Lowered seizure threshold

*There is variability in the potential for a specific cyclic antidepressant to interact with the drugs listed.

QUICK REFERENCE
Medications for Treating Depression (SSRIs)

Generic Name	Brand Name	Average Daily Dosage Range (mg/day)	Side Effects (usually diminish; may require attention if persist)	Side Effects Requiring Immediate Attention	Significant Drug Interactions* (not all-inclusive)
Citalopram	Celexa	10-40	▪ Anxiety	▪ Bleeding, especially gastrointestinal	▪ Amphetamines
Escitalopram	Lexapro	5-20	▪ Blurred vision	▪ Bruising	▪ Anti-arrhythmic drugs
Fluoxetine	Prozac	20-80	▪ Change in appetite	▪ Chills or fever	▪ Anticoagulants (blood thinners)
Fluvoxamine	Luvox	50-300	▪ Change in weight	▪ Extreme eye or skin sensitivity to sunlight	▪ Anticonvulsants
Paroxetine	Paxil	20-60	▪ Dizziness	▪ Seizures	▪ Antipsychotics
Sertraline	Zoloft	50-200	▪ Drowsiness	▪ Shortness of breath	▪ Aspirin
Vilazodone	Viibryd	10-40	▪ Dry mouth	▪ Skin rash or hives	▪ Benzodiazepines
			▪ Headache	▪ Swelling of the hands or feet	▪ Beta blockers
			▪ Insomnia		▪ Buspirone
			▪ Mild to moderate constipation		▪ Cimetidine
			▪ Nausea		▪ Diet pills
			▪ Sexual problems		▪ Drugs that depress the CNS (antihistamines, narcotics, muscle relaxants, and barbiturates)
			▪ Sweating		▪ HIV protease inhibitors
			▪ Stimulation		▪ Lithium
			▪ Teeth grinding		▪ MAOI antidepressants (phenelzine, isocarboxazid, and tranylcypromine
			▪ Tremor of the hands		▪ MAOI drugs (selegiline, isoniazid, linezolid)
			▪ Yawning		▪ NSAIDs
					▪ Products containing L-tryptophan
					▪ Serotonin precursors and serotonin agonists (triptans, tramadol)
					▪ Saint-John's-wort
					▪ Some nonsedating antihistamines
					▪ TCA antidepressants

Warnings/Precautions

- ▪ Not indicated during pregnancy or while breastfeeding
- ▪ Liver or kidney impairment may require dosage adjustment or discontinuation of treatment
- ▪ Can trigger mania/hypomania
- ▪ May increase the risk of suicidal thinking in young adults, adolescents, and children
- ▪ Withdrawal reactions
- ▪ Serotonin syndrome
- ▪ Hyponatremia
- ▪ Amotivational syndrome

*There is variability in the potential for a specific SSRI to interact with the drugs listed.

QUICK REFERENCE
Medications for Treating Depression (SNRIs)

Generic Name	Brand Name	Average Daily Dosage Range (mg/day)	Side Effects (usually diminish; may require attention if persist)	Side Effects Requiring Immediate Attention	Significant Drug Interactions* (not all-inclusive)
Desvenlafaxine **Duloxetine** **Venlafaxine**	**Pristiq** **Cymbalta** **Effexor**	**50-400** **40-60** **75-350**	■ Anxiety ■ Blurred vision ■ Change in appetite ■ Change in weight ■ Dizziness ■ Drowsiness ■ Dry mouth ■ Headache ■ Insomnia ■ Mild to moderate constipation ■ Nausea ■ Sexual problems ■ Sweating ■ Stimulation ■ Teeth grinding ■ Tremor of the hands ■ Yawning	■ Bleeding, especially gastrointestinal ■ Bruising ■ Chills or fever ■ Increased blood pressure ■ Increased heart rate ■ Seizures ■ Shortness of breath ■ Skin rash or hives ■ Swelling of the hands or feet	■ Anticoagulants (blood thinners) ■ Anti-arrythmics ■ Antipsychotics ■ Cimetidine ■ Diet pills ■ Drugs that depress the CNS (anti-histamines, narcotics, muscle relaxants, and barbiturates) ■ Lithium ■ MAOI antidepressants (phenelzine, isocarboxazid, and tranylcypromine ■ MAOI drugs (selegiline, isoniazid, linezolid) ■ Products containing L-tryptophan ■ Quinolones ■ Serotonin precursors and serotonin agonists (triptans, tramadol, Saint-John's-wort) ■ TCA antidepressants

Warnings/Precautions

- Not indicated during pregnancy or while breastfeeding
- Liver or kidney impairment may require dosage adjustment or discontinuation of treatment
- Can trigger mania/hypomania
- May increase the risk of suicidal thinking in young adults, adolescents, and children
- Withdrawal reactions
- Serotonin syndrome
- Hyponatremia
- High blood pressure, additional monitoring as necessary
- Increased intraocular pressure
- Orthostatic hypotension

*There is variability in the potential for a specific SNRI to interact with the drugs listed.

194   *Handbook of Clinical Psychopharmacology for Therapists*

Generic Name	Brand Name	Average Daily Dosage Range (serum levels)	Side Effects (usually diminish; may require attention if persist)	Side Effects Requiring Immediate Attention	Significant Drug Interactions (not all-inclusive)
Bupropion	Wellbutrin	150-300mg	▪ Blurred vision ▪ Constipation ▪ Diarrhea ▪ Dizziness ▪ Dry mouth ▪ Hand tremor ▪ Increased appetite ▪ Nausea ▪ Sexual dysfunction ▪ Weight gain	▪ Blood pressure changes ▪ Confusion ▪ Difficulty breathing ▪ Excitation ▪ Extreme constipation ▪ Irregular heartbeat ▪ Problems with urination (difficult or painful urination; unable to urinate) ▪ Seizure ▪ Significant drowsiness ▪ Skin rash or hives ▪ Swelling of the feet or hands ▪ Yellow eyes or skin	▪ Anti-arrythmics ▪ Antipsychotics ▪ Beta blockers ▪ Caffeine in arge amounts ▪ Carbamazepine ▪ Drugs that depress the CNS (antihistamines, narcotics, muscle relaxants, and barbiturates) ▪ Drugs that lower seizure threshold ▪ Duplicative bupropion products ▪ HIV protease inhibitors ▪ Levodopa ▪ MAOI antidepressants ▪ Other drugs with MAOI properties such as selegiline, isoniazid, lirezolid, triptans ▪ SSRI antidepressants ▪ Tricyclic antidepressants
Warnings/Precautions ▪ Not indicated during pregnancy or while breastfeeding ▪ Liver or kidney impairment may require dosage adjustment or discontinuation of treatment ▪ May increase the risk of suicidal thinking in young adults, adolescents, and children ▪ Lowered seizure threshold					
Mirtazapine	Remeron	15-45mg	▪ Constipation ▪ Dizziness ▪ Dry mouth ▪ Increased appetite ▪ Weight gain	▪ Blood pressure changes ▪ Chills or fever ▪ Confusion ▪ Difficulty breathing ▪ Excitation ▪ Extreme constipation ▪ Irregular heartbeat ▪ Seizure ▪ Significant drowsiness ▪ Skin rash or hives ▪ Swelling of the feet or hands	▪ Drugs that depress the CNS (antihistamines, narcotics, muscle relaxants, barbiturates, and other psychiatric medications) ▪ MAOI antidepressants ▪ Other drugs with MAOI properties such as selegiline, isoniazid, linezolid, triptans
Warnings/Precautions ▪ Not indicated during pregnancy or while breastfeeding ▪ Liver or kidney impairment may require dosage adjustment or discontinuation of treatment ▪ May increase the risk of suicidal thinking in young adults, adolescents, and children ▪ Lowered seizure threshold ▪ Diabetes mellitus					

Generic Name	Brand Name	Average Daily Dosage Range (serum levels)	Side Effects (usually diminish; may require attention if persist)	Side Effects Requiring Immediate Attention	Significant Drug Interactions (not all-inclusive)
Isocarboxazid	Marplan	10-40mg	■ Blurred vision ■ Constipation ■ Dizziness ■ Dry mouth ■ Hand tremor ■ Increased appetite ■ Sexual dysfunction ■ Weight gain	■ Changes in blood pressure ■ Excitation or mania ■ Extreme constipation ■ Extreme eye or skin sensitivity to sunlight ■ Extreme sedation ■ Irregular heart rate ■ Problems with urination (difficult or painful urination; unable to urinate) ■ Seizure ■ Severe headache ■ Shortness of breath ■ Extreme sweating ■ Yellow skin or eyes	■ Antidiabetic agents ■ Bupropion ■ Buspirone ■ Carbamazepine ■ Cyclic antidepressants ■ Dextromethorphan ■ Drugs that depress the CNS (antihistamines, narcotics, muscle relaxants, and barbiturates) ■ Drugs used during surgery ■ Ephedrine ■ Levodopa ■ L-tryptophan ■ Meperidine (Demerol) ■ Other drugs with MAOI properties such as selegiline, isoniazid, linezolid, triptans ■ Phenylephrine ■ Phenylpropanolamine ■ Pseudoephedrine ■ SSRI antidepressants ■ Stimulants ■ Tyramine
Phenelzine	Nardil	30-90mg			
Selegiline	Emsam (patch)	6-12mg			
Tranylcypromine	Parnate	20-60mg			

Warnings/Precautions

■ Not indicated during pregnancy or while breastfeeding
■ Liver or kidney impairment may require dosage adjustment or discontinuation of treatment
■ Can trigger mania/hypomania
■ May increase the risk of suicidal thinking in young adults, adolescents, and children
■ Cardiac and blood pressure monitoring as indicated
■ Lowered seizure threshold
■ Pheochromocytoma
■ Hyperthyroidism
■ Orthostatic hypotension
■ Tyramine restrictions and dietary adherence

17

Bipolar Medications

For treating bipolar disorder, pharmacotherapy is unquestionably the mainstay of treatment. Although medication options over the last thirty years have grown more plentiful, they also have become more complex. The initial treatment of choice for mania was lithium. The anticonvulsants, carbamazepine and valproic acid (also known as divalproex), also became established as effective agents. For many years medication regimens included one or a combination of these three agents.

However, within the last several years, drug selection trends have changed. Routinely, medication regimens include multiple mood stabilizers, concurrent antidepressant therapy, and adjunctive agents, such as benzodiazepines and/or antipsychotics. These emerging patterns of drug use are necessary due to the severity of symptom presentation and the complicated course of illness for many patients. Even with these substantial treatment options, poor response or treatment resistance is not uncommon. In this chapter we address in detail lithium, divalproex, carbamazepine, and lamotrigine. General reference information is also provided for other agents you may encounter in your practice or which are often referenced in research articles. The atypical antipsychotic olanzapine is FDA-approved for use in bipolar disorder and is covered in chapter 19 of this book.

Throughout this book, the authors use the term *mood stabilizer* to describe medications used in the treatment of bipolar disorder. However, this term is not officially recognized by the U.S. Food and Drug Administration (FDA), and experts have not yet agreed upon other terminology. In the American Psychiatric Association's "Practice Guideline for the Treatment of Patients with Bipolar Disorder" (Revision) (APA 2002), the term "mood stabilizer" was eliminated. Until such time that replacement language is adopted by experts, this edition of the *Handbook* will contain both terms, "mood stabilizer" and "bipolar medications," since readers may be familiar with both.

Special mention is necessary regarding medication treatment for bipolar II. Several clinical questions have arisen. First, is there a difference in responsiveness to the various mood stabilizers between bipolar I and bipolar II? Second, what is the role of antidepressants in bipolar II, especially as monotherapy? Regarding the preferred mood stabilizer in bipolar II, studies are inconclusive, although lithium, carbamazepine, divalproex, and lamotrigine have all been found to be effective. As to the role of antidepressants, few definitive studies have been conducted, but preliminary results suggest that antidepressants may be safe and effective, and may not present a high risk for manic and hypomanic switching.

Although guidelines are not in agreement on antidepressant monotherapy (without a mood stabilizer), some practitioners advocate that many patients do not require a mood stabilizer. Due to the high morbidity and mortality associated with bipolar II, the decision to exclude a mood stabilizer must be made on a case-by-case basis. Further study is needed to confirm these initial findings, and until such time that clear guidelines exist, medication decisions should be given careful and individual consideration (MacQueen and Young 2001).

Review of Treatment Guidelines

A number of well-known treatment guidelines for bipolar disorder have been developed in the last decade. In 2000, Goldberg provided a comprehensive review of relevant guidelines current to that time. Many of these guidelines have been periodically reassessed as shown below:

- The Expert Consensus Guideline Series (1996, 2000, 2004)

- Clinical Practice Guidelines for Bipolar Disorder from the Department of Veterans Affairs (1999)

- The Texas Medication Algorithm Project (1998, 2004, 2006 [Bipolar I])

- The Canadian Network for Mood and Anxiety Treatment (1997, 2005, 2006)

- American Psychiatric Association's "Practice Guidelines for Treatment of Patients with Bipolar Disorder" (1994, 2002)

- International Consensus Group on Bipolar I Depression Treatment Guidelines (2004)

Notable in these revisions are recommendations for:

- Rational inclusion of anticonvulsants and second-generation antipsychotics

- Recognition and management of side effects, particularly metabolic syndrome with second-generation antipsychotics

- Systematic use of combination therapies

- Maintenance treatment

- Treatment of bipolar depression

- Relapse prevention and prophylaxis

- Commentary on the effectiveness of the guidelines in terms of adherence and outcomes

In treating bipolar disorder, as in other medical conditions, adhering to basic principles of medication use is particularly important for positive outcomes. Certainly, some newer anticonvulsants and second-generation antipsychotics have demonstrated efficacy. Others have yet to be rigorously evaluated. First-line agents should be used before drugs with little or no evidence of effectiveness.

Lithium

The use of lithium in psychiatry has varied historically. In the nineteenth century, lithium salts were employed in the treatment of anxiety, as well as for gout and seizures. The importance of lithium's antimanic actions was indirectly discovered, in 1949, with observations that it produced a calming effect in animals. Human testing in agitated or manic patients followed, with encouraging results. However, lithium's use did not gain acceptance in American medicine until 1970, due to safety concerns following reports of toxicity in cardiac patients who were using lithium chloride as a salt substitute. Lithium is now firmly established as a safe and effective treatment for acute mania and for the prevention of manic-depressive episodes, with response rates in typical bipolar disorder estimated at 60 to 80 percent. However, lithium's mechanism of action remains to be identified. Except for mild cognitive and motor slowing in healthy individuals, lithium does not share the sedating or euphoriant properties of other psychotropics.

Most treatment guidelines consider lithium and divalproex as first-line agents. Many physicians select divalproex over lithium because of concerns about side effects and toxicity. Other prescribers prefer lithium and, when therapeutic guidelines are followed, believe it is the most effective agent for many patients. Regardless of the indication, safe and effective use of lithium requires close monitoring of blood levels and management of side effects; this chapter covers those aspects of therapy in detail.

Lithium is the lightest of the solid elements, is widely found in nature, and, because of its chemical activity, will combine with other ions to form lithium salts (Gennaro 1980). Lithium salts share some, but not all, properties of sodium and potassium. The two therapeutically available forms are lithium carbonate and lithium citrate.

Lithium demonstrates a narrow *therapeutic window*—the therapeutic dose is very close to the toxic dose. (See also "Therapeutic Index" in appendix A.) Consequently, lithium is prescribed not only by dose and stage of symptoms but also by concentration in the blood (see figure 17-A). Side effects are often indicative of blood level but not always. During acute states, daily doses of 1200 to 2400 mg of lithium are required, with most patients needing less after stabilization (600 to 1800 mg per day). Also, as the acute episode resolves, many patients will become more intolerant of side effects, necessitating a dosage reduction. The onset of action of lithium occurs in five to fourteen days, although full stabilization may take up to several months.

Dosage Guidelines for Lithium		
Stage	Dosage Range (mg/day)	Serum Level (mEq/l)
Acute mania	1200–2400	0.8–1.5
Maintenance	600–1800	0.6–1.2

Figure 17-A

Side Effects and Their Management

Lithium produces a distinct continuum of side effects that range from relatively benign, transient symptoms to toxicity that can be fatal. The most significant side effects fall into the following categories:

Gastrointestinal

Nausea, vomiting, and diarrhea can occur to varying degrees at any time during treatment. These side effects may appear at the beginning of treatment or upon dosage increases. *However, GI symptoms may also be one of the critical indicators of lithium toxicity.* Obtaining a lithium blood level in response to the appearance of these symptoms is important. After ruling out an elevated lithium level as a cause of GI symptoms, changing from one dosage form to another, especially to a long-acting or liquid preparation, is often helpful. Lithium may also be administered after meals, or the total daily dosage may be divided into smaller doses to alleviate the nausea.

Nervous system and neuromuscular

Initial complaints, which usually diminish with time, include headache, lethargy, and muscle weakness. Nearly half of patients experience a fine hand tremor at some time during lithium treatment. For most people, this initial symptom remits; however, for 10 percent of patients, it is a continuing side effect (American Society of Health System Pharmacists 2000). Often the tremor becomes worse when the individual reaches for something. Sustained tremor, at therapeutic levels, can be managed with reassurance and by limiting stimulants, such as caffeine, which may exacerbate the tremor. Sometimes this tremor is treated with beta blockers, usually propranolol (Inderal).

Not all neurologic side effects are benign; sometimes they are indicators of toxicity. *Worsening of tremor, confusion, stupor, and slurred speech are warning signs that require a lithium blood level to be taken to rule out toxicity.* Severe lithium toxicity can result in seizures, CNS depression, irregular heartbeat, decreased kidney function, coma, or death. Although various emergency measures, including dialysis, can be employed in lithium intoxication, there is no antidote. An episode of severe lithium intoxication will resolve as the drug is eliminated from the body, usually over several days. A small number of patients are left with permanent neurological impairment following acute or chronic dosage excesses.

Endocrine

Thyroid hormones are frequently affected by lithium but rarely in a clinically significant way. Changes in certain laboratory tests of thyroid function are common but seldom require discontinuation of treatment. The two significant endocrine effects attributed to lithium therapy are clinical hypothyroidism (1 to 4 percent) and goiter (5 percent) (American Society of Health System Pharmacists 2000). Several potential risk factors have been identified, including age, gender (more prevalent in women), and familial history of hypothyroidism (Johnston and Eagles 1999; Kleiner et al. 1999). Several treatment options for hypothyroidism are utilized depending on the clinical situation. Periodic thyroid function monitoring is important, not only from a safety standpoint but to rule out (in the bipolar individual with depressed or mixed-state features) hypothyroidism as the cause of symptoms.

Renal

The pharmacokinetics of lithium are important in understanding its kidney-related side effects. Lithium, unlike most other medications, relies only on the kidney for elimination from the body, without any liver metabolism. Therefore, adequate kidney function is critical for safe lithium use. *Interference or alteration in normal kidney functioning can potentially lead to a buildup of lithium.* Lithium use usually should be avoided in the presence of renal disease. Also, since elderly people in general show age-related decreases in kidney function, lithium should be prescribed cautiously and with appropriately reduced dosages.

Additionally, lithium excretion is directly related, in an inverse way, to sodium excretion. Conditions leading to excess sodium elimination will cause a corresponding increase in the amount of lithium retained in the body. Excessive sodium loss occurs from diarrhea, vomiting, fever, dehydration, profuse sweating, diuretic medications, and severely salt-restricted diets.

The benign effects of lithium on the kidney will be experienced by the majority of patients as increased thirst (polydipsia) and increased urination (polyuria). To ensure adequate lithium excretion, patients must be advised to maintain fluid intake, even in the presence of polyuria.

Since the inception of its use, there has been debate about the long-term effects of lithium on the kidney. After initiation of treatment, 30 to 50 percent of patients experience a decrease in the ability of the kidney to concentrate urine. This effect persists in 25 percent of patients after one to two years of treatment (American Society of Health System Pharmacists 2000). Conclusions about whether lithium causes structural changes in the kidney are confounded by findings that such changes occur in bipolar patients independent of lithium treatment (Gitlin 1999). Progressive deterioration in kidney function, although potentially very serious, is a rare occurrence and is likely related to additional factors, such as lithium intoxication, high serum levels, interacting drugs, age, or concurrent medical conditions (Johnson 1998).

Hematological

A benign, reversible increase in white blood cell (WBC) count occurs frequently with lithium treatment. This is clinically nonsignificant and does not require discontinuation of treatment.

Cardiovascular

It is not unusual for lithium to induce some minor changes on electrocardiogram (EKG) studies. However, serious cardiac problems are rare at therapeutic levels.

Dermatological

The more common dermatological effects of lithium treatment are rash and acne-like lesions. Whether to stop lithium therapy is determined by the severity of either of these conditions.

Weight gain

Various mechanisms have been proposed, without conclusion, for this relatively common side effect, estimated at up to twenty pounds in at least 20 percent of patients (Vestergaard, Amdisen, and Schow 1980). Supervised caloric restriction may be helpful.

Teratogenicity

Lithium carries risk during pregnancy, especially the first trimester, due to congenital abnormalities, most notably of the heart. In rare situations, it may be necessary to continue lithium treatment in the pregnant patient, with dosage adjustments as necessitated by pregnancy-induced changes in kidney function.

Monitoring blood levels

Laboratory monitoring is necessary throughout lithium treatment to determine a safe and therapeutic dose and to limit side effects. The especially critical times to obtain a lithium level are during initiation, with dosage changes, with breakthrough symptoms, and any time toxicity is suspected (see figure 17-B). In the presence of severe side effects, the prescriber will often discontinue lithium, pending laboratory results. Even though side effects and serum levels are not absolutely correlated in all patients, there is a general association (see figure 17-C).

Mechanism of Action

Decades of research have yet to provide a clear understanding of the exact mechanism of action of lithium. Multiple sites of action within the CNS have been identified, none of which fully explain lithium's action on both mania and depression. Since neurotransmitter production, release, and reuptake rely on various ions (sodium, calcium, potassium, and magnesium), lithium's ionic properties may affect neurotransmitter-mediated depression and mania. Another potential mechanism of action of lithium is linked to its ability to stabilize cell membranes, via activity at sodium and potassium channels.

Lithium's benefit in mania may be linked to effects on dopamine and norepinephrine, possibly by preventing dopamine receptor supersensitivity in the manic individual. Additionally, lithium blocks some cocaine- and amphetamine-induced

---

Recommended Lithium Monitoring

Reason	Frequency
Initiation of treatment	Every 3 to 7 days for first several weeks
	Once monthly for 3 to 6 months
Routine	Every 1 to 3 months in stable patient
With dosage change	Within 3 to 5 days
Signs of toxicity	Immediate
Symptoms of mania or depression	Immediate
Addition or discontinuation of interacting meds	Within 3 to 5 days
In presence of medical conditions resulting in dehydration	Immediate
Suspected pregnancy	Immediate

Figure 17-B

Mild	Moderate	Severe
(Lithium level up to 1.5)	(Lithium level 1.5–2.5)	(Lithium level above 2.5)
Increased thirst	Recurring, persisting, or	Decreased urine output
Increased urination	worsening nausea,	Stupor
Weight gain	vomiting, or diarrhea	Seizure
Nausea, vomiting,	Coarse tremor	Cardiovascular collapse
diarrhea	Muscle twitching	Coma, death
Fine hand tremor	Confusion	
Muscle weakness	Slurred speech	
Drowsiness		
Lethargy		

Figure 17-C

symptoms of mania, which are thought to be mediated by stimulant-related increases in CNS dopamine concentration. The action of lithium on norepinephrine is variable, causing an initial prolonged increase in reuptake, although this effect is not evident with long-term administration (American Society of Hospital Pharmacists 2000).

Lithium's serotonergic activity is postulated to be responsible for its role in preventing depressive episodes of bipolar disorder. Some bipolar patients demonstrate low CNS concentrations of serotonin. Lithium may contribute to serotonin production by increasing the uptake of the tryptophan, a serotonin precursor (American Society of Health System Pharmacists 2000).

Since the early 1990s it has been suggested that lithium's actions inside neuronal cells explain its therapeutic effects, specifically reducing overactivity of second messenger systems (Weber, Saklad, and Kastenholz 1992). Evidence has continued to be gathered supporting that theory, and broadened in scope. Current concepts imply that chronic lithium administration alters the function of three signaling pathways, G protein, protein kinase A, and protein kinase C. In addition, it is now postulated that lithium possesses neuroprotective properties. Chronic lithium administration increases the amount of neuroprotective substances in the brain (Manji 2001; Chang 2000). Neuroprotective proteins are thought to protect against the destructive consequences of certain biochemical processes in the brain. For instance, it is postulated that there may be neuroanatomical changes associated with mood disorders, such as a reduction in CNS neuron quantity and cell volume. Another theory is that glutamate and NDMA receptor activation may result in cellular damage. There is evidence to suggest that the neuroprotective proteins mitigate some of this damage. Although this line of research is relatively new, it holds great promise for maximizing drug therapies, as well as for uncovering crucial information regarding the etiology of bipolar disorder.

Anticonvulsants

Three anticonvulsants, carbamazepine (Tegretol), divalproex (Depakote), and lamotrigine (Lamictal), have demonstrated efficacy for the treatment of bipolar disorder. Depakote, Lamictal, and a sustained-release form of carbamazepine (Equetro) are FDA-approved. Carbamazepine and divalproex have been widely used for many years, while lamotrigine is a newer agent. Various treatment guidelines generally agree that divalproex is one of the first-line agents for mania. It is believed by some to be the preferred agent for rapid cycling, although this is not a universal recommendation. For mixed episodes, divalproex is recommended as one of the first-line agents. Carbamazepine is generally considered a second-line agent for mania, and a first- or second-line agent for mixed episodes. Lamotrigine is approved for acute and maintenance therapy and is generally considered a first-line agent for the treatment of bipolar depression. Lamotrigine is a second-line agent for rapid cycling.

Like lithium, the exact mechanisms of action have yet to be identified for the anticonvulsants. It is noteworthy that several anticonvulsants, including divalproex, lamotrigine, and topirimate, have demonstrated some of the same neuroprotective effects as lithium (Li, Ketter, and Frye 2002). Carbamazepine is thought to work by prolonging the inactivation of sodium ion channels or by potentiating the action of GABA, the primary inhibitory neurotransmitter in the CNS. Divalproex appears to work via both of these mechanisms. Most anticonvulsants possess common mechanisms of action. Although not proven, one of the properties that may explain lamotrigine's effectiveness in bipolar disorder is the inhibition of the actions of glutamate, an excitatory neurotransmitter (Korn 2000; Ketter, Manji, and Post 2003).

Side Effects and Their Management: Carbamazepine and Divalproex

There are important therapeutic and side-effect differences between carbamazepine and divalproex. Side effects are experienced by about 30 percent of patients treated with carbamazepine (Hollister 1992). Central nervous system effects are common; they include sedation, dizziness, drowsiness, blurred vision, and incoordination. Gastrointestinal side effects include nausea, vomiting, diarrhea, and abdominal pain, all of which may be alleviated by taking the medication with food or milk. Many of the CNS and GI side effects are often dose-related and can be minimized by small dosage increases during titration or dosage reduction. Dermatological side effects can manifest with a red, itching rash or hives; they often necessitate discontinuation of treatment. Carbamazepine should be administered with caution to patients with a history of cardiac problems and liver disease.

Carbamazepine can induce decreases in white blood cell (WBC) count. These changes may be slight, especially during the first few weeks of treatment, and do not absolutely warrant stopping the medication. However, with a significant reduction in WBC or related components, most clinicians will consider discontinuing the medication and further evaluate these hematological changes.

Divalproex is tolerated slightly better than carbamazepine relative to nervous system side effects, notably in fewer complaints of fatigue and dizziness. Gastrointestinal side effects of nausea, vomiting, and indigestion are common, although these are usually transient. Use of sustained-release tablets (Depakote) may reduce these effects. Divalproex can occasionally interfere with the normal blood-clotting cycle. Potential liver damage is also possible with valproate, although this effect has primarily been demonstrated in children taking multiple anticonvulsant medications.

Blood level monitoring is required for carbamazepine and divalproex, utilizing therapeutic anticonvulsant ranges (see figure 17-D). While there are not established ranges for antimanic effects, performing routine monitoring will identify potentially toxic levels. Levels should be taken weekly for the first month and every one to three

Dosage Guidelines for Anticonvulsants*

Drug	Dosage Range[a] (mg/day)	Serum Level[b] (mcg/ml)
Carbamazepine	600–1600	4–10+
Divalproex	750–1500	50–100
Lamotrigine	50–400	c
Topiramate	50–300	c

a Serum levels are based on established anticonvulsant use. Mood-stabilizing response may fall above or below these values.

b Dosage requirements may be less for patients on multiple psychotropics.

c Serum monitoring may not be necessary.

* For doses for children and adolescents, see appendix B.

Figure 17-D

months thereafter. Excessively elevated serum levels (overdoses) of the anticonvulsants are potentially life-threatening. Associated with carbamazepine toxicity are neurologic and cardiac malfunctions, while divalproex overdose may produce somnolence and coma. To promptly achieve therapeutic serum levels of divalproex, a loading dose has been suggested (Keck et al. 1993). This strategy employs a rapid titration, based on body weight, over the first one to five days of treatment. Side-effect intolerance or potential for drug interactions may limit the application of this regimen.

Side Effects and Their Management: Lamotrigine

Lamotrigine is generally well tolerated, with the most common side effects being CNS, GI, and dermatologic. Common CNS side effects are dizziness, headache, ataxia, drowsiness, and tremor. These are frequently dose-related. Nausea and vomiting are the most common dose-related GI side effects.

Rare, serious, and potentially life-threatening dermatologic reactions, including Stevens-Johnson syndrome, are associated with lamotrigine. Prescribers are advised to inform patients of this risk and to seek immediate medical advice upon the appearance of rash. Rash occurs in about 10 percent of patients, is usually benign, and is most common during the initial titration phase, although it can emerge at any time during treatment. Concurrent divalproex therapy increases the likelihood of serious rash. At onset, there are no distinguishing features between benign and serious rashes. Following the recommended slow titration schedule reduces the risk of serious rash.

Although there are no recommendations currently for routine ophthalmologic screening, prescribers are advised of the potential for lamotrigine to bind with melanin-containing ocular tissue.

Other Anticonvulsants

Based on overlapping pharmacologic properties, in clinical practice other anticonvulsants are sometimes prescribed for refractory bipolar disorder, despite the lack of well-controlled premarketing studies to support their use. Over time, some of these agents prove to be effective and ultimately are incorporated into expert guidelines and/or receive FDA approval. For other anticonvulsants, their effectiveness fails to be demonstrated, either in practice or through postmarketing studies. A list of other anticonvulsants and comments as to their documented efficacy are provided below:

- Topiramate (Topamax): Well-controlled studies are lacking. However, some prescribing of topiramate for bipolar disorder occurs. Weight loss is a side effect of topiramate, and this may be beneficial in some cases.

- Oxcarbazepine (Trileptal): Structural variant of carbamazepine. Theoretical advantage over carbamazepine due to better tolerability and more favorable drug interaction profile.

- Tiagabine (Gabitril): No evidence to support use.

- Levetiracetam (Keppra): No evidence to support use.

- Gabapentin (Neurontin): Although heavily promoted by the manufacturer and widely used when first released, there is no evidence to support use in treating bipolar disorder.

- Pregabalin (Lyrica): Chemically similar to gabapentin. No evidence to support use.

Second-Generation Antipsychotics

Antipsychotics have long been established as adjunctive agents in the treatment of bipolar disorder. Historically, the first-generation antipsychotics were used to treat agitation and aggressive behavior. In the past few years, the second-generation antipsychotics have become established as primary agents in the treatment of acute mania and mixed mania (Perlis 2007). Aripiprazole, olanzapine, quetiapine, risperidone, and ziprasidone are all FDA approved for acute mania, and all but quetiapine are approved for mixed mania. At this time, only aripiprazole and olanzapine are approved for maintenance therapy. Quetiapine and olanzapine combined with fluoxetine are approved for bipolar depression (Facts and Comparisons 2008). FDA indications are subject to change so the manufacturer's product insert and the FDA website are alternative sources of information.

While the second-generation antipsychotics pose less risk for extrapyramidal side effects, consideration must be given to other potentially serious side effects, such as seizures, cardiac arrhythmias, hypertension, and metabolic syndrome (increased weight, type II diabetes mellitus, and hyperlipidemia). See chapter 19 for a full discussion of these medications.

Combinations of Medication

Patients with bipolar disorder frequently require multiple medications or changes in therapy. For example, antianxiety agents are helpful in reducing anxiety and agitation, especially in patients who refuse antimanic or antipsychotic agents. Likewise an added antipsychotic is more effective than a mood stabilizer alone in acute manic episodes that include significant psychomotor activity and delusions or hallucinations. Ongoing treatment with antipsychotics after the manic episode is resolved is often not necessary. However, it is not uncommon for a refractory patient to require a combination of mood stabilizers, an antidepressant, and an antipsychotic.

For patients with bipolar depression, the role of antidepressant therapy remains controversial. Certainly there is a risk of triggering a manic switch, but recent concerns have surfaced about whether antidepressants actually can induce rapid cycling. Likewise, length of treatment with antidepressants is debated, ranging from six weeks to six months. Practice patterns are likely to reflect this controversy. As to the choice of antidepressants in bipolar depression, the guidelines are mostly in agreement that bupropion, venlafaxine, or an SSRI is preferred.

The systematic Treatment Enhancement Program for Bipolar Disorder (STEP-BD) attempted to answer the questions of whether antidepressants improve outcomes in bipolar depression and whether they increase the risk of mania (Sachs et al. 2007). This large NIMH-sponsored project included over 4,000 community patients at twenty-two sites, and was conducted between 1995 and 2005. Over 4,000 patients constituted the population, of which 366 enrolled in the study. Patients were randomized to receive placebo, paroxetine, or buproprion. The mood stabilizer that patients were taking prior to enrollment was continued and was usually lithium or valporate. Recovery rates were 23.5 percent with antidepressant and 27.3 percent with placebo. Affective switch rates were 10.1 percent with antidepressant and 10.7 percent with placebo. The differences in these rates were not statistically significant.

A notable limitation is the 10 percent recruitment rate, which was a small percentage of the overall population. However, investigators also obtained similar results from a quasi-experimental analysis of 335 STEP-BD patients who did not participate in the study. A second limitation was that patients with a history of antidepressant-induced mania were not enrolled under the direction of their treating provider. Lastly, the antidepressants used in the study are associated with low switch rates, limiting conclusions about treatment-emergent mania with other antidepressants.

Although the STEP-BD study does not resolve the controversy regarding antidepressant treatment in bipolar depression, it is the largest and most recent study of this nature and provides a basis for further research.

Length of Treatment

Patients with bipolar disorder face long-term (lifetime) treatment with medications. Although use of antidepressants and antipsychotics may be limited to specific periods, a mood stabilizer is considered routine maintenance therapy in most patients. Medication-free periods are seldom beneficial and often result in symptom relapse. If evidence continues to mount that mood stabilizers have neuroprotective effects, maintenance treatment becomes even more important to achieve positive outcomes.

Patient Education

Comprehensive patient education is critical in ensuring compliance and in ultimately limiting the devastating effects of bipolar disorder. Perhaps the most difficult fact for the patient to accept is the need for long-term treatment. In addition, patients must become active participants in identifying target symptoms and critical side effects, especially with lithium.

The first year after diagnosis can be an extremely difficult time for the patient and is often marked by treatment noncompliance and relapse. Thus patient education should include a discussion of the serious implications of medication noncompliance. Some individuals may naively (or out of denial) view periodic manic episodes as relatively benign occurrences, when in fact these are times of increased mortality risk. Patients should be informed that recurring manic episodes may increase susceptibility to future episodes. Additionally, some patients may actually become less responsive to mood-stabilizing treatment with repeated episodes of mania. The therapist can be instrumental in helping patients recognize that continued medication noncompliance may actually contribute to a progressive worsening of their disorder.

Psychotherapeutic Issues

Professional opinions about lithium vary by discipline and by individual clinician. Some therapists find it easier to support the use of a "natural" substance, whereas others have been influenced by reports of side effects and toxicity. While the acutely manic patient is most often hospitalized, patients with hypomania or cyclothymia may be initiated on medications as outpatients, making the therapist an important part of the stabilization process. In this role, the therapist can assist the patient in assessing response and identifying side effects.

Patients will often resist mood stabilizers because of concerns not only about side effects but about therapeutic effects. What is clinically considered a symptom may be a desired state for the patient: a higher lever of energy, creativity, and confidence. It is important to explore with the patient the sense of loss bipolar patients typically feel when valued conditions are diminished. For the bipolar patient, the desire for the manic "high" can be quite strong, not unlike the craving a drug addict experiences during the initial stages of recovery. This analogy may be helpful to patients who are struggling to accept the disease. The therapist can provide support and reassurance by acknowledging that mania is indeed a powerfully reinforcing "intrinsic high" but eventually the longing to be manic will diminish.

Psychotherapy is not only possible but also can be very productive with the bipolar patient. Miklowitz (1996), in addressing combined psychotherapy and medication treatment for bipolar disorder, offers a comprehensive and detailed description of two approaches, family psychoeducation and individual therapy. The latter incorporates elements of interpersonal therapy for affective disorders with strategies to stabilize social rhythms. However, the therapist must be skilled at identifying symptoms of hypomania, mania, and depression, and the necessity for medication adjustment referrals. The therapist can be tested especially by the effects of medication noncompliance, when symptoms return, and judgment and insight diminish.

Drug therapy is increasingly being advocated for an expanded spectrum of cylic mood symptoms, such as premenstrual syndrome, personality disorders, and temperamental disorders (Jacobsen 1993; Deltito 1993; Akiskal 1996; Akiskal and Bowden 2000). Although these presentations are inherently difficult for the treating clinician, there are no evidence-based guidelines directing medication use. The therapist is likely to encounter patients being treated with mood stabilizers who do not meet the *DSM-IV-TR* criteria for bipolar I, bipolar II, or cylcothymia. As with all medication therapy, it is important to identify target symptoms and expected response indicators before these medications are prescribed.

Generic Name	Brand Name	Average Daily Dosage Range (serum levels)	Side Effects (usually diminish; may require attention if persist)	Side Effects Requiring Immediate Attention	Significant Drug Interactions* (not all-inclusive)
Carbamazepine	Tegretol Equetro	600-1600mg (4-10+ mcg/ml)	■ Constipation ■ Dry mouth ■ Mild diarrhea ■ Mild dizziness ■ Mild hand tremor ■ Mild nausea	■ Back-and-forth movement of the eyes ■ Black stools ■ Bleeding or bruising ■ Blood in the urine ■ Blurred or double vision ■ Confusion ■ Difficulty breathing ■ Extreme diarrhea ■ Extreme eye or skin sensitivity to sunlight ■ Irregular heartbeat ■ Problems with urination (difficult or painful urination; unable to urinate) ■ Significant drowsiness ■ Skin rash or hives ■ Swelling of the feet or hands ■ Yellow eyes or skin	■ Anticoagulants (blood thinners) ■ Anticonvulsants ■ Antipsychotics ■ Birth control pills ■ Buspirone ■ Calcium channel blockers ■ Cimetidine ■ Drugs that depress the CNS (antihistamines, narcotics, muscle relaxants, and barbiturates) ■ Grapefruit juice ■ HIV protease inhibitors ■ Isoniazid ■ Lithium ■ Macrolide antibiotics ■ MAOI antidepressants ■ Oral antifungal agents ■ SSRI antidepressants ■ Tricyclic antidepressants

Warnings/Precautions

■ Not indicated during pregnancy or while breastfeeding
■ Liver or kidney impairment may require dosage adjustment or discontinuation of treatment
■ Suicidality
■ Anemia
■ Diabetes mellitus
■ Hyponatremia
■ Increased intraocular pressure
■ Cardiac toxicity

*There is variability in the potential for a specific mood stabilizer to interact with the drugs listed.

Generic Name	Brand Name	Average Daily Dosage Range (serum levels)	Side Effects (usually diminish; may require attention if persist)	Side Effects Requiring Immediate Attention	Significant Drug Interactions* (not all-inclusive)
Divalproex	Depakote	750-1500 mg (50-100 mcg/ml)	■ Constipation ■ Dry mouth ■ Hair loss ■ Mild diarrhea ■ Mild dizziness ■ Mild hand tremor ■ Mild nausea ■ Weight gain	■ Bleeding or bruising ■ Confusion ■ Significant drowsiness ■ Yellow eyes or skin ■ Severe abdominal pain	■ Anticoagulants (blood thinners) ■ Anticonvulsants ■ Aspirin or nonsteriodal anti-inflammatory drugs ■ Drugs that depress the CNS (antihistamines, narcotics, muscle relaxants, and barbiturates)
Warnings/Precautions ■ Not indicated during pregnancy or while breastfeeding ■ Liver or kidney impairment may require dosage adjustment or discontinuation of treatment ■ Suicidality ■ Anemia ■ Pancreatitis ■ Polycystic ovarian syndrome					
Lamotrigine	Lamictal	50-500 mg	■ Mild dizziness ■ Blurred vision ■ Fatigue ■ Insomnia ■ Mild nausea ■ Vomiting ■ Dry mouth ■ Headache	■ Bleeding or bruising ■ Skin rash or hives ■ Fever ■ Shortness of breath or difficulty breathing ■ Mood changes ■ Dark-colored urine	■ Anticonvulsants ■ Birth control pills containing estrogen ■ Drugs that depress the CNS (antihistamines, narcotics, muscle relaxants, and barbiturates)
Warnings/Precautions ■ Not indicated during pregnancy or while breastfeeding ■ Liver or kidney impairment may require dosage adjustment or discontinuation of treatment ■ Suicidality ■ Stevens Johnson Syndrome					

*There is variability in the potential for a specific mood stabilizer to interact with the drugs listed.

Generic Name	Brand Name	Average Daily Dosage Range *(serum levels)*	Side Effects *(usually diminish; may require attention if persist)*	Side Effects Requiring Immediate Attention	Significant Drug Interactions* *(not all-inclusive)*
Lithium	Eskalith Lithonate	600-2400 mg *(0.6-1.5 mEq/L)*	■ Acne ■ Hair loss ■ Increased frequency of urination ■ Mild diarrhea ■ Mild hand tremor ■ Mild nausea ■ Sensitivity to cold ■ Thirst ■ Weight gain	■ Clumsiness ■ Confusion ■ Difficulty breathing ■ Irregular heartbeat ■ Loss of appetite ■ Muscle weakness ■ Seizure ■ Severe diarrhea ■ Severe nausea ■ Significant drowsiness ■ Blurred vision ■ Slurred speech ■ Swelling of the hands or feet ■ Trembling	■ ACE inhibitors ■ Antipsychotics ■ Calcium channel blockers ■ Carbamazepine ■ Diuretics ■ Drugs that depress the CNS (antihistamines, narcotics, muscle relaxants, and barbiturates) ■ Metronidazole ■ Nonsteroidal anti-inflammatory drugs ■ SSRI antidepressants ■ Theophylline

Warnings/Precautions
■ Not indicated during pregnancy or while breastfeeding
■ Kidney impairment may require dosage adjustment or discontinuation of treatment
■ Cardiac monitoring as indicated
■ CBC as indicated
■ Urinalysis as indicated
■ Thyroid function monitoring
■ Renal function monitoring

*There is variability in the potential for a specific mood stabilizer to interact with the drugs listed.

18

Antianxiety Medications

The first benzodiazepine synthesized was chlordiazepoxide (Librium), in 1957. Since then, many others have been developed and are available in the United States. These medications are used both for anxiety (sedatives) and insomnia (hypnotics). Additional uses are as anesthetics and as aids in handling withdrawal from other drugs. Some are used primarily as hypnotics (flurazepam, temazepam, and triazolam), but they differ little, other than by use, from the other benzodiazepines. When benzodiazepines were first developed, they represented a significant improvement over the previously available antianxiety agents: the barbiturates, meprobamate (Equanil, Miltown), tybamate (Tybatran), glutethimide (Doriden), methyprylon (Noludar), and ethchlorvynol (Placidyl). The benzodiazepines had better antianxiety specificity and were much less lethal in overdose.

These medications have been very widely used (and abused) because anxiety and insomnia are very common and because these drugs are very effective and well tolerated. Within twenty to thirty minutes after an oral dose, the effects can be felt. Benzodiazepines can cause sedation, slurred speech, incoordination, prolonged response time in higher doses (or when the person is very sensitive to the drug), and sometimes a lessening of inhibitions, as with alcohol.

The main differences between the different drugs are their pharmacodynamics: especially half-life and metabolism (see figure 18-A). Those with a longer half-life tend to build up in the system—even if taken only once a day. Most are metabolized by the liver and therefore can build up in the system when the liver is impaired, as with alcoholic liver disease. The three least dependent on the liver are lorazepam, temazepam, and oxazepam. The ones with a very short half-life (triazolam, midazolam, and, to a lesser degree, lorazepam) can cause anterograde amnesia: loss of memory for a short period after the drug has worn off.

Half-Lives of Benzodiazepines

- More than 24 hours:
  Diazepam
  Chlordiazepoxide
  Flurazepam
  Prazepam
  Clorazepate

- 18–24 hours:
  Clonazepam

- 8–16 hours:
  Temazepam
  Lorazepam
  Alprazolam
  Oxazepam
  Zolpidem

- Less than 6 hours:
  Triazolam
  Midazolam
  Zaleplon*
  Eszopiclone*

* These two prescription sleeping pills are technically not benzodiazepines, but they are often mentioned alongside benzodiazepines due to their use as prescription sleeping medications.

Figure 18-A

Types of Antianxiety Drugs

Benzodiazepines

The benzodiazepines work by interacting with benzodiazepine receptors, of which there are three types. Most current benzodiazepines show little selectivity for these receptor types; however, those developed in the future may have greater selectivity and possibly less sedation or dependence potential. Benzodiazepine receptors are co-located with GABA receptors, which usually function as presynaptic inhibiting receptors. The benzodiazepine receptors have a high density in the limbic system. Binding of a benzodiazepine at the BZ receptor enhances the effect of GABA and increases the influx of chloride ions (see figure 18-B; also see chapter 9 for a more detailed discussion of the biological basis of anxiety disorders). Figure 18-C gives the dosage range for benzodiazepines.

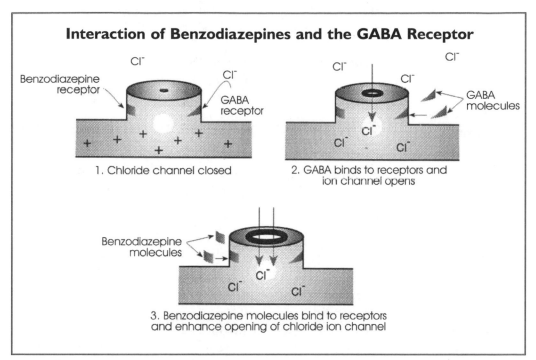

Interaction of Benzodiazepines and the GABA Receptor

1. Chloride channel closed

2. GABA binds to receptors and ion channel opens

3. Benzodiazepine molecules bind to receptors and enhance opening of chloride ion channel

Figure 18-B

Atypical Benzodiazepines

There are several new benzodiazepine derivatives being used as hypnotics (see figure 18-C). Estazolam (ProSom) is a triazolobenzodiazepine with a rapid onset of action, intermediate half-life, and no significant active metabolites; thus it does not have a tendency to lead to drug accumulation and daytime sedation. Quazepam (Doral) has the same active metabolite as flurazepam and has similar properties. Zolpidem (Ambien) and eszopiclone (Lunesta) are short-acting nonbenzodiazepines. Zaleplon (Sonata), with a half-life of one hour, is the shortest-acting nonbenzodiazepine hypnotic. Some studies suggest these medications may be associated with less cognitive impairment and reduced risk of dependency. This is likely due to their greater specificity in interacting preferentially with only one of the three benzodiazepine receptors. Most benzodiazepines tend to suppress REM sleep and Stage III and IV (delta) sleep (Nishino, Mignot, and Dement 1998), thereby altering "sleep architecture" and producing a less restful sleep. This can lead to daytime fatigue and impaired concentration. However, zolpidem, eszopidone, and zaleplon have been shown to have little, if any, effect on sleep architecture and are therefore preferable as hypnotics.

Buspirone

Buspirone is a unique antianxiety agent. It acts at the 5-HT 1A receptor; however, its exact mechanism of action is not fully understood. Buspirone tends to have a delayed onset of action—similar to the antidepressants. A typical starting dose is 5 mg two or three times per day; typically patients require 20 to 40 mg per day in divided doses (see figure 18-C). Reduced anxiety is seen within one or two weeks.

Dosages of Antianxiety Agents*

Generic Name	Brand Name	Single-Dose Dosage Range (mg)	Usual Dosage Range (mg/day)
Benzodiazepines			
Diazepam	Valium	2–10	4–40
Chlordiazepoxide	Librium	10–50	15–100
Flurazepam	Dalmane	15–60	15–60
Prazepam	Centrax	5–30	20–40
Clorazepate	Tranxene	3.75–15	7.5–60
Clonazepam	Klonopin	0.5–2	1–8
Temazepam	Restoril	15–30	15–60
Lorazepam	Ativan	0.5–2	1.5–6
Alprazolam	Xanax and	0.25–2	0.5–6
	Xanax XR	0.5–3	0.5–6
Oxazepam	Serax	10–30	30–90
Triazolam	Halcion	0.125–0.5	.125–0.5
Midazolam	Versed (injectable only)		
Atypical and Nonbenzodiazepines			
Estazolam	ProSom	1.0–2.0	1.0–2.0
Zolpidem	Ambien and	5–10	5–10
	Ambien CR	6.25–12.5	6.25–12.5
Zaleplon	Sonata	5–10	5–10
Eszopiclone	Lunesta	1–3	1–3
Other Antianxiety Agents			
Buspirone	BuSpar	5–20	10–40
Hydroxyzine	Atarax, Vistaril	10–50	30–200
Diphenhydramine	Benadryl	25–100	75–200
Propranolol	Inderal	10–80	20–160
Atenolol	Tenormin	25–100	25–100
Clonidine	Catapres, Kapvay	0.1–.3	0.2–0.9
Doxepin	Silenor	3–6	3–25

* For doses for children and adolescents, see appendix B.

Figure 18-C

The advantages of buspirone over benzodiazepines are that it is not associated with tolerance or dependence, it does not interact with other CNS depressants (such as alcohol), and it is not associated with impaired psychomotor function. The drug's disadvantages are its delayed onset of action and that it is not always effective, especially in people who have used benzodiazepines. The most common side effects of buspirone are nausea, dizziness, and, paradoxically, anxiety.

Antihistamines

Certain antihistamines are frequently used in the treatment of anxiety: hydroxyzine (Vistaril, Atarax) and diphenhydramine (Benadryl) (see figure 18-C). They act by blocking histamine receptors in the CNS, causing sedation and thereby reducing anxiety. They can also cause drowsiness and impaired performance. They work within twenty to thirty minutes and last four to six hours. They are not habit-forming, but have the disadvantages that tolerance can develop to their anxiolytic (antianxiety) effects and they tend to have a narrow therapeutic window between reducing anxiety and producing sedation.

Beta Blockers

Beta blockers are medications that act by blocking the effects of norepinephrine at the receptor. They are very effective at reducing the peripheral manifestations of anxiety (increased heart rate, sweating, tremor), but are not very effective at blocking the internal experience of anxiety. They are used very effectively for the treatment of performance anxiety, such as that caused by public speaking. The most commonly used beta blocker is propranolol (Inderal), but atenolol (Tenormin) and several others are also used (see figure 18-C). Beta blockers can cause dizziness and lowered blood pressure (in fact, their main use is as antihypertensives), and can cause depression if used over a long period of time. They have been used with some benefit as adjunctive agents in the treatment of panic disorder. Beta blockers are not habit-forming, but should be discontinued slowly to avoid rebound elevation of blood pressure.

Clonidine

Clonidine (Catapres and Kapvay) is an alpha-2 adrenergic agonist, which thereby functions as a presynaptic inhibitor of norepinephrine release. It is usually used to treat hypertension (like the beta blockers) but has been used to treat anxiety disorders with some success. It is also used to treat opiate withdrawal. A typical starting dose is 0.1 mg two to three times daily (see figure 18-C). It is also available as a transdermal patch.

Tiagabine

Tiagabine (Gabitril) is an anticonvulsant that has shown some promise in the treatment of anxiety disorders. It is a selective GABA reuptake inhibitor. Currently, there are few controlled studies, but there have been several clinical trials for treatment of PTSD and panic disorder (Rosenthal 2003; Taylor 2003). The usual dosage range reported was 4 to 12 mg per day. Further studies are necessary to define its clinical usefulness.

Length of Treatment

Antianxiety medications, especially benzodiazepines, can provide relief of anxiety regardless of the cause: situational stress, hyperthyroidism, or manic excitement (see figure 18-D). Of course, it is crucial to recognize and treat the underlying disorder. The use of benzodiazepines should be avoided until other measures have been tried (such as psychotherapy and relaxation training) or if anxiety is severe.

Benzodiazepines are very safe and effective in the short-term treatment of anxiety. However, prolonged use (over six months) may lead to tolerance and dependence. There have been several waves of public alarm about the abuse potential of benzodiazepines. Over ten years ago, there was much concern about Valium abuse, as portrayed in the book *I'm Dancing as Fast as I Can* (Gordon 1990). More recently, there has been much concern about abuse of Xanax, and memory impairment due to Halcion.

Because of the potential for dependence and abuse, it is best to try to use benzodiazepines only for short-term treatment. (One bad experience with someone who abuses these drugs is enough to make you vow to never prescribe them long-term again.) The problem lies in identifying beforehand that small percentage of people at high risk for abuse. A prior history of substance abuse is, of course, a good predictor but is not always present. On the other hand, many people take moderate doses of benzodiazepines for years without escalation in dose or any deleterious side effects. And some patients with panic disorder or other anxiety disorders who do not tolerate or respond to other forms of treatment (such as antidepressants or buspirone) do well on long-term maintenance with benzodiazepines without abuse developing. However, long-term benzodiazepine treatment is presently, and probably will remain, controversial.

Benzodiazepine Withdrawal

Minor tranquilizers and sedative-hypnotics are widely used in general medical practice and psychiatry. Although the benzodiazepines as a class are much safer than earlier medications (there is less risk of dependency and abuse, and withdrawal symptoms are generally much less dangerous than with barbiturates), problems do exist

---

Indications for Antianxiety Agents

- Adjustment reaction

- Phobic disorders

- Panic disorders

- Generalized anxiety disorder

- Obsessive-compulsive disorder

- Post-traumatic stress disorder

- Psychophysiological disorders related to anxiety (somatization disorder)

- Other disorders with prominent anxiety or agitation

Figure 18-D

when patients begin to reduce doses, especially if they discontinue rapidly or "cold turkey." Benzodiazepine withdrawal syndromes are encountered frequently. They cause considerable patient distress, can be dangerous at times, and are almost always avoidable if the clinician follows the discontinuation guidelines carefully.

When patients are treated daily for more than a few weeks, especially in moderate to high doses, the nervous system adapts to the presence of the drugs (tolerance develops) such that any rapid drop in blood levels of the medication can precipitate a withdrawal syndrome. Symptoms of withdrawal include the following (Smith and Wesson 1983):

Mild to Moderate	Severe
Anxiety	Seizures
Restlessness	High fever
Insomnia	Psychosis
Nightmares	Death

Typically, antianxiety medications with short half-lives (see figure 18-A) are more likely to produce withdrawal symptoms (since the medications are more rapidly eliminated from the system). However, clearly, withdrawal can occur with all minor tranquilizers and sedative-hypnotics (with the exception of buspirone and possibly zolpidem, which are chemical compounds unrelated to the benzodiazepines).

Often anxiety symptoms occur after medications are discontinued. It is sometimes difficult to distinguish between anxiety symptoms attributed to withdrawal, per se, and a reemergence of the primary anxiety associated with the original anxiety disorder. One defining feature is that symptoms that continue longer than two weeks tend to indicate the persistence of the underlying disorder. In such cases, discontinuation is premature (since the underlying disorder has not yet resolved) and continued treatment is warranted. However, withdrawal symptoms may mimic the anxiety symptoms, especially in panic disorder.

When symptoms are determined to be withdrawal, the medication should be restarted or returned to the dosage level previously used for chronic treatment. Then a *very gradual* withdrawal regime can be initiated, a 5 to 10 percent reduction of the daily dosage per week. With the shorter half-life tranquilizers, often the pace of medication discontinuance must be even more gradual; that is, a longer time must be allowed between progressive decreases in dose.

For reasons that are not well understood, many patients find that it is especially difficult to discontinue the very last dose, even if discontinuation has proceeded well up to that point. For example, many patients have problems discontinuing the final dose of alprazolam (e.g., 0.25 mg twice a day). It is advisable to not rush this final stage of drug phaseout. It may be wise to take an additional month or two to gradually discontinue the medication, or in some cases you may want to consider ongoing treatment with what amounts to microdoses of these medications. If there are no noticeable side effects, there are really no contraindications for prolonged treatment with very low doses of minor tranquilizers.

Finally, severe cases of drug dependence (high doses) are most safely detoxed in the hospital. Anticonvulsants, such as carbamazepine, are effective in controlling withdrawal symptoms, but a long-acting benzodiazepine, such as diazepam, may also be used.

Patient Education

Patients who have been prescribed antianxiety medications should be cautioned about the risk of dependence, the dangers of combining these drugs with alcohol (the story of Karen Ann Quinlan can be helpful in this regard), and the possible impairment of coordination (including driving a car). You may find it helpful to have an agreement with your client that he or she will use the medications only for a specific length of time, such as one month. Some patients are too quick to ask for antianxiety medications, and some are too reluctant. Both of these represent problems that need to be dealt with. For example, some patients have severe, disabling anxiety or insomnia and need to be encouraged to take antianxiety medications for a short period of time. They need to be reassured that they will not become addicted after a few days of treatment.

Similarly, people taking buspirone often need a lot of encouragement to keep taking the medication long enough to get benefit. This is especially the case for those looking for a "quick fix." Studies show that the benefits of buspirone are still increasing after three to six months of use.

Patients who have been on the medications for some time need to be advised against abrupt discontinuation, which can lead to a severe withdrawal syndrome and possible convulsions. A reduction in dose is likely to lead to a reemergence of the anxiety symptoms for which the person is being treated, such as panic attacks. If this is due only to drug withdrawal, the symptoms usually subside within two weeks. For this reason, as stated above, it is best to taper off benzodiazepine dosage very slowly after prolonged use.

Generic Name	Brand Name	Average Dosage Range	Side Effects (usually diminish; may require attention if persist)	Side Effects Requiring Immediate Attention	Significant Drug Interactions* (not all-inclusive)
Antianxiety Agents		**Single Dose**	■ Blurred vision ■ Dizziness ■ Nausea	■ Amnestic effects ■ Confusion ■ Excessive drowsiness ■ Excitation ■ Severe weakness ■ Shortness of breath ■ Skin rash or hives ■ Slurred speech ■ Swelling of the hands or feet	■ Beta blockers ■ Birth control pills ■ Calcium channel blockers ■ Carbamazepine ■ Digoxin ■ Disulfiram ■ Drugs that depress the CNS (antihistamines, narcotics, muscle relaxants, and barbiturates ■ Grapefruit juice ■ HIV protease inhibitors ■ Isoniazid ■ Levodopa ■ Macrolide antibiotics ■ Oral antifungal agents ■ Propoxyphene ■ SSRI antidepressants ■ Valproic acid
Alprazolam	Xanax	0.25-2mg			
Chlordiazepoxide	Librium	10-50mg			
Clonazepam	Klonopin	0.5-2mg			
Clorazepate	Tranxene	3.75-15mg			
Diazepam	Valium	2-10mg			
Lorazepam	Ativan	0.5-2mg			
Oxazepam	Serax	10-30mg			
Sedative Hypnotics		**Daily Dose**			
Estazolam	ProSom	1-2mg			
Flurazepam	Dalmane	15-60mg			
Quazepam	Doral	7.5-15mg			
Temazepam	Restoril	15-30mg			
Triazolam	Halcion	0.25-0.5mg			

Warnings/Precautions

■ Not indicated during pregnancy or while breastfeeding
■ Liver or kidney impairment may require dosage adjustment or discontinuation of treatment
■ Increased intraocular pressure
■ Tolerance/dependence
■ Withdrawal seizures after rapid dosage reduction or abrupt discontinuation of treatment

*There is variability in the potential for a specific benzodiazepine to interact with the drugs listed.

19

Antipsychotic Medications

Antipsychotic medications have truly revolutionized the treatment of psychotic disorders. Their effectiveness is so vastly superior to previous treatments that they have ushered in a new era in the treatment of severe mental illnesses. Chlorpromazine (Thorazine) was first used in 1952 as a postoperative sedative. It was subsequently used as a sedative for psychiatric patients, and it was soon discovered that it had antipsychotic properties. Soon other "phenothiazines" were developed.

When these drugs were first used in clinical settings, the mechanism of action was unknown, although the medications were clearly quite successful in reducing psychotic symptoms. Later research determined that antipsychotic medications acted by producing a chemical blockade of dopamine D2 postsynaptic receptors and that their clinical potency correlated with their degree of dopamine blockade. This led to the dopamine hypothesis of schizophrenia (see chapter 11).

Other, chemically distinct dopamine blockers were then developed, such as thiothixene, haloperidol, loxapine, molindone, and pimozide. All of these antipsychotics are potent dopamine blockers and collectively were called neuroleptics (now called first-generation antipsychotics) because they inadvertently cause certain neurological side effects (discussed next). More recently, second-generation antipsychotics have been developed (clozapine, olanzapine, and others), which are effective antipsychotics yet are weak dopamine blockers and cause minimal neurological side effects. This group, which has revolutionized the treatment of psychosis, is discussed separately later in this chapter.

First-Generation Antipsychotics

The phenothiazines and similar antipsychotics can be divided into high-potency and low-potency groups (see figure 19-A). In addition, they can be ranked according to their tendency to produce extrapyramidal symptoms (EPS) versus sedation and anticholinergic side effects (see figure 19-B).

Side Effects and Their Management

All first-generation antipsychotics (FGA), to a greater or lesser degree, produce the following side effects, which can be classified into five groups.

Extrapyramidal

The first-generation antipsychotics produce extrapyramidal side effects due to the blocking of dopamine receptors. In addition to producing a reduction in positive psychotic symptoms by blocking dopamine in the mesolimbic region, they unfortunately produce extrapyramidal symptoms by dopamine blockade in the basal ganglia. There are three types of acute extrapyramidal symptoms: Parkinsonian side effects are those that resemble Parkinson's disease, with slowed movements, decreased facial expression, resting tremor, and a shuffling gait. Dystonic symptoms involve sustained muscle spasms, usually of the neck or shoulder (such as torticollis) and can be quite frightening and painful. Akathisia refers to an intense feeling of restlessness. At times this side effect can be confused with psychotic agitation and thus mistakenly result in the physician increasing the dose of medication, which results in increased akathisia. Severe akathisia can be very uncomfortable and is associated with increased noncompliance and increased risk of suicide.

Anticholinergic

Antipsychotic medications block acetylcholine receptors and thereby affect the parasympathetic nervous system. This leads to dry membranes (especially mouth and eyes), blurred vision (especially near vision), intestinal slowing (constipation), difficulty urinating, sedation, and sexual dysfunction. These symptoms may be very mild or, depending on the type of medication, quite severe and disabling.

Antiadrenergic

Antipsychotic medications produce an alpha-adrenergic blockade, which leads to orthostatic hypotension. This means that when the person stands up, blood pressure drops precipitously, leading to a transient light-headedness and potentially a fall and injury.

Tardive dyskinesia

All of the above side effects appear within the first few hours or days of treatment or with increases in dose. In contrast, the tardive dyskinesias (disorders involving involuntary movements) appear late in the course of treatment or when the medication is reduced or discontinued. These movements usually improve slowly over time, but they may persist for years even after the medication is discontinued.

Dosages of Antipsychotic Medications*

Generic Name	Brand Name	Dosage Range (mg/day)	Equivalence[a] (mg)
Low-Potency			
Chlorpromazine	Thorazine	50–1500	100
Thioridazine	Mellaril	150–800	100
High-Potency			
Fluphenazine	Prolixin[b]	3–45	2
Haloperidol	Haldol[b]	2–40	2
Loxapine	Loxitane	50–250	10
Perphenazine	Trilafon	8–60	10
Pimozide	Orap	1–10	1
Thiothixene	Navane	10–60	5
Trifluoperazine	Stelazine	10–40	5
Second-Generation			
Aripiprazole	Abilify	10–30	10
Asenapine	Saphris	5–20	10
Clozapine[c]	Clozaril	300–900	50
Iloperidone	Fanapt	12–24	1-2
Lurasidone	Latuda	40–80	10
Olanzapine[c]	Zyprexa[b]	1–2	5–20
Paliperidone	Invega[b]	3–12	1–2
Quetiapine	Seroquel	300–750	0
Risperidone[c]	Risperdal[b]	4–16	1–2
Ziprasidone	Geodon	40–160	10
Antiparkinsonian/ Anticholinergic Drugs			
Amantadine	Symmetrel	100–300	
Benztropine mesylate	Cogentin	1–8	
Biperiden	Akineton	2–8	
Trihexyphenidyl	Artane	5–15	

* For doses for children and adolescents, see appendix B.

a Dose required to achieve efficacy of 100 mg chlorpromazine

b Available in time-release IM formulation

c Second-generation antipsychotic

Figure 19-A

Side Effects of Antipsychotic Medications

Medication	Sedation	Extrapyramidal[a]	Anticholergenic[b]
Aripiprazole	+	+/0	0
Asenapine	+	+	+
Chlorpromazine	++++	++	++++
Clozapine	++++	0	+++++
Fluphenazine	+	+++++	++
Haloperidol	+	+++++	+
iloperidone	++	+/0	++
Loxapine	+	+++	++
Lurasidone	+	+/–	0
Olanzapine	+	+/0	+
Paliperidone	+	+	+
Perphenazine	++	+++	++
Pimozide	+	+++++	+
Quetiapine	+	+	0
Risperidone	+	+	+
Thioridazine	++++	+	+++++
Thiothixene	+	++++	++
Trifluoperazine	+	++++	++
Ziprasidone	+	+/0	++

a Acute: Parkinson's dystonias, akathisia. Does not reflect risk for tardive dyskinesia.

b All first-generation antipsychotics may cause tardive dyskinesia.

Figure 19-B

Atypical side effects

As with all medications, certain people may have allergic reactions to antipsychotic medications. Weight gain is a common side effect. Agranulocytosis, a very serious blood disorder, was reported in the past, but it now appears to have been caused by a contaminant in some drug preparations and has not been reported recently. Hepatitis, similarly, has not been reported recently. Since the antipsychotics lower the seizure threshold, they may lead to grand mal seizures. They also interfere with temperature regulation and may lead to hyperthermia, especially when the person exercises during warm weather. Antipsychotics raise prolactin levels, and this may cause lactation. Neuroleptic malignant syndrome (NMS) is a rare but potentially fatal reaction to antipsychotic medication. It is characterized by fever, confusion, and rigidity. If not recognized and treated promptly, it can lead to irreversible coma and death.

Symptoms that require immediate medication reevaluation are these:

Side Effects Calling for Medication Reassessment

- Confusion
- Falls
- Inability to urinate
- Prolonged or severe constipation
- Rash
- High fever (may be due to agranulocytosis or NMS)
- Involuntary movements
- Jaundice (yellowish discoloration of skin, including eyes)
- Severe sedation
- Severe restlessness
- Muscle spasm (such as torticollis)

Management

Many of the side effects of antipsychotic medications can be managed so that they are less troublesome to patients. This ensures that patients are more willing to comply in taking them. Some side effects, such as sedation, can be managed by reducing the dose or by switching to a less sedating antipsychotic. (One should always use the lowest effective dose—although determining that dose is not always easy.) Extrapyramidal side effects can be reduced by switching to a less potent (and more sedating) antipsychotic. Additionally, extrapyramidal side effects typically are managed by the addition of an antiparkinsonian drug (such as benztropine, trihexyphenidyl, or biperiden; see figure 19-A). However, these medications also have side effects (dry mouth, blurred vision, and constipation), but are usually fairly well tolerated. Akathisia may be treated with antiparkinsonian drugs, beta blockers (such as propranolol), benzodiazipines, or a combination of these. Usually by adjusting the dose, changing medications, and/or adding adjunctive medications (such as an antiparkinsonian), the side effects of the antipsychotic medications can be reduced to a tolerable level.

Second-Generation Antipsychotics

In contrast to the first-generation antipsychotics, the second-generation antipsychotics (SGA) are strong serotonin (5-HT2A and 5-HT2C) blockers and produce varying degrees of dopamine (D2) blockade. Clozapine is the prototypical agent. It is effective for both positive and negative symptoms, and studies have shown that as many as 40 percent of those who have failed to respond to haloperidol and chlorpromazine respond to clozapine.

Clozapine has a very low incidence of extrapyramidal side effects and very few cases of tardive dyskinesia. It is very sedating and has some anticholinergic and antiadrenergic side effects (see figure 19-B). Sedation is the most troublesome side effect. Clozapine lowers the seizure threshold and can cause hepatitis. The most serious side effect, however, is a severe blood disorder, agranulocytosis, which has caused several deaths in the United States. These deaths have occurred despite the mandatory weekly monitoring of white blood cell count. (Note: After six months with normal blood counts, monitoring can then take place on a biweekly basis.) Clozapine can cost as much as $10,000 per year because of the need for weekly blood tests, although this cost is offset by reduced hospitalizations. Also, there have been a few sudden deaths associated with clozapine, presumably cardiac in nature.

Since the release of clozapine, researchers have sought to develop a second-generation antipsychotic without the side effects of clozapine (especially agranulocytosis). As of this writing, six other atypical agents have been released: risperidone, paliperidone, olanzapine, quetiapine, aripiprazole, and ziprasidone, and several others may soon be released. These agents vary somewhat in their pharmacological profile and, as a group, may revolutionize the treatment of schizophrenia, and possibly affective psychoses.

The benefits of the second-generation antipsychotics include better tolerability by patients, significantly reduced risk of tardive dyskinesia, reduction of negative symptoms, improved cognition, and reduced neuroanatomical changes (enlargement of lateral ventricles). Their use has led to a renewed emphasis on rehabilitation.

Aripiprazole (Abilify), like Geodon, is less sedating and less prone to cause weight gain. It can cause nausea and anxiety, especially initially.

Olanzapine (Zyprexa) has a very low tendency to cause extrapyramidal side effects. However, it is sedating and tends to cause weight gain and problems in carbohydrate metabolism.

Paliperidone (Invega) is a metabolite of risperidone, which is being marketed separately. It has the same side effects as risperidone but may be better tolerated because of the extended-release formulation.

Quetiapine (Seroquel) has a low incidence of extrapyramidal side effects. It is sedating and can cause dry mouth.

Ziprasidone (Geodon) is less sedating and causes less weight gain but can cause extrapyramidal side effects. It may have more effect on cardiac conduction (QT prolongation) than the other second-generation antipsychotics, and its use should be avoided in patients with significant cardiovascular disease.

Risperidone (Risperdal) was the first second-generation antipsychotic after Clozapine. It is a very potent dopamine blocker, with significant risk of causing extrapyramidal side effects, and minimal sedation.

Asenapine (Saphris) has an advantage in that it can be administered sublingually, adding to compliance (e.g., in hospital settings, patients cannot "cheek" their medicine). It can also be used on a prn (as needed) basis.

Iloperidone (Fanapt) is an effective antipsychotic that can cause hypotension but has very little, if any, extrapyramidal and metabolic side effects. Dosing must be started at a low level (1 mg) and titrated slowly (up to 12 mg).

Lurasidone (Latuda) has the advantage of reduced side effects. It must be taken with food.

Other Side Effects

Recent concern about the use of second-generation antipsychotics has focused on their tendency to produce weight gain, an alteration of carbohydrate metabolism similar to diabetes, and an alteration of lipid metabolism. There have been cases in which this was not discovered until the patient developed diabetic coma. Also, sometimes the diabetes did not resolve after the medication was discontinued. The elevation of serum lipids may lead to an increased risk of heart disease and stroke (Lindenmayer et al. 2003; Wirshing et al. 2002). The magnitude of this risk was discussed at a joint conference of the American Diabetes Association, American Psychiatric Association, and the American Association of Clinical Endocrinologists (*Journal of Clinical Psychiatry* 2004). Their conclusion was that clozapine and olanzapine appear to have significant metabolic effects, risperidone and quetiapine appear to have lower metabolic effects, and ziprasidone and aripiprazole appear to have minimal metabolic effects (although they have been less studied). They recommend that all patients on these medications should have their weight, blood sugar, and lipid levels monitored.

Choice of Medication

The antipsychotic medications tend to be effective in the treatment of psychotic symptoms, regardless of the disorder. They can be effective in substance-induced delusional disorders, delirium, schizophrenia, mania, delusional disorder, and so on. First-generation antipsychotics tend to be effective for positive symptoms but do little to improve negative symptoms. The newer, second-generation antipsychotics are more effective for negative symptoms, although they are clearly not a panacea since they are successful in only about 30 percent of cases. Both the CATIE study (Lieberman et al. 2005) and a recent meta-analysis (Leucht et al. 2009) concluded that olanzapine is more effective than other second-generation antipsychotics, but also has more metabolic side effects. In choosing an antipsychotic, one must weigh efficacy against side effects.

The choice of medication is generally based on three factors:

- If an antipsychotic medication has been used with success in the past, generally the same medication is again prescribed.

- The patient's motor state is important to consider. Typically, very agitated patients may be given a more sedating (low-potency) medication, whereas markedly regressed or withdrawn patients will be given a less sedating (high-potency) drug.

Special Considerations in Choosing an Antipsychotic

Patient Type	Medication Choice
Child	Low dose
Elderly	High-potency, low dose or second-generation antipsychotic[a]
Anxious or agitated	Zyprexa, Seroquel
Bipolar, manic	Second-generation antipsychotic[b]

a The use of second-generation antipsychotics in the elderly has been shown to be associated with increased mortality. On the other hand, the use of first-generation antipsychotics is associated with EPS and the development of tardive dyskinesia. The choice of medication must be made after weighing these risks.

b Use caution when combining with lithium (may produce encephalopathy).

Figure 19-C

- The side-effect profile of the drug chosen must be considered in relation to the individual patient (see figure 19-C). For example, in the elderly, drugs high in anticholinergic side effects are likely to increase confusion and memory problems, thus high-potency drugs are often used, such as haloperidol or perphenazine.

Individual differences in drug metabolism vary considerably and the dosage ranges are quite broad, thus it is always difficult to know what dose will be required. People are usually started on a low dose and gradually titrated upward depending on clinical response and side effects. In the past, the use of high doses of antipsychotic medications, referred to as *rapid neuroleptization*, was popular. However, more recent studies have shown that moderate doses will produce the same eventual outcome (after ten days) with fewer side effects.

Length of Treatment

All psychotic symptoms do not respond in the same time frame when treated with antipsychotic medications. Typically, severe restlessness, agitation, and marked confusion may subside after a few hours or a few days of treatment. However, longer periods of treatment are generally necessary to resolve symptoms such as delusions, hallucinations, and thought disorder. Some patients may show improvement in these symptoms within a week or two, but in some chronic schizophrenics, many weeks of treatment may be required to gradually reduce these positive symptoms.

The length of treatment also depends on the type of disorder. In substance-induced psychoses, delirium, or brief reactive psychosis, the medication usually can

---

AIMS
(Abnormal Involuntary Movement Scale)

Rate the presence of involuntary movements in the following areas according to severity: 1 = none, 2 = minimal, 3 = mild, 4 = moderate, 5 = severe.

Muscles of facial expression	1 2 3 4 5
Lips and perioral area	1 2 3 4 5
Jaw	1 2 3 4 5
Tongue	1 2 3 4 5
Upper extremities	1 2 3 4 5
Lower extremities	1 2 3 4 5
Trunk	1 2 3 4 5
Overall severity of abnormal movements	1 2 3 4 5
Incapacitation due to abnormal movements	1 2 3 4 5
Distress due to abnormal movements	1 2 3 4 5
Problems with teeth or dentures	Yes/No
Usually wears dentures	Yes/No

Source: US Department of Health, Education, and Welfare

Figure 19-D

be discontinued after the acute phase. In schizophreniform disorder and atypical psychosis, it is often necessary to continue the medication for six months in order to avoid relapse. As mentioned previously, many studies have shown that discontinuation of medication in schizophrenia is associated with higher relapse rates. The general rule is to continue treating schizophrenics for at least one year following the remission of psychotic symptoms to prevent relapse. However, because of the risk of tardive dyskinesia, this judgment must be based on the patient's prior history and ongoing assessment of emerging side effects. Abnormal movements, which may signal the emergence of TD, should be checked at least every six months, for example, by using the AIMS scale (see figure 19-D).

Patient Education

Psychotic disorders are always accompanied by significant functional impairment and great personal suffering. A very common problem, especially with schizophrenia, is relapse. Most often, relapse can be traced to noncompliance with the medication regime. Thus patient education becomes a very important part of treatment. Education involves helping patients to recognize prodromal symptoms of their illness (which may necessitate a dosage increase). Often it is helpful to discuss the prodromal period prior to a psychotic episode in detail to emphasize the particular symptoms that may serve as warning signs for that person. It is also vital that both patients and their families be educated about the effects and side effects of antipsychotic medications—particularly tardive dyskinesia—so that side effects can be properly managed. They should be reassured that most side effects can be reduced to tolerable levels.

Helping patients understand the reasons for taking the medication and the need to manage side effects is an important part of ensuring compliance. Education of the patient's spouse and family is also very important in this regard. Often family members are the first to notice a change in the patient's behavior necessitating a medication adjustment. The patient's physician and psychotherapist play a crucial role in helping to educate the patient and in detecting early symptoms of relapse.

Psychotherapeutic Issues

Several issues are important in doing psychotherapy with someone with schizophrenia, where medication compliance is often an issue and where medication noncompliance is usually, eventually, associated with relapse. One goal is to recognize and take measures to minimize side effects. Several studies have shown that akinesia and akathisia are associated with medication noncompliance. Another issue is making the schizophrenic symptoms ego-dystonic to the patient. This may be a long process, involving repeatedly pointing out the ways in which the symptoms are dysfunctional in the patient's life.

Medication may be seen by the patient as intrusive and controlling or, alternatively, as comforting—a transitional, object-like extension of the therapist. Patients will be prone to interpret the medication in psychotic ways, especially when they are more symptomatic (and more in need of medication). When compliance remains a significant problem, consideration may be given to using one of the long-acting injectable forms of the antipsychotics (risperidone microspheres, haloperidol decanoate, or fluphenazine decanoate).

QUICK REFERENCE
Medications for Treating Psychosis (First-generation Antipsychotics)

Generic Name	Brand Name	Average Daily Dosage Range (mg/day)	Side Effects (usually diminish; may require attention if persist)	Side Effects Requiring Immediate Attention	Significant Drug Interactions* (not all-inclusive)
Chlorpromazine	Thorazine	50-1500	■ Breast enlargement	■ Bleeding or bruising	■ Amphetamines
Fluphenazine	Prolixin	3-45	■ Discharge from the breast	■ Changes in blood pressure	■ Anticonvulsants
Haloperidol	Haldol	2-40	■ Dizziness	■ Confusion	■ Beta blockers
Loxapine	Loxitane	50-250	■ Dry mouth	■ Discoloration of skin or eyes	■ Drugs that depress the CNS (antihistamines, narcotics, muscle relaxants, and barbiturates)
Molindone	Moban	20-225	■ Mild to moderate constipation	■ Excitation or mania	■ HIV protease inhibitors
Perphenazine	Trilafon	8-60	■ Nasal congestion	■ Extreme constipation	■ Levodopa
Thioridazine	Mellaril	150-800	■ Salivation	■ Extreme eye or skin sensitivity to sunlight	■ Lithium
Trifluoperazine	Stelazine	10-40	■ Sexual problems	■ Extreme sedation	■ Tricyclic antidepressants
			■ Tremor of the hands	■ Fever	■ SSRI Antidepressants
			■ Weight gain	■ Irregular heart rate	
				■ Problems with urination, (difficult or painful urination; unable to urinate)	
				■ Seizure	
				■ Shortness of breath	

Warnings/Precautions

- Not indicated during pregnancy or while breastfeeding
- Liver or kidney impairment may require dosage adjustment or discontinuation of treatment
- Can trigger mania/hypomania
- Cardiac monitoring as indicated
- Increased intraocular pressure
- Orthostatic hypotension
- Lowered seizure threshold
- Routine vision exams
- Metabolic syndrome (increased blood pressure, diabetes mellitus, elevated cholesterol, weight gain)
- EPS, acute reactions (akathisia, dystonia, parkinsonian symptoms)
- Tardive dyskinesia or tardive dystonia
- Neuroleptic malignant syndrome
- Hyperpyrexia

*There is variability in the potential for a specific first-generation to interact with the drugs listed.

QUICK REFERENCE
Medications for Treating Psychosis (Second-generation Antipsychotics)

Generic Name	Brand Name	Average Daily Dosage Range (mg/day)	Side Effects (usually diminish; may require attention if persist)	Side Effects Requiring Immediate Attention	Significant Drug Interactions* (not all-inclusive)
Aripiprazole	Abilify	15–30	▪ Breast enlargement	▪ Bleeding or bruising	▪ Amphetamines
Asenapine	Saphris	10–20	▪ Discharge from the breast	▪ Changes in blood pressure	▪ Anti-arrhythmics or other drugs that can affect the heartbeat
Clozapine	Clozaril	300–900	▪ Dizziness	▪ Confusion	▪ Anticonvulsants
Iloperidone	Fanapt	12–24	▪ Dry mouth	▪ Discoloration of skin or eyes	▪ Caffeine
Lurasidone	Latuda	40–80	▪ Mild to moderate constipation	▪ Excitation or mania	▪ Cimetidine
Olanzapine	Zyprexa	5–20	▪ Nasal congestion	▪ Extreme constipation	▪ Drugs that depress the CNS (antihistamines, narcotics, muscle relaxants, and barbiturates)
Paliperidone	Invega	3–12	▪ Salivation	▪ Extreme eye or skin sensitivity to sunlight	▪ HIV protease inhibitors
Quetiapine	Seroquel	300–750	▪ Sexual problems	▪ Extreme sedation	▪ Levodopa
Risperidone	Risperdal	4–16	▪ Tremor of the hands	▪ Fever	▪ Lithium
Ziprasidone	Geodon	60–160	▪ Weight gain	▪ Irregular heart rate	▪ Macrolide antibiotics
				▪ Priapism	▪ Oral antifungal agents
				▪ Problems with urination, (difficult or painful urination; unable to urinate)	▪ SSRI antidepressants
				▪ Seizure	▪ Tricyclic antidepressants
				▪ Shortness of breath	

Warnings/Precautions

▪ Not indicated during pregnancy or while breastfeeding
▪ Liver or kidney impairment may require dosage adjustment or discontinuation of treatment
▪ Can trigger mania/hypomania
▪ Cardiac monitoring as indicated
▪ Increased intraocular pressure
▪ Orthostatic hypotension
▪ Lowered seizure threshold
▪ Routine vision exams
▪ Metabolic syndrome (increased blood pressure, diabetes mellitus, elevated cholesterol, weight gain)
▪ EPS, acute reactions (akathisia, dystonia, parkinsonian symptoms)
▪ Tardive dyskinesia or tardive dystonia
▪ Neuroleptic malignant syndrome
▪ Hyperpyrexia
▪ CBC as required for clozapine

*There is variability in the potential for a specific second-generation antipsychotic to interact with the drugs listed.

Antipsychotic Medications 233

20

Over-the-Counter Dietary Supplements and Herbal Products

In 1998, Eisenberg and colleagues reported on the increasing use of complementary and alternative medicine (CAM) in the United States between 1990 and 1997. Herbal medication use by respondents increased from 2.5 percent in 1990 to 12 percent in 1997. At that time, it was estimated that American consumers were spending 4 billion dollars per year on herbal products. A follow-up review for the years 1997 to 2002 by Tindle et al. (2005) revealed that in 2002 the use of herbal products had increased to 15 percent of respondents. In a recent 2007 survey, nearly 18 percent of respondents reported use of herbal products (National Institutes of Health 2008). Although these surveys were not identical, they nonetheless provide a compelling picture of the increasing use of herbal products in the United States.

Between 1990 and 1997 the most rapidly growing segment of the market was for products used to treat or prevent psychiatric symptoms, including Saint-John's-wort, kava kava, ginkgo, and valerian (Beaubrun and Gray 2000). Sales of mood-altering herbals approached the $400-million-per-year mark in the year 2000 (*Consumer Reports* 2000). Worldwide, 80 percent of people use botanical products, and an estimated 40 percent of U.S. citizens have turned to alternative medicines (LaFrance et al. 2000).

There were, however, some notable changes between 2002 and 2007 in the use of specific products. When looking at the top ten products in 2002, ginkgo and Saint-John's-wort were second and sixth respectively. In 2007, ginkgo was seventh, and Saint-John's-wort was not among the top ten.

The therapist is likely to encounter patients who are already taking herbal remedies or who are seeking information about them. Questions about the use of these products should be part of the diagnostic workup. This chapter provides an overview of the relevant issues surrounding these products, especially safety, efficacy, and psychosocial implications.

In Germany, the government has attempted to regulate the use of herbal products, and has done so by promoting research, public education, and medical education. However, in the United States, herbal and other over-the-counter (OTC) products are neither approved prior to marketing nor regulated for efficacy by the FDA. The only limitation imposed upon the manufacturers of these products is that they cannot advertise that they prevent or treat certain diseases. Claims can be made, however, for use in nondisease conditions or physical functions.

Although some herbal products do have documented effectiveness in treating some psychiatric conditions, their use also can be problematic or even, at times, dangerous for the following reasons:

- No assurances of strength or potency. Some products have been shown to have absolutely none of the particular substances listed on the label. There are currently no standardization requirements for herbal products.

- Some products have been shown to contain impurities or contaminants, such as arsenic, mercury, and lead. Potent pharmaceuticals have been discovered in these products, such as digitalis and estazolam (Harris 2000).

- Products with the following seal appearing on the label have been independently tested: USP (US Pharmacopia). This organization tests over-the-counter products to determine if they are free from contaminants and whether or not they include the actual advertised ingredients and the advertised dose. They do not ensure efficacy but do help the consumer to obtain products that are free from contaminants.

- Serious adverse reactions can occur with these products, yet safety monitoring is nearly nonexistent. The FDA can request that one of these products be withdrawn from the market, but manufacturers are not required to comply unless consumers are faced with an "imminent hazard."

- Some herbals (most notably Saint-John's-wort) have significant effects on liver metabolism and pose dangers of potentially harmful drug-drug interactions. Although some documentation exists regarding drug interactions, there is a relative lack of accurate information available. There is currently no systematic process in place to assess and report drug interactions with herbals. Many products contain multiple ingredients, making the precise identification of drug interactions difficult.

- Seventy percent of people in the United States who use herbal products never inform their doctors (LaFrance et al. 2000), increasing the likelihood that an adverse reaction or drug interaction will occur and be misidentified.

In addition to the informational and regulatory challenges associated with herbals, the therapist also encounters the psychosocial implications of their use. The following is a summary of the key points offered by Cauffield (2000) and Harris (2000) that are relevant to therapists:

- Some of the demographics of herbal users overlap with those of psychotherapy patients, increasing the possibility that issues regarding their use will surface. These characteristics include higher levels of education and income, as well as an association between an interest in alternative therapies and a commitment to personal growth.

- The conditions cited by users of herbals are often chronic, difficult to treat by conventional methods, and associated with complicated lifestyle features. Examples are chronic pain, anxiety, insomnia, depression, fatigue, and memory problems. These are representative of what therapists routinely treat.

- Alternative therapies with an established role in medicine and psychiatry include relaxation techniques, chiropractic care, biofeedback, and hypnosis. Less established is the role of herbal and high-dose vitamin regimens. It can be difficult for patients and practitioners to differentiate between these realms when determining a course of treatment. Additionally, while certain alternative therapies are sometimes covered under insurance, herbals are almost always excluded, resulting in higher out-of-pocket costs for the patient.

The Promise of Herbal Remedies

It is important to keep in mind that a number of important and highly effective pharmaceuticals originally were derived from botanic sources. The list includes poppy (morphine), willow bark (aspirin), belladonna tops (atropine), and foxglove leaf (digitalis). It is certainly reasonable to assume that other botanicals may prove to be safe and effective treatments for certain psychiatric disorders as well.

However, progress in this area is impeded by two significant factors: First, because herbs are not patentable, there is a decreased incentive for pharmaceutical companies to pour the millions of dollars into the type of research that is required to bring prescription drugs to market. The result is a paucity of well-controlled research. Single-case reports and testimonials do not constitute solid scientific evidence. For many of the products, the active ingredient or ingredients has not even been determined. The second problem is the lack of oversight by the FDA. This has resulted in misleading claims or outright false advertising. As the philosopher David Hume stated, "Extraordinary claims require extraordinary evidence," and solid research is often lacking in this area. This is especially problematic, as noted above, when it comes to the issue of drug-drug interactions. Medical catastrophes and deaths most surely have occurred when people unknowingly mixed certain herbal products with prescription drugs.

We need to be watchful and cautious as the evidence regarding OTC herbal products (both pro and con) continues to accumulate. And remember, "natural" does not mean safe. Some so-called natural products can, in fact, be deadly.

OTC Products with Some Research Documenting Efficacy

Product	Conditions Treated	Usual Adult Daily Dose	Side Effects	Drug-Drug Interactions[a]
Saint-John's-wort (hypericum perforatum)	Depression	900–1800 mg	Minimal nausea Insomnia Hypomania/mania Photosensitivity Interference with certain lab tests	Significant[b]
SAM-e (s-adenosyl-methionine)	Depression	400–1600 mg	GI symptoms Hypomania/mania Serotonin syndrome	Not well established
Omega-3 fatty acids	Mood disorders Affect instability	1–9 grams	GI upset	None
Folic acid	Mood disorders	400–500 mcg	None	None

OTC Products That May Be Beneficial

Product	Conditions Treated	Usual Adult Daily Dose	Side Effects	Drug-Drug Interactions
Melatonin	Sleep disturbance	0.5 mg	Sedation; at higher doses may aggravate depression	Not well established
Ginkgo Biloba	Cognitive impairment	20–240 mg	GI problems Headache Dizziness Bleeding Interference with certain lab tests	Not well established[c]

OTC Products That *May* Increase Psychiatric Symptoms or Be Dangerous (Not Recommended)

Product	Intended Effects	Adverse Psychiatric Effects
Yohimbine	Treatment of impotency	Anxiety
Kava Kava[d]	Decrease anxiety	Associated with toxicity

a For details on drug-drug interactions, see Ayd (2000); Fugh-Berman (2000); derMarderosian and Beutler (2008).

b Significant due to hepatic enzyme induction. Do not use with birth control pills, protease inhibitors, immuno-suppressants (e.g., cyclosporine), asthma medications (e.g., theophylline), SSRIs, MAOI antidepressants, venlafaxine, mirtazapine, tricyclic antidepressants, amphetamines, anticonvulsants, levodopa, warfarin, and digoxin. Other, as yet undiscovered, interactions may also exist.

c May cause bleeding in people taking aspirin. Do not use with divalproex, anticoagulants, moderate-to-high intake of caffeine. May induce seizures.

d May potentiate effects of alcohol, benzodiazepines, barbiturates, and antipsychotics (side effects); adverse effects also seen with cimetidine and levodopa.

21

Medication Discontinuation

It is generally best to taper off a medication slowly, usually over several weeks or months, depending on the medication and the length of time a person has been taking it. With some medications the consequences of stopping abruptly can be very problematic, but with others they can be serious, even life threatening. When any psychotropic medication is discontinued, clinicians should be particularly watchful for changes or worsening of mental status. It is important to note that discontinuation symptoms are sometimes experienced during dosage reductions or when changing from a longer to a shorter half-life form of the medication. Also, with certain classes of medications, after discontinuation of a medication a patient may become unresponsive to that medication. For example, a person who is stable on lithium for treatment of bipolar disorder and develops a manic episode following discontinuation of lithium may not respond to lithium when it is restarted (Post, 2011). This has also been reported anecdotally with antidepressants and antipsychotics (Shore, Matthews, Cott, & Lieberman, 1995; Fava et al., 2002), though the evidence is not conclusive. It is thought that each episode, whether it is mania, depression, or psychosis, has a neurophysiological effect on the brain (i.e., damage to brain structures and nerve cells) that may make it unresponsive to a medication that was previously effective.

While the discussion is beyond the scope of this book, special precautions may be necessary for monitoring and managing discontinuation or withdrawal symptoms in newborns if the mother was on chronic therapy with certain psychotropic medications, such as psychostimulants or benzodiazepines.

Antidepressants

While antidepressants are not considered habit forming, or addictive, abrupt discontinuation can cause significant symptoms. Certain discontinuation symptoms may occur with all antidepressants, while others are specific to a given class of antidepressant.

There is a potential for relapse into depression or, paradoxically, mania when an antidepressant is withdrawn too quickly. This can usually be avoided by tapering the antidepressant slowly, e.g., 25 to 50 percent of the current dose per month. For example, if a person is taking 40 mg of citalopram (Celexa) daily, it can be tapered by taking 30 mg per day for one month, then 20 mg per day for a month, then 10 mg per day for a month, and then stopped. Or, if the person is taking 20 mg per day, it would be reduced to 10 mg daily for one month and then stopped. The more slowly it is tapered, the less the likelihood of relapse and/or withdrawal symptoms.

Discontinuation symptoms vary by antidepressant class as follows:

- *Heterocyclic antidepressants:* Dizziness, nausea, vomiting, headache, malaise, sleep disturbances, increased body temperature, or irritability.

- *SSRIs and SNRIs:* Agitation, anxiety, tremulousness, dizziness, tinnitus, dysphoria, headache, insomnia, nightmares, irritability, lethargy, gastrointestinal disturbances, or sensory sensations described as "electric shocks." Discontinuation symptoms tend to be more severe with shorter half-life agents, such as venlafaxine and paroxetine.

- *MAOIs:* Irritability, pressured or slurred speech, muscle rigidity, increased body temperature, insomnia, nightmares, muscle spasms, painful muscle contractions, ataxia, electric shock sensations, or hallucinations.

Again, discontinuation symptoms can usually be avoided by tapering slowly, as shown previously. These symptoms may persist for two or three weeks after the medication is stopped. One strategy for managing persistent symptoms is to have the patient take a single dose every few days when the symptoms recur.

Psychostimulants

When discontinuing psychostimulants after long-term use, clinicians should monitor for signs of unmasked depression, dysphoria, sleep disturbances, difficulty concentrating, fatigue, and irritability. These symptoms usually resolve within a week, with the exception of unmasked depression, which may require treatment in some cases. Generally, psychostimulants can be tapered over several weeks to a month, depending on the medication, dosage form, and half-life. Concerns about dependence or addiction with psychostimulants are greater for patients with a history of alcohol or drug dependence.

Hypnotics

Benzodiazepine and non-benzodiazepine hypnotics have the potential to be habit forming and produce tolerance and dependence. Hypnotics can best be tapered by skipping days, e.g., going from daily dosing to every other night, then every third night, and then as needed or once a week. Discontinuation symptoms include dysphoria and rebound insomnia. Withdrawal symptoms can include abdominal cramps, vomiting, sweating, muscle pain, tremors, and seizures. The withdrawal symptoms from having developed a dependence on the medication will resolve in about two weeks. Even after withdrawal symptoms have resolved, insomnia or rebound insomnia may persist.

Mood Stabilizers

Mood stabilizers should be tapered slowly, similarly to antidepressants. Abrupt discontinuation of any type of mood stabilizer can precipitate a manic episode and/or cause mood instability. Other discontinuation reactions for each type of mood stabilizer are summarized below:

- *Lithium:* Discontinuation may precipitate a manic episode or other mood instability.

- *Anticonvulsant mood stabilizers:* Abrupt discontinuation can cause a seizure. Other potential discontinuation symptoms include headache, dizziness, and shakiness.

- *Second-generation antipsychotics:* Discontinuation may lead to a manic episode or mood instability. Also, sometimes *withdrawal dyskinesias* will appear, involving involuntary movements of the hands, limbs, or face, but they usually resolve within a few weeks to a few months.

It is usually safe to reduce the dose at intervals of one to two weeks, as long as the mood disorder is still being treated. That is, slow tapering of a mood stabilizer is not likely to cause discontinuation symptoms, but taking a person with bipolar disorder off all medications is likely to lead to the reemergence of symptoms of bipolar disorder.

Antianxiety Medications (Benzodiazepines)

Benzodiazepine antianxiety medications are the most difficult to discontinue, because abrupt discontinuation can cause severe withdrawal symptoms, including seizures. Also, a rapid dosage reduction can lead to severe anxiety and/or panic attacks. Therefore, these medications need to be reduced very gradually. One tapering regimen is to decrease the dose by about 10 percent per week, recognizing that the last step, reducing to zero, can be very difficult and often takes longer than a week. So, for example, a current daily dose of 6 mg of alprazolam would be decreased by 0.5 mg each week. This is usually best done by first switching to the long-acting form, or clonazepam, in order to avoid peaks and valleys of blood level, which can worsen withdrawal symptoms.

Antipsychotics

Antipsychotics are not associated with significant discontinuation or withdrawal symptoms. However, abruptly stopping antipsychotics can cause physical symptoms of gastrointestinal problems, dizziness, headache, or insomnia. Of greatest concern when reducing or discontinuing antipsychotics is the recurrence of psychotic symptoms. Therefore, dosage reductions must be done slowly and carefully, with incremental dose reductions at one- to six-month intervals. Unfortunately, sometimes abrupt discontinuation is necessary, such as when clozapine causes a dangerous drop in the white blood cell count. In this situation, the risk of psychosis can be reduced by using a different antipsychotic.

22

Red Flags: When to Reevaluate

Previous chapters have discussed the diagnostic phase of treatment, in which the clinician makes initial decisions regarding possible referral for medication treatment. We have also outlined basic treatment strategies and medication doses. The nonmedical therapist is crucially involved in monitoring patient response to medications: noting signs of symptomatic improvement, the emergence of adverse effects, and, at times, exacerbation of symptoms. Knowing what to look for and when to direct the patient back to the prescribing physician is an important task. In this chapter, we will address six important conditions or circumstances in which a re-referral is indicated: failure to respond, need for dosage adjustment, unexplained relapse, the onset of new medical conditions, side-effect problems, and discontinuation of medication treatment.

Failure to Respond

As noted in earlier chapters, a positive medication response is rarely immediate. Most psychotropic medications require a number of days or weeks to reach adequate blood levels and produce physiologic changes that yield symptomatic improvement. Also, there exists tremendous variability from patient to patient regarding absorption and metabolism of medications, which affects the ultimate response time. Initial doses often must be raised gradually, as tolerance for side effects is achieved and blood levels of the medication approach therapeutic levels.

Critical to appropriate treatment is conducting an *adequate trial*. Adequate trials must assume that the correct diagnosis has been made and the patient has actually taken the medication as prescribed. Beyond this, the two most important variables to consider are dosage and length of treatment. A general rule with all psychotropics is to use the lowest dose that is effective, although at the same time not to undertreat. The clinician must be willing to increase doses in order to achieve meaningful results, while continuously monitoring for the emergence of side effects.

Generally, if patients have been treated with moderate to high doses of psychotropic medications (or at adequate blood levels) for four or five weeks without noticeable improvement, a re-referral should be made for dosage increase, augmentation, or perhaps a change to another class of medication. It is not unusual to encounter patients who have been treated for months (or even years!) on a particular drug or dose without symptomatic improvement. This is not appropriate. Any condition that warrants medication treatment is undoubtedly causing considerable suffering. There is no justifiable reason to mistreat or undertreat for a long period of time without carefully reevaluating the current treatment and making necessary adjustments.

Need for Dosage Adjustment

In addition to patients' failure to respond, therapists commonly encounter situations in which the patient has shown a positive response, but the symptomatic improvement is only partial. Many patients who show partial response can experience enhanced improvement when doses are increased or medications are augmented. In such cases of partial response, a re-referral is warranted.

Unexplained Relapse

Sometimes a patient who has responded well to psychotropic medication treatment will, at some point, experience the reemergence of symptoms—even when medications are continued. When this occurs, the clinician should consider the following common reasons:

- Failure to comply with treatment; for example, the patient has not been taking medication as prescribed.

- The patient has started to drink alcohol excessively, which may exacerbate depression or anxiety symptoms, interferes with sleep, and may also interfere with metabolism of the psychotropic medication. Other substance abuse may account for increased symptomatology (e.g., caffeine disrupting sleep).

- The patient has experienced a significant increase in psychosocial stressors.

- A medical condition has developed that may contribute to the development of psychiatric symptoms, such as thyroid disease.

- "Breakthrough symptoms": At times the underlying neurochemical disorder or metabolic activity of the individual undergoes a change that results in a reemergence of symptoms. In many cases of breakthrough symptoms, a dosage adjustment (usually an increase in dose) may be successful.

- Tolerance to the drug can develop. This is uncommon; however, there is increasing evidence that some medications work well in early stages of some biologically based mental illnesses but are not as successful in later phases of the illness. For example, lithium is very effective in early episodes of bipolar disorder but is less effective after a number of episodes. This probably does not represent true "tolerance" but, rather, a change in the underlying pathophysiology or neurochemical substrate.

Onset of New Medical Conditions

A patient may initially be able to tolerate and safely take psychotropic medications; however, the onset of certain physical conditions can change this, necessitating a re-referral. Such conditions include pregnancy, epilepsy, certain types of glaucoma, and physiological changes associated with aging and kidney disease. Another time to reevaluate medications occurs when the patient has an upcoming surgery, since psychotropics can interact with anesthetics administered before or during surgery and may also inhibit the healing process. Likewise, new prescription and over-the-counter medications added to cope with coexisting medical problems can cause drug interaction problems (see appendix C). This is frequently seen in elderly patients, who often have a host of medical problems and take many medications.

Side-Effect Problems

All psychotropic medications have side effects to a greater or lesser degree. Some side effects are minor, benign, and transient. Others are quite unpleasant and at times dangerous. Summarized in figure 22-A are the most common side effects associated with the various classes of psychotropic medications. These are classified into three groups:

- Minor or benign: Many of these side effects diminish or disappear with continued treatment as tolerance develops.

- Troublesome side effects: These can cause moderate levels of discomfort and may result in poor compliance.

- Potentially serious side effects: These may cause excessive discomfort and can actually be dangerous.

A re-referral is warranted in cases where side effects are troublesome or potentially serious, or when clinical signs of drug toxicity appear (see figure 22-B).

When It Is Time to Discontinue

Once a patient has fully recovered, the question of when to stop medication arises. Often, even if the patient is asymptomatic, an abrupt discontinuation of medications can result in either relapse or withdrawal symptoms. The matter of when to stop is highly individual and depends heavily on three factors:

- The patient's history of previous episodes

- Your assessment of the patient's vulnerability to relapse

- The patient's feelings about discontinuing medications. Figure 22-C provides *very general* guidelines for length of treatment; each case must be evaluated individually.

It is important to note that people treated with benzodiazepines will develop a tolerance to the medication, and if it is abruptly discontinued, they *will* have withdrawal symptoms—some of which can be serious. Slow tapering of doses is required and almost always can be safely accomplished (see "Benzodiazepine Withdrawal" in

Side Effects of Psychotropic Medications

Medication Class	Mild or Benign	Troublesome	Potentially Serious
Antidepressants			
Tricyclics	Dry mouth Constipation Nasal congestion Mild sedation	Oversedation Sexual dysfunction Weight gain Hypotension Tremor Blurred vision Rash Urinary retention	Dizziness or falls, especially in the elderly Seizures Photosensitivity Cardiac arrhythmias Mania or hypomania Glaucoma Urinary retention Low white blood cell count Fever Sudden high fever with jaundice Priapism High white blood cell count Swollen lymph nodes Respiratory distress
SSRIs	Sweating Nausea or gas Diarrhea Constipation Dry mouth Sedation	Headache Anxiety Insomnia Weight loss Rash Sexual dysfunction Apathy Amotivation Emotional blunting Weight gain	Mania or hypomania
MAOIs	Headaches Dizziness Dry mouth Constipation Nausea Diarrhea	Increased heart rate Blurred vision Weight gain Anxiety Sexual dysfunction	Low blood pressure Falls Muscle spasms Hallucinations Hypertensive crisis Mania or hypomania

Figure 22-A

Handbook of Clinical Psychopharmacology for Therapists

Side Effects of Psychotropic Medications *(continued)*

Medication Class	Mild or Benign	Troublesome	Potentially Serious
Antipsychotics	Mild sedation Tremor Dry mouth Blurred vision Increased perspiration Constipation Nasal congestion	Rigidity Sexual dysfunction Oversedation Low blood pressure Extrapyramidal symptoms Breast enlargement	Agranulocytosis Urinary retention High blood pressure Severe rigidity, especially with fever, jaundice Abnormal movements Falls Confusion Liver toxicity Cardiac arrhythmia Photosensitivity Impaired temperature regulation
Mood Stabilizers			
Lithium	Nausea Tremor	Weight gain Memory problems Sedation Muscle weakness Vomiting Diarrhea	Oversedation Confusion Incoordination
Anticonvulsants	Sedation Nausea Vomiting Headache Tremor	Muscle twitching Rash Blurred vision Dizziness Weight gain	Confusion Urinary retention Bone marrow depression
Antianxiety Agents			
Benzodiazepines	Mild sedation Constipation	Oversedation Confusion (especially in the elderly) Parodoxical stimulation	Dizziness or falls Low blood pressure
Buspirone	Dizziness Nausea Headaches	Insomnia Nervousness Dysphoria	
Antihistamines	Drowsiness GI upset	Dry mouth Sexual dysfunction Low blood pressure	Difficulty breathing Urinary retention

Figure 22-A *continued*

Signs of Toxicity or Overdose

Antidepressants[a]:
- Oversedation
- Cardiac arrhythmia
- Falls
- Dilated pupils
- Confusion
- Psychosis
- Seizures
- Coma
- Agitation

Lithium[b]:
- Oversedation
- Confusion
- Incoordination
- Seizure
- Coma

Anticonvulsants:
- Oversedation
- Confusion
- Incoordination
- Cardiac arrhythmia

Antipsychotics:
- Oversedation
- Hyperthermia
- Restlessness or agitation
- Seizures
- Rigidity
- Coma
- Falls
- Cardiac arrhythmia
- Confusion

Antianxiety Agents:
- Confusion
- Slurred speech
- Incoordination
- Falls
- Oversedation
- Coma

a Severe tricyclic overdoses oftentimes are fatal. SSRIs, venlafaxine, and bupropion: low degree of toxicity.

b Severe overdoses oftentimes are fatal.

Figure 22-B

chapter 18). In general, it is wise to withdraw *all* psychotropic medications gradually; for example, antidepressants should be withdrawn gradually over a period of four to eight weeks. A re-referral to the prescribing physician is warranted when, in your judgment, it is time to begin discontinuing treatment.

Finally, from start to finish, ongoing collaboration and communication between psychotherapist and physician is important. Even at times when no problems exist, you may simply want to update the physician on the patient's progress.

Length of Continued Treatment After Patient Becomes Asymptomatic

Disorder	Time Frame
Major depression	
First episode	6–12 months
Subsequent episodes	12–36 months or possibly indefinitely
Panic disorder	
First episode	6 months
Subsequent episodes	12–24 months
Psychotic disorder	
Brief psychotic episode (remitting quickly)	3 months
Schizophrenia and schizophreniform disorder	
First episode	12 months
Subsequent episodes	24 months to indefinite
Bipolar disorder	Generally requires ongoing prophylactic treatment
Obsessive-compulsive disorder	6 months[a]
Post-traumatic stress disorder	6 months[a]
Borderline personality disorder	6 months[a]

a The time frame for discontinuing has not been firmly established.

Figure 22-C

23

Child and Adolescent Psychopharmacology

Previous chapters have covered the basics of clinical psychopharmacology as it applies to older adolescents and adults. In this chapter we will focus on issues related to the treatment of children and younger adolescents. The organization of this chapter differs in that it will include both diagnostic and treatment considerations.

Issues in Diagnosing and Initiating Pharmacologic Treatment of Children and Adolescents

If one looks at the literature in child psychiatry prior to fifteen years ago, it would appear that children were seen as being quite similar to adults with respect to both diagnostic and treatment issues. Although there is some degree of overlap, there are also significant features that distinguish psychiatric syndromes and pharmacologic treatments in children and adults.

It is likely that the majority of emotional suffering experienced by youngsters is related to situational stresses and responds best to nonmedical, psychological treatments (e.g., family therapy). However, it is also becoming increasingly clear that many major mental illnesses begin in childhood (e.g., 33 percent of cases of obsessive-compulsive disorder and up to 27 percent of cases of bipolar disorder have childhood or early adolescent onset). Not only do these disorders cause considerable suffering in young children, but they also can markedly interfere with normal social and academic developmental experiences. For example, more than one-half of children experiencing major depression continue to be symptomatic for two or more years. During depressive episodes, many experience significant social withdrawal and academic failure, often due to an impaired ability to concentrate. Even if they recover, many of these children find it hard to ever "catch up" academically or in terms of developing age-appropriate social skills.

There is also increasing evidence that some psychiatric disorders are subject to progressive neurobiological impairment if they go untreated (the kindling model of disease progression). Toxic levels of neurotransmitters (e.g., glutamate) or stress hormones (e.g., cortisol) may damage neural tissue (see figure 23-A). Pharmacologic treatment of these disorders may not only be successful in terms of improving symptoms, but may also be *neuroprotective* (i.e., medication treatment may either protect against brain damage or promote normal neuromaturation).

Disorders with Evidence of Progressive Neurobiological Impairment

■ Bipolar illness

■ Attention-deficit/hyperactivity disorder

■ Schizophrenia

■ Some cases of recurrent, unipolar depression

■ Some cases of post-traumatic stress disorder

Figure 23-A

In addition to clinical considerations, there are other unique challenges in the prescribing of psychotropic medications for children. With children, there is no true *informed consent* since parents are the ones who usually make the decision whether or not to allow medication treatment. At least three concerns arise regarding this: (1) Parental fears about drug use (or possible addiction) may lead them to withhold treatment from some children who need it. (2) Some parents may adopt a view of psychiatric drug treatment in which they see the disorders simply as a "chemical imbalance," and they may think pills will fix the problem and ignore psychological factors (e.g., dysfunctional family dynamics) as a focus for treatment. (3) The young person may be left out of the loop (i.e., not spoken to or allowed to discuss in detail how he or she feels about medication treatment).

Most child clinicians agree that children (ages seven and older) should be included in discussions about psychiatric medication treatment. This is important in order to encourage the child to voice concerns about treatment (e.g., many children conclude that if they need medicine, it must mean that they are very ill or "crazy"). Also, these early experiences with psychiatric treatment, if perceived to be positive by the child, may go a long way to instill positive attitudes about mental health treatment. This is critical since many of the more severe disorders that warrant medical treatment during childhood are the first manifestations of what may be lifelong mental illnesses. Including the child in discussions regarding medication treatment can often foster a positive relationship with the therapist, as the child feels respected enough to be included.

Parents need to devote a good deal of time to addressing all of their concerns about drug treatment. Parents who do not wholeheartedly endorse treatment will often sabotage treatment. Informed consent should also include the risks of not treating certain disorders.

Medication Metabolism in Young Clients

The normal rate of hepatic (liver) metabolism is high in children until the time of puberty. The result is that most medications are aggressively metabolized in the liver and rapidly excreted. Thus dosing for prepubertal children requires doses that may approach or equal adult dosing (because what ultimately matters is how much drug enters circulation). The use of seemingly high doses for young children may be counterintuitive for many parents, thus it will be helpful to explain to them the role of increased rates of drug metabolism in children.

During a period of time (two to four months) surrounding the entry into puberty, the rate of hepatic metabolism significantly slows. For this reason, youngsters who have been maintained on a dose of psychiatric medication, tolerating it well, may begin to show increasing side effects when this change in metabolic rate occurs (and as more of the drug begins to escape the liver and enter circulation). Dosage adjustments may then be required to minimize side effects.

Drug Research and Outcome Studies

As important as efficacy studies are, there is a paucity of good studies in child psychopharmacology (with one notable exception: there are numerous well-controlled studies of the treatment of ADHD with stimulants). Historically, pharmaceutical companies did not conduct tests of psychiatric drugs on children. However, in 1998 the Food and Drug Administration mandated that safety studies be carried out for new psychiatric drugs with child subjects. Recently the FDA offered financial incentives (by way of extensions of patents) if efficacy studies are done with children. Thus in very recent times, better-controlled studies have been initiated; however, many of these are not yet published. In the next few years the database of well-done studies should increase significantly.

Another issue regarding research in this area is that many studies do not include severely ill children (the reason for this is that it is not judged to be ethical to expose severely disturbed children to placebos over a period of months). Thus in research in some areas of child psychiatry, groups of subjects (e.g., those with major depression) often include only mild-to-moderately severe cases. Information about treatment outcomes for severely ill kids is often limited to case studies. It is important to keep these research limitations in mind when evaluating the outcomes of medication studies.

Fears Regarding Drug Addiction

Many parents are understandably concerned about the use of habit-forming drugs to treat their children. It is important to talk openly with parents about these concerns (even if they do not initiate the conversation, since many do harbor fears). Among psychiatric medications, only two classes of drugs are potential drugs of abuse: stimulants (e.g., Ritalin) and benzodiazepines (e.g., antianxiety drugs such as Xanax). However, the vast majority of children with psychiatric disorders do not abuse these medications. For instance, although stimulants can be abused by those genetically predisposed to substance abuse, such drugs generally do not produce euphoria in ADHD children. In fact, many children with ADHD experience stimulants as causing mild dysphoric effects. Additionally, data now exists to strongly indicate that among those with ADHD, the use of stimulants actually decreases the risk of substance abuse (when compared to drug-abuse rates, which are high among untreated ADHD subjects) (Biederman et al. 1999; Kuczenski et al. 2002).

Substance abuse by children and adolescents is a common and serious concern in our society. It must also be kept in mind that untreated mental illnesses result in significant emotional suffering and contribute to a much higher likelihood of drug abuse. Low self-esteem, depression, anxiety, and a sense of alienation often prompt the use of illicit drugs as a form of self-medication. Thus any risk-benefit assessment of medication treatment and drug abuse must certainly take into consideration the risks of failure to treat the psychiatric disorder.

Attention-Deficit/Hyperactivity Disorder (ADHD)

ADHD affects approximately 5 to 7 percent of children. With neurologic maturation, most teenagers with ADHD will experience a noticeable reduction in motoric restless-ness or hyperactivity, but the core symptoms of ADHD (e.g., impulsivity, impaired attention, and lack of intrinsic motivation) continue through adolescence and on into adulthood. Most experts agree that about one-third of ADHD children completely outgrow the disorder by early adulthood (likely due to the ongoing maturation of the prefrontal lobes, which may continue until the late twenties or early thirties). Two-thirds of children with ADHD experience ongoing symptoms throughout life.

Diagnostic Issues

It is very important to emphasize that most psychiatric disorders in childhood present with some degree of motoric restlessness and inattention. Thus these out-wardly observable behaviors absolutely do not automatically lead to a diagnosis of ADHD. Figure 23-B lists those disorders that must be considered in any comprehensive evaluation of children with hyperactivity and inattention.

The diagnosis of ADHD is based largely on three sources of data: family history (since ADHD is considered to be a genetically transmitted disorder and thus often runs in families), a very careful history detailing the nature and onset of behavioral symptoms, and a description of current symptoms (especially as they vary across situations). It is also a diagnosis of exclusion (one must always first rule out those disorders listed in figure 23-B).

The most common presentation for ADHD is an early onset (often present in infancy) of restlessness, unstable sleep patterns, affective lability (in particular, crying a lot and difficulty in being soothed). Most true ADHD children are identified in pre-school when they have their first sustained contact with other children and encounter social standards (expectations to control behavior, follow rules, and stay on task in age-appropriate ways). There is some controversy among experts, but general agree-ment that this *very early onset* of significant behavioral problems is very characteristic of ADHD. However, there is emerging data to suggest that some children destined to have bipolar disorder may show early-onset behaviors that are ADHD-like (i.e., prodromal symptoms of bipolar).

During childhood, the following symptoms predominate: hyperactivity, impulsiv-ity, impaired self-control, difficulties staying on task, and limited ability for intrinsic motivation (e.g., motivation to stay focused, especially on mundane, unexciting, or low-stimulus-value tasks). Such symptoms are often highly context-dependent; that is, most noticeable in situations requiring that the child remain still and quiet (e.g., in the

Differential Diagnosis of Childhood Onset Psychiatric Disorders Presenting with Hyperactivity and Inattention
■ Diffuse brain damage (e.g., commonly seen in fetal alcohol syndrome)
■ Anxiety disorders (e.g., separation anxiety)
■ Agitated depression
■ Situational stress
■ Bipolar mania
■ Prepsychotic conditions
■ Impaired affect regulation associated with severe early abuse or neglect (see chapters 12 and 13)
■ Boredom (especially likely in bright children who are academically understimulated)

Figure 23-B

classroom), yet may not be as noticeable when in an environment that is inherently exciting, novel, or stimulating (e.g., playing video games).

With adolescence, as noted above, motoric hyperactivity often is reduced, but core symptoms remain. Disorganization (manifest in messy lockers, notebooks, and bedrooms) often is pronounced in the ADHD adolescent, as are increasing problems adapting to society's and school's demands for independent task performance and self-control.

It is important to note that the so-called "inattentive type" of ADHD appears to be a totally unrelated neurologic disorder (children with this disorder do show impaired attention; however, they are neither hyperactive nor impulsive). This fundamental difference is also underscored by the failure of stimulants to treat the inattentive subtype (except in rare instances).

Neurobiology

Numerous studies suggest impaired frontal lobe functioning in people suffering from ADHD (evident in studies of metabolic functioning, e.g., SPECT and PET scans). In addition, abnormalities have been shown in the dopamine neurotransmitter system. Likewise, dopamine agonists (e.g., stimulants or bupropion) are effective medications for reducing ADHD symptoms. Minor structural abnormalities have also been found in the brains of ADHD subjects (e.g., smaller cerebellar volumes, smaller volumes of frontal and temporal areas, and a smaller caudate nucleus).

Appropriate treatment with stimulants may not only reduce symptoms, but also may normalize the chemical microenvironment of the developing brain and ensure more normal brain maturation. Castellanos et al. (2002) demonstrated that ADHD children have smaller cerebral and cerebellar volumes than age-matched controls. The degree of reduction in frontal, temporal, cerebellar, and white-matter volumes correlated significantly with parent and teacher ratings of ADHD symptom severity. Unmedicated ADHD subjects exhibited strikingly smaller white-matter volumes compared to both controls and medicated ADHD children (treated with stimulants). This suggests that appropriate treatment may be neuroprotective.

Psychopharmacology of ADHD

There are three classes of medications with empirical support of efficacy in the treatment of ADHD: stimulants, certain antidepressants, and alpha-2 adrenergic agonists.

Stimulants

The mechanism of action of stimulants is inhibition of dopamine reuptake (additionally, amphetamines promote increased release of dopamine from vesicles). Figure 23-C lists currently available stimulants. There are different ways to categorize stimulants, either by the onset of action or duration of action. In general, most of these agents have a moderately rapid onset, with symptom reduction occurring thirty to forty-five minutes after ingestion and a duration of action ranging from four to twelve hours. Depending on the formulation, dosing is two to three times daily, with some

Stimulants	
Immediate-Release	**Typical Daily Doses**
Methylphenidate	
Ritalin	10–60 mg
Metadate	10–60 mg
Methylin	10–60 mg
Concerta	18–54 mg
Dexmethylphenidate (Focalin)	5–20 mg
Dextroamphetamine	
Dexedrine	5–40 mg
Amphetamines	
Amphetamine mixed salts (Adderall)	5–40 mg
Methamphetamine (Desoxyn)	5–25 mg
Extended-Release	**Typical Daily Doses**
Methylphenidate	
Ritalin SR	20–60 mg
Ritalin LA	20–60 mg
Metadate ER	10–60 mg
Metadate CD	20–60 mg
Methylin ER	20–60 mg
Concerta	18–54 mg
Daytrana (transdermal patch)	10–30 mg
Dextroamphetamine	
Dexedrine spansules	5–40 mg
Amphetamine	
Adderall XR	5–40 mg
Lisdexamphetamine	
Vyvanse	30–70 mg

Figure 23-C

long-acting products providing once-daily dosing. What is most important is to find the best possible dose and dosing schedule for a given patient.

There are over 200 well-controlled studies of stimulant use, and outcomes are significantly positive. Assuming an accurate diagnosis and appropriate dosing, any one stimulant taken results in approximately a 70 percent response rate. Although the stimulants are similar, there are differences. Thus, if a trial with one stimulant (e.g., methylphenidate) is less than optimal, then it is advisable to conduct a trial on another stimulant (e.g., dextroamphetamine). If systematic trials are conducted on each of the three classes of stimulants, good outcomes are seen in about 90 percent of patients treated (Barkley 2000). Across studies, effect sizes generally are 1.0 (Walkup 2003).

The following briefly highlight important issues regarding stimulant treatment:

- Very low risk of abuse in ADHD patients.

- ADHD affects all aspects of life, not just academic performance. Thus it is often best to administer medications each day (i.e., not just on school days).

- Start treatment with immediate-release formulations and then switch to extended-release preparations, if tolerated and effective.

- Stimulants work only for a short period of time, and the positive effects wear off in the late afternoon or evening. Thus coadministration of antidepressants (see below) may be an option for targeting symptoms later in the day.

- Most children successfully treated with stimulants will require ongoing medication treatment well into adolescence and possibly into adulthood.

- Side effects:

  - Initial insomnia (if taken later in the day)

    - Solutions: earlier dosing; clonidine or trazodone given at bedtime

  - Anorexia: generally affects the patient only when the drug is active (i.e., usually only interferes with appetite at lunchtime). Has not been associated with significant problems obtaining adequate nutrition. Focalin may have less of this effect.

  - Stomachache

    - Solution: give with food

  - Mild dysphoria

    - Solutions: switch classes of stimulants; add an antidepressant such as bupropion

  - Lethargy, sedation, or impaired concentration: usually indicates that the dose is too high

  - Failure to accurately diagnose and treat with stimulants can have very adverse consequences (see figure 23-D)

Alpha-2 adrenergic agonists

Clonidine (Catapres, Kapvay) and guanfacine (Tenex, Intuniv) may be used to treat core ADHD symptoms (see figure 23-E); however, they are most effective in reducing irritability, aggression, and impulsivity and in promoting sedation (to treat initial insomnia). Alpha-2 agonists are also the treatment of choice for comorbid tics.

Consequences of Misdiagnosis and Stimulant Treatment	
Diagnosis	**Consequences**
Anxiety disorder	Increased anxiety
Agitated depression	Increased agitation
Preschizophrenic	Psychosis
Bipolar disorder	Increased manic symptoms *may* cause cycle acceleration
Situational stress	Failure to address psychological issues

Figure 23-D

Alpha–2 Adrenergic Agonists		
Generic	**Brand Name**	**Typical Doses**
Clonidine	Catapres, Kapvay	0.15–0.4 mg[a]
Guanfacine	Tenex, Intuniv	0.25–1.0 mg[b] 0.05–0.12 mg per kg[c]

a Three to four times a day
b Two to three times a day
c One time a day

Figure 23-E

There have been three reported cases of death in children taking clonidine in conjunction with a stimulant. However, the FDA has conducted an investigation and failed to find any significant cause for concern in coadministering these drugs. Combined use of alpha-2 agonists and stimulants is a common practice (both for treating ADHD and comorbid ADHD and tics) (Walkup 2003).

Antidepressants

Twenty percent of ADHD children will experience co-occurring depression. Antidepressants certainly may be helpful in reducing mood symptoms. However, beyond this use of antidepressants, certain classes of antidepressants have been shown to have positive effects on core ADHD symptoms. Not all antidepressants treat ADHD; only those that increase the availability of dopamine or norepinephrine are useful (thus SSRIs, although often a good adjunct for treating anxiety or depression, are not effective in treating core ADHD symptoms). Antidepressants that have evidence of efficacy in treating ADHD are listed in figure 23-F.

Treatment outcomes with antidepressants are not as robust as those seen with stimulants, but they afford several advantages:

- Once-a-day dosing

- No need for triplicate prescription

Antidepressants Used to Treat ADHD		
Generic	**Brand Name**	**Typical Daily Dosage**
Bupropion	Wellbutrin SR/LA	150–300 mg
Atomoxetine	Strattera	1.2–1.8 mg/kg

Figure 23-F

- No addiction potential
- Clinical effects (generally seen within five to forty days after initiating treatment) typically last twenty-four hours a day
- Can treat comorbid depression

Depression

Serious depression in children and young adolescents likely heralds the onset of severe and highly recurrent unipolar depressions (35 percent) or bipolar disorder (48 percent) (Geller et al. 2002; Geller and DelBello 2003). Seventy percent of people with prepubertal bipolar disorder initially present with depression, and on average have between two and four depressive episodes prior to their first mania. There has been growing concern that the use of antidepressants may be risky in bipolar patients (potentially exacerbating a manic episode or causing cycle acceleration). Thus the clinician must conduct a comprehensive evaluation to rule out potential bipolarity in all depressed children and teenagers. The following history and clinical features should alert the clinician to a higher risk of bipolar disorder:

- Atypical depressive symptoms (e.g., hypersomnia, severe fatigue, increased appetite, and weight gain)
- Seasonal (winter) depressions
- History of separation anxiety disorder
- History of ADHD or ADHD-like symptoms
- Positive family history of bipolar disorder
- History of hypomania

Diagnostic Issues

Although there are similarities between childhood-onset and adult-onset major depression, there are also notable differences. Using standard *DSM-IV-TR* criteria for diagnosing major depression failed to accurately diagnose 76 percent of young children judged to be suffering with major depression (Luby et al. 2002). For more diagnostic precision, these authors recommend modified *DSM-IV-TR* criteria using the following instead.

- Depressed or irritable mood for more days than not
- Plus four of the following (versus five required for adults):
  - Anhedonia
  - Significant weight loss or gain
  - Insomnia or hypersomnia more days than not
  - Psychomotor agitation or retardation
  - Fatigue more days than not
  - Feelings of worthlessness or excessive guilt
  - Impaired concentration
  - Recurrent thoughts of death or suicide

Also, in children, irritable and anhedonic mood is more common than a sad or depressed mood. See figure 23-G for a list of additional depressive symptoms.

Diagnostic Signs and Symptoms of Major Depression in Children

Most Common Symptoms
- Irritability
- Anhedonia
- Play themes of death, suicide, or self-destruction
- Social withdrawal
- Low self-esteem
- Vegetative symptoms (e.g., sleep disturbance)

Common Symptoms
- School failure
- Sadness
- Loneliness
- Low energy

Associated Signs and Symptoms
- Vague, nonspecific physical complaints
- Being bored
- Reckless behavior; acting out
- Substance use/abuse
- Running away from home
- Extreme sensitivity to rejection or failure
- Difficulty with relationships

Figure 23-G

Psychopharmacology of Depression

Early case reports and clinical experience have shown that *very severely depressed, hospitalized* children and adolescents often did respond to treatment with tricyclic antidepressants (Walkup 2004). However, tricyclics are plagued by significant side effects, they are very toxic in overdoses, and there have been six cases of sudden death in children (due to cardiac effects with the tricyclic desipramine). Thus, in this chapter we will address only the newer antidepressants, which are much safer and have more benign side effects.

To date, the double-blind, placebo-controlled studies of antidepressants in the treatment of major depression have been limited to SSRIs and one study of venlafaxine (although drugs such as bupropion are in common use and other classes of drugs are undergoing trials). Placebo responses in these child studies are higher than those seen in adult studies (in most adult studies, placebo response rates are about 25 percent, and placebo rates in child studies, typically, are 35 percent). Thus, to be judged to be statistically significantly better than placebo, the drug must have a very high level of demonstrated efficacy and large sample sizes. The limited studies in this area of investigation reveal that SSRIs are much better tolerated than tricyclics and are significantly more effective than either placebos or tricyclics (Emslie and Mayes 2001; Wagner et al. 2003; March et al. 2004; Whittington et al. 2004). However, the effect sizes are small. A meta-analysis of studies by Jureidini et al. (2004) shows an effect size across six randomized, placebo-controlled studies of just 0.26. This is a very small effect size and *may* suggest that antidepressant efficacy is only slightly superior to placebos.

However, it is important to note that most of the studies reviewed in this meta-analysis suffered from significant methodological flaws (Walkup 2004). These studies were supported by pharmaceutical companies and done largely in response to an FDA incentive: "Companies could extend their patents for a drug for six months by testing it on children ... whether the trial demonstrated that the drug worked or not. There was, in other words, a powerful incentive to do the trials, but no incentive to do them well" (Mahler 2004, 59).

A more recent, large-scale, federally funded program, Treatments for Adolescents with Depression Study (TADS) has addressed many of the methodological issues raised in other studies. The sample included 432 adolescents (ages twelve to seventeen) suffering from major depression. The subjects were randomly assigned to one of four groups. After twelve weeks of treatment, the percentages of responders were placebo: 35 percent, cognitive-behavioral therapy (CBT): 43 percent, fluoxetine (Prozac): 61 percent, and combination CBT and fluoxetine: 71 percent. Here drug treatments were significantly better than placebo or psychotherapy alone. The effect sizes were 0.8 and 0.6 for the combination treatment and fluoxetine

Antidepressants, Children, Teens, and Suicidality

There has been a good deal of media attention regarding potential risks of antidepressants and increased suicidality (especially in children and adolescents). The initial concern came from studies in England that raised concerns about increased suicidality in young patients treated with the antidepressant Paxil. In this study, which included 1,300 patients, Paxil was compared to placebo, and reports of increased suicidality were seen in 1.2 percent of placebo and 3.4 percent of Paxil-treated subjects (unpublished data referred to in Aursnes et al. 2005). This difference is statistically significant. It is important to note that there were no actual suicides in this group of youngsters and a number of so-called suicidal "events" occurred in the Paxil group when the children *stopped* taking the medication (data continued to be collected for a period of twenty-eight days following discontinuation).

In trying to understand and address this issue, one significant problem is that the concept of "suicidality" has been very loosely defined in this and other studies. Most times it include reports of increased thoughts about suicide, suicide gestures, non–lethal-intent self-mutilation (as is often seen in borderline personality disorders), and, in one instance, even a report of a child slapping herself qualifying as a suicide attempt (Brown University 2004). Of course, actual suicides and lethal attempts are also included under this umbrella of *suicidality*.

Concerns regarding increased suicidality have had a significant impact. Currently, the United Kingdom Committee on Safety of Medications has banned the

continued

use of all antidepressants in patients under age eighteen, with the exception of fluoxetine (Prozac). In the United States, the FDA has also responded to concerns about increased suicidality by requiring drug companies to issue warnings about the use of these drugs with younger clients. They also initiated a study to investigate the data: They are currently evaluating a database of 4,400 teenagers treated with antidepressants, and final conclusions are pending. It is interesting to note that in this large group of adolescents treated with SSRIs, there have been no suicides. It has also been documented that in geographic areas where antidepressants are in widespread use, suicide rates have dropped among adolescents (Mahler 2004).

Even though the likelihood of increased suicidality may be low in large group studies, the clinician must be on the lookout for the emergence of suicidal tendencies in all patients who suffer from major depression. It is certainly possible that in some cases the drug can contribute to this problem. The following may account for increased suicidality seen in some individuals treated with antidepressants:

- Activation and increased restlessness may add to a general sense of emotional discomfort.

- Antidepressants can provoke dysphoric mania in some youngsters who, in fact, have bipolar disorder (this may be one of the more common reasons for treatment-emergent suicidality).

- Increased energy may occur before a decrease in dysphoric mood (the person then has the energy to carry out a suicide attempt).

continued

alone, respectively (March et al. 2004; Glass 2004). These results, obviously, are more promising.

In evaluating the commonly found high placebo response rates, it is very important to keep in mind that although acute treatment placebo responses in children are generally high, no study has evaluated the ability of placebos to prevent breakthrough symptoms or to reduce recurrence. Currently available efficacy studies are limited in duration (eight to eighteen weeks), and there is an absence of long-term follow-up. Typically, positive placebo responses, if they occur, tend to be time-limited. Owing to the highly recurrent nature of depression in youngsters, the issue of longer-term effects is crucial, although no systematic data exist to address this issue.

Two findings that are important to note from these empirical studies and clinical experience appear to be that (1) the time to onset of positive mediation effects may be longer for children than for adults (with children, although symptomatic improvement may be noted within four weeks, in some instances an adequate trial of eight to twelve weeks may be required); and (2) a syndrome of apathy/amotivation or emotional disinhibition, sometimes seen in adults on chronic SSRI treatment, is more commonly encountered in children (Walkup 2004; Barnhart, Makela, and Latocha 2004).

With children, treatment is started with low doses for the first week or two and then, if tolerated, gradually increased. The reason for a low starting dose is that approximately 5 percent of children have a condition referred to as 2D6 hypometabolism. The liver enzyme 2D6 is responsible for metabolizing a number of antidepressant (and other) drugs. In these children, there is inadequate first-pass metabolism resulting in high blood levels of a drug (and thus, very significant side effects). Were they to be started on higher doses, the initial side effects could be overwhelming, thus the starting low-dose strategy. This is especially important not only because of the need to reduce the unpleasantness of side effects. Additionally, if parents notice acute onset side effects happening with their children, they may (and often do) conclude that psychiatric medications are dangerous or too problematic for their child, and they may never again be open to the notion of psychiatric medication treatments.

In other respects, the treatment with children and adolescents is similar to that with adults (see chapter 16).

Bipolar Disorder

The average age of onset of bipolar disorder is nineteen years of age (APA 2002, 386). However, it is becoming clear that there are cases of childhood onset. This is an area of investigation where the jury is still out. A good deal of controversy exists about the prevalence of very-early-onset bipolar disorder, but it may be that up to 27 percent of cases first emerge in late childhood or early adolescence.

Diagnostic Issues

As mentioned above, 70 percent of cases of early-onset bipolar illness first become manifest in major depressive episodes; 30 percent begin with mania or hypomania. The signs and symptoms of childhood-onset mania (figure 23-H) differ from the adult presentation of the disorder (the more typical, adult version generally is seen to emerge as early as ages fifteen to sixteen).

An important and often difficult differential diagnosis to make is childhood mania versus ADHD. This is complicated by the likelihood that, although bipolar and ADHD may represent distinct disease entities, there is a considerable amount of symptom overlap (see figure 23-I).

Possible diagnoses of comorbidities may exist, including:

■ ADHD and bipolar disorder are two separate diagnoses that are comorbid in some children.

■ In *some presumably* ADHD children, the symptoms may be a prodrome of bipolar disorder (i.e., may be an early manifestation of the disorder). Note:

■ Noncompliance.

■ Patient-initiated discontinuation: There are two common, problematic results that might account for increased suicidality; antidepressant withdrawal symptoms and/or the loss of what had been a positive antidepressant effect, plunging the patient back into depression.

What is clear is that untreated major depression carries significant risks of potential suicide, antidepressants take several weeks of treatment before the first signs of clinical improvement, and depression can worsen during this start-up period of treatment. In evaluating these kinds of concerns, it is always important to differentiate between media hype and scientific data. For parents who may be interested in this issue, refer them to the NIMH website: www.nimh.nih.gov.

Signs and Symptoms of Early-Onset Bipolar Mania
(Papolos and Papolos 2007)

■ Nonepisodic (more continuous)
■ Mixed mania is most typical with marked dysphoria and irritability
■ Intense rage episodes
■ Severe oppositional behavior
■ Ultrarapid cycling (extreme emotional lability)

Figure 23-H

Symptomatic Similarities: ADHD and Childhood-Onset Mania

- Irritability
- Inattention
- Hyperactivity
- Impulsivity
- High level of energy
- Pressured speech
- Chronic and nonepisodic

Figure 23-I

Most ADHD children do not go on to develop bipolar illness, and most bipolar patients do not have early ADHD-like symptoms. Thus there may be a subtype of bipolar illness that simply presents with early signs that mimic ADHD.

- Baroni and colleagues (2009), acknowledging that there is debate about the clinical manifestations and differential diagnosis between ADHD and bipolar disorder, reviewed the literature to seek further clarity on this diagnostic distinction. One of the conclusions is that a diagnosis of mania must include a distinct change in mood along with cognitive and behavioral changes. In other words, ADHD symptoms, such as distractibility and agitation, should not be considered in making a diagnosis of mania unless those symptoms increase over baseline at the same time there is a change in mood.

Differentiating Bipolar Disorder from ADHD

Symptoms common to bipolar but very rare with ADHD[a,b]:

- Decreased need for sleep without daytime fatigue
- Intense, prolonged rage attacks (lasting two to four hours)
- Hypersexuality
- Flight of ideas
- Morbid nightmares[b]
- Psychotic symptoms

Family history of clear-cut bipolar disorder or one or more of the following in blood relatives:

- Suicide
- Severe alcohol/drug abuse
- Multiple marriages
- Starting numerous businesses
- Hyperthymia (a form of chronic hypomania characterized by high energy and productivity, gregariousness, impulsive behavior, and decreased need for sleep)

a Geller, Craney, et al. (2003), 25–50
b Popper (2004)

Figure 23-J

- Childhood-onset bipolar disorder may be related to other bipolar spectrum conditions but represents a particular subtype of mood disorder (i.e., it is in some ways different from adult-onset bipolar conditions).

An accurate diagnosis is important because inappropriate medical treatment may worsen the clinical condition (e.g., stimulants or antidepressants may cause cycle acceleration in bipolar patients). Figure 23-J lists clinical features and other factors that help to differentiate ADHD from bipolar illnesses.

Psychopharmacology of Bipolar Disorder

The choice of treatment will depend on the current clinical presentation.

Major depression where bipolar disorder is suspected

- Since antidepressants may provoke switching or cycle acceleration, they should be avoided as a monotherapy.

- Mood stabilizers (see chapter 17) that have some antidepressant actions should be used first (e.g., lithium, quetiapine, or olanzapine-fluoxetine combination. Note: lamotrigine is an effective treatment for bipolar depression, but owing to an increased risk of severe rashes, it may not be a first-line medication for children).

- Combinations of mood stabilizers (e.g., lithium and divalproex).

Mania

- If there is a very severe agitation, benzodiazepines or second-generation antipsychotics may be administered. Lithium and anticonvulsant mood stabilizers often take seven to fourteen days to begin reducing symptoms. Benzodiazepines and second-generation antipsychotics may begin to work in several hours.

- Head-to-head comparisons of mood stabilizers fail to show that any one mood stabilizer is superior (at least in group studies). Thus the choice of treatment often is based on the side-effect profile of the medication. Ultimately, the majority of children with mania must be treated with two or more mood stabilizers in combination to achieve a good outcome (Kowatch et al. 2000; Emslie and Mayes 2001; Geller, Biederman et al. 2003).

- Second-generation antipsychotics (e.g., olanzapine) may also be added to mood stabilizers.

- Although widely used, gabapentin is an ineffective monotherapy for mania. It may, however, be useful as an add-on drug, especially in reducing anxiety.

- Atypical antipsychotics may also be used, usually added to other agents. Patients should be monitored for side effects, especially metabolic syndrome (weight gain, type II diabetes mellitus, and hyperlipidemia).

- The antipsychotic quetiapine is FDA approved for treating both mania and bipolar depression in adults and has recently been shown to have efficacy in the treatment of childhood-onset bipolar disorder.

Comorbid ADHD and bipolar disorder

■ Initiate treatment with mood stabilizers.

■ Once stability has been achieved, stimulants may be gradually added.

Details regarding side effects and drug interactions for what is often very complex polypharmacy are beyond the scope of this book. However, we would like to highlight some side effects and drug interactions that can be especially problematic for children and teenagers.

Lithium

■ Increased thirst, urination, and bedwetting

■ Weight gain (seen in 30 to 40 percent of patients)

■ Aggravation of acne

■ Tremor

■ Cognitive impairment

■ Sedation

■ Frequent blood tests are required, which may be very hard for young children to tolerate

Mood-stabilizing anticonvulsants

■ Weight gain (especially with carbamazepine and divalproex)

■ Menstrual irregularities

■ Polycystic ovaries (with divalproex)

■ Tremor

■ Sedation

Interactions

■ Be especially alert to the likelihood that carbamazepine, oxazepine, and topiramate can reduce levels of birth control pills, rendering them ineffective.

Childhood-onset bipolar disorder may be a more severe version of the disorder. Early recognition, accurate diagnosis, appropriate acute treatment, and ongoing maintenance treatment are necessary not only for reducing the intense suffering, but also to prevent kindling and suicide (which is an all-too-common outcome of untreated or poorly treated bipolar disorder in young people).

Anxiety Disorders

Anxiety disorders are the most common psychiatric conditions in childhood, affecting 5 to 18 percent of children (Pine et al. 1998). They not only cause significant emotional suffering but can often markedly interfere with academic performance, the development of peer relationships, the acquisition of social skills, and interpersonal competency. Anxiety disorders arising in childhood and early adolescence frequently herald the onset of what may become lifelong psychiatric disorders, and they are often comorbid with other psychiatric illnesses (especially common with bipolar disorder and ADHD).

Diagnostic Issues

In most children experiencing clinically significant anxiety, the cause is situational stress (e.g., parents going through a divorce, exposure to domestic violence, witnessing parental arguments, sexual abuse, or the effects of a parent abusing alcohol or other drugs). In most instances, these types of anxiety reactions respond best to psychotherapeutic interventions, where medication treatment is not necessary.

Other anxiety disorders that arise in childhood or early adolescence include:

- Inhibited temperament: A genetically influenced temperamental style that affects 10 to 15 percent of children (Kagan 1998) and can lead to:

  - Timidity and anxiety in novel situations

  - Behavioral inhibition

  - Persistent vigilance

  - Heightened autonomic arousal

  - A clinically significant anxiety disorder later in life for approximately one-third of children born with this temperamental style.

- Obsessive-compulsive disorder: The lifetime prevalence rate is 2.5 percent (APA 2000, 460) with one-third having childhood onset. The symptoms in children are essentially the same as seen in adults with OCD.

- Separation anxiety disorder: The prevalence rate is 4 percent of children and young adolescents (APA 2000, 123). This is manifest by significant distress when away from home or separated from parents or other major attachment figures. It often also presents as school avoidance and somatic complaints (e.g., stomachaches).

- Social phobia/social anxiety disorder: Lifetime prevalence rates may be as high as 13 percent, with most cases beginning in mid-adolescence (APA 2000, 453). A critical factor for children is that this form of anxiety almost invariably leads to social withdrawal, and children thus miss out on a number of important experiences necessary for the development of social skills. Loneliness, low self-esteem, depression, and substance use or abuse are common consequences of untreated social phobia.

- Generalized anxiety disorder (includes overanxious disorder of childhood): Lifetime prevalence is 5 percent, one-half with childhood or adolescent onset (APA 2000, 474). As with adults, GAD is characterized by excessive worry.

- Post-traumatic stress disorder: Prevalence rates in children and young teenagers are not well established. In addition to typical PTSD symptoms (see chapter 12), young children often present with the following (APA 2000, 466):

  - Generalized nightmares of monsters or of being threatened

  - Tendency to represent the trauma in repetitive play

- Stomachaches and headaches

- Specific phobias: Most are not severe and are time limited. However, it is important to note that with clinically significant specific phobias, 70 percent of youngsters have another comorbid psychiatric disorder, which may at first not be readily apparent (Walkup 2002). Thus it is important to be watchful for coexisting psychopathology.

- Panic disorder: Very rare in children and young teenagers. Generally, panic disorder may first be seen in older adolescents (APA 2000, 436). If isolated panic attacks are seen in children and younger teens, it is important to inquire about possible, significant psychological stressors.

Psychopharmacology of Anxiety Disorders

The research on medication treatment for anxiety disorders in children is sparse (with the exception of treatment of obsessive-compulsive disorder). Thus this overview is limited. (For more extensive reviews, see Coghill 2003).

Obsessive-compulsive disorder

- Serotonin reuptake inhibitors are the standard first-line treatment (sertraline, fluvoxamine, and clomipramine are FDA-approved for use in children) (Geller, Biederman et al. 2003; March et al. 1998). A meta-analysis of twelve studies (total N = 1044) reveals a positive but modest effect size (0.46) for treatment with SSRIs and clomipramine (Geller, Biederman, et al. 2003).

- The response to medication treatment is gradual and improvement may be expected to continue during the first twelve months. Symptomatic improvement generally plateaus at about twelve months (see figure 23-K).

- Treatment-resistant cases sometimes respond to SSRIs augmented with low doses of clomipramine (e.g., 10 to 50 mg a day), lithium, or second-generation antipsychotics (e.g., risperidone).

Symptomatic Improvement of OCD Symptoms in Medication Responders with Treatment with SSRIs

Duration of Treatment	% of Symptom Reduction
6–10 weeks	25–30%
18–24 weeks	40–50%
52 weeks	>50%

Source: Walkup (2002); Cook et al. (2001); Thomsen, Ebbesen, and Persson (2001)

Figure 23-K

Separation anxiety disorder, social anxiety disorder, generalized anxiety disorder

■   These three disorders may be related. Not uncommonly, children with separation anxiety later go on to develop social anxiety and/or generalized anxiety disorder.

■   If school refusal is a part of the presenting problem, often short-term use of a benzodiazepine can be helpful (antidepressants, discussed below, require several weeks of treatment before the onset of symptoms reduction). Generally, the longer children avoid school, the more difficult it is to return. Thus benzodiazepines can provide almost immediate relief and may help the child re-enter school quickly. Antidepressants are coadministered, with the onset of symptom reduction generally occurring in four to eight weeks. Once the SSRI provides benefits, the benzodiazepine can be gradually discontinued.

■   SSRIs appear to be very robust in treatment effects. In a large randomized, placebo-controlled study (Walkup et al. 2001), 128 children (ages six to seventeen) with a diagnosis of separation, social, or generalized anxiety disorder were treated with the SSRI fluvoxamine (for eight weeks at a maximum dose of 300 mg per day). Seventy-six percent of the fluvoxamine group had significant improvement, with an effect size of 1.1 (this is considered to be an impressive response and among the highest effect sizes reported in the treatment of any pediatric psychiatric disorder). Other SSRIs must be subjected to systematic research, but such treatment is quite promising.

Post-traumatic stress disorder

■   Well-controlled research in this area of pharmacologic treatment with children is lacking. Typically SSRIs are used as a first-line agent with positive outcomes similar to those seen in adults (Donnelly 2003; Seedat et al. 2002); however, these findings are based on case reports and open-label studies.

Specific phobias

■   As noted above, if phobias are severe, always look carefully for underlying comorbidity. Most phobias can be treated with standard exposure-based cognitive-behavioral treatment. For conditions that require urgent attention (e.g., fears of dental procedures), benzodiazepines can be used. See chapter 12 for additional, basic treatment guidelines.

Panic disorder

■   See guidelines outlined in chapters 9, 16, and 18.

Miscellaneous Disorders

Psychotic Disorders

Early-onset schizophrenia is rare. There is increasing evidence that psychotic symptoms in children and younger adolescents are much more likely to be associated with mood disorders. Thus, in such cases, effective medication treatment must always include the use of antidepressants and/or mood stabilizers. However, psychotic symptoms in young people, regardless of the specific diagnosis, are generally treated with second-generation antipsychotics. Traditional antipsychotics are associated with significant side effects, including tardive dyskinesia. Newer-generation antipsychotics (olanzapine, ziprasidone, paliperidone, aripiprazole, risperidone, paliperidone, and quetiapine) are much better tolerated. However, it must be noted that weight gain and extrapyramidal side effects (such as dyskinesias) are more common in children and young adolescents than in adults. Most studies, to date, have been open-label studies (risperidone and olanzapine) that have indicated positive outcomes in the treatment of psychosis in children (American Academy of Child and Adolescent Psychiatry 2001). There are also reports of the use of clozaril in treating treatment-refractory cases; however, the frequent blood draws and monitoring for agranulocytosis are difficult for children to tolerate, thus clozaril should be seen as a treatment of last resort (Coghill 2003).

Autism Spectrum Disorders (Autism and Asperger's Syndrome)

No medication has been found that treats core symptoms of these developmental disorders. However, certain associated target symptoms may respond to pharmacologic interventions (see figure 23-L). Several agents, including fenfluramine, secretin, naltrexone, vitamin B_6, and corticosteroids, have been purported to be effective but have not been found to be effective in cross-validation studies.

The hormone oxytocin has been shown to be effective in treating autistic spectrum disorders in experimental subjects. More studies are needed, but this appears to be a medication that holds promise for treating this very difficult to treat set of disorders.

Medication Treatment for Target Symptoms Associated with Autism Spectrum Disorders

Symptoms	Medication
Aggression	Second-generation antipsychotics[a, b, c]
Self-injurious behaviors	Second-generation antipsychotics[a, b, c]
Hyperactivity	Alpha-2 agonists; stimulants[d]
Repetitive behaviors, rituals, compulsions	SSRIs, clomipramine[e, f]
Pro-social behavior	oxytocin[g]

a Hardan et al. (1996); b Nicolson, Awad, and Sloman (1998); c McCracken et al. (2002); d Quintana et al. (1995); e McDougle et al. (1996); f Coghill (2003); g Hollander et al. 2007; Kosfeld et al. 2005; Petrovic et al. 2008

Figure 23-L

Medications for Treating Children and Adolescents (Psychostimulants)

Generic Name	Brand Name	Average Daily Dosage Range[a] (mg/day)	Side Effects (usually diminish; may require attention if persist)	Side Effects Requiring Immediate Attention	Significant Drug Interactions[b] (not all-inclusive)
Amphetamine	Amphetamine	5–70	■ Dizziness	■ Agitation	■ Anticoagulants
Amphetamine mixture	Adderall	5–40	■ Nervousness	■ Bruising or bleeding	(blood thinners)
Atomoxetine	Strattera	40–100	■ Blurred vision	■ Confusion	■ Anticonvulsants
Dexmethylphenidate	Focalin	5–40	■ Difficulty	■ Dark-colored urine	■ Beta blockers
Dextroamphetamine	Dexedrine	5–40	sleeping	■ Excitation or mania	■ Caffeine
Lisdexamfetamine	Vyvanse	30–70	■ Decreased	■ Extreme eye or skin sensi-	■ Digoxin
Methylphenidate	Ritalin	5–50	appetite	tivity to sunlight	■ MAOI
	Concerta	5–54	■ Weight loss	■ Fast or irregular heart rate	antidepressants
	Metadate	5–50	■ Headache	■ Fatigue or weakness	■ Other stimu-
			■ Nausea	■ Fever, or flu-like symptoms	lant medications
			■ Dry mouth	■ Increased blood pressure	(decongestants, diet
				■ Persistent throbbing	pills, some asthma
				headache	medications)
				■ Seizures	■ SSRI antidepressants
				■ Shortness of breath	■ Thyroid medications
				■ Skin rash or itching	■ Tricyclic
				■ Sore mouth, gums, or throat	antidepressants
				■ Splotchy purplish darkening	
				of the skin	
				■ Swelling of the face	
				■ Tics	
				■ Mood or behavior changes	
				■ Vomiting	
				■ Yellow eyes or skin	

Warnings/Precautions

■ Not indicated during pregnancy or while breastfeeding
■ Liver or kidney impairment may require dosage adjustment
  or discontinuation of treatment
■ Can trigger mania/hypomania
■ Height/Weight monitoring in children
■ Alcohol/substance abuse
■ Cardiac monitoring as indicated
■ Increased intraocular pressure
■ Lowered seizure threshold
■ Tourette syndrome
■ Hyperthyroidism

a There are numerous products and dosage forms and strengths available for psychostimulants.
b There is variability in the potential for a specific stimulant to interact with the drugs listed.
c Atomoxetine (Strattera) is technically an antidepressant, not a stimulant, but it is FDA approved for the treatment of ADHD.

Epilogue

On the Horizon

These are exciting times in mental health and the neurosciences: new discoveries are being made each month. As this book goes to press, no less than two dozen new psychotropic medications are in the various phases of prerelease investigation and research. There is great promise for continued breakthroughs: new medications that may provide more safe, effective, and selective treatments for mental disorders.

There have been many advances in psychopharmacology over the past fifty years and new treatments that have progressively resulted in decreases in emotional despair in many millions of people suffering from psychiatric disorders. Yet, in closing, we want to strongly underscore the importance of the human relationship in psychiatric treatment. Ultimately, loneliness, alienation, hopelessness, and demoralization are not to be cured with chemicals but, rather, must be addressed in the arena of human contact and understanding. This is what psychotherapists do best. And, in collaboration with our medical colleagues, we can make a real difference in the lives of our clients.

Appendix A

Pharmacokinetics

This appendix provides an expanded discussion of the pharmacokinetics of psychotherapeutic agents presented in chapter 4. It is intended for therapists with a special interest in this area or for those who actively comanage medication-treated patients.

Absorption

Absorption is important not only as the initial step in the pharmacokinetic process, but also as a determinant of a crucial clinical parameter called *bioavailability*, defined as the amount of drug reaching systemic circulation (Winter 1988). The amount of the drug that is bioavailable is usually expressed as a percentage of the administered dose. Medications directly injected into a vein (intravenous) are nearly 100 percent bioavailable, whereas orally administered drugs produce variable patterns of bioavailability. For instance, demonstrated oral bioavailability for some antipsychotics and certain tricyclic antidepressants ranges from 30 to 60 percent (Hollister 1992). Bioavailability may be decreased by a physiological process called the *first-pass effect*, in which a significant amount of the drug is metabolized before reaching the bloodstream. Most tricyclics undergo extensive first-pass metabolism, contributing to their relatively low bioavailability.

The therapist may encounter the clinical ramifications of bioavailability in regard to the issue of generic medications. Bioavailability is the benchmark measurement for determining bioequivalence between brand name and generic products. With many medications, generic formulations meet bioavailability standards and can provide economical alternatives to brand-name products. This can be an important issue for psychiatric patients with limited financial resources, who often will simply quit taking their medications because of the expense or will take them sporadically to "make them last longer."

However, absolute bioequivalence is not guaranteed for all generic products. Although the active ingredient may be quantitatively the same as in the brand-name product, there may be differences in the manufacturing process or in the physical properties of the final preparation that can affect the rate and extent of drug absorption. From a practical standpoint, the patient may experience a variable or inadequate response from the generic product. Although this does not occur frequently, it is a factor to consider when a patient responds atypically to a drug—especially with medications that have a narrow therapeutic index, such as anticonvulsants and tricyclic antidepressants. Psychotropics with periodic reports of generic unequivalence include nortriptyline and carbamazepine. Advise patients taking these medications to avoid frequent switches from brand to generic preparations and changes between generic manufacturers.

Distribution

Distribution of a medication throughout the body is a two-phase process. Initially, distribution is preferential for organs with a rich supply of blood flow, such as the kidney, liver, heart, and brain. In the second phase, the drug moves into areas with less extensive circulation, such as muscle and fat tissue. In chapter 4 these latter areas of the body are referred to as *reservoirs*, sometimes called *compartments*. Eventually (usually within several minutes), equilibrium is established. At equilibrium, the process of drug distribution is completed, and the flow of the drug between compartments is relatively stable. When, as for most drugs, equilibrium is reached rapidly, the body as a whole is considered to be a single compartment, and the distribution pattern is referred to as a *single-compartment model*. In this case it is assumed that the drug is uniformly distributed throughout the body; in other words, the serum level of the drug is equal to the concentration in organs and tissues.

Some psychotherapeutic medications, however, demonstrate "two-compartment" distribution. In the two-compartment model, equilibrium is reached more slowly because of significant movement of the drugs into muscle and fat cells. Also distribution is not uniform throughout the body. Depending on the physical or chemical properties of the drug, and upon the physiological state of the patient, the drug can be unequally distributed between organs and reservoirs. Ultimately, large concentrations of medications can accumulate in deep reservoir areas.

Due to individual physiologic differences, there can be wide variations in effective dosages of the same medication from patient to patient. Also, when a medication is stopped (by either therapeutic plan or noncompliance), complete elimination of the drug does not occur immediately, or even within known half-life parameters. This partially explains why recurrence of psychosis may not immediately appear in the noncompliant schizophrenic and why depressive symptoms reemerge weeks (or days) after an antidepressant is discontinued. (The therapist can help educate the patient as to the potential consequences of medication discontinuation.)

Circulating in the plasma are various proteins to which medications can attach. This process is called *protein binding* and provides another reservoir area for drugs. Only the unbound, or "free," molecules of a drug are able to cross cell membranes and reach an eventual site of action; thus a bound drug is inactive, whereas an unbound drug is active. Most psychotropic medications are bound extensively to serum proteins, usually albumin. Laboratory monitoring results typically indicate a total concentration that includes both bound and unbound drug molecules.

Metabolism

Metabolism (biotransformation) of most drugs primarily occurs through the action of enzymes located predominately in the liver. Metabolic enzymes are also found in the gastrointestinal tract (in bacteria and intestinal tissue), the kidney, the lung, and the placenta. This system, comprised of more than thirty related enzymes, is called the *mixed function oxidase* (MFO) or *cytochrome P450 system*. These enzymes are iron-containing proteins, located in the endoplasmic reticulum, that serve to mediate the process of electron and proton transfer during drug metabolism. The intended result of drug metabolism is the transformation of the original compound into one that is more readily eliminated by the kidney. In general, this means converting drugs that are more lipid-soluble to ones that are more water-soluble. The most common enzymes involved in drug metabolism are known by the following designations: 1A2, 2A6, 2C9, 2C19, 2D6, 2E1, and 3A4. The majority of drugs and naturally occurring compounds are metabolized by the CYP3A4 isoenzyme, both in the liver and in the gastrointestinal tract (Benet, Kroetz, and Sheiner 1996; Michalets 1998).

Drug metabolism takes place through a series of chemical reactions, categorized as phase I and phase II. Specific types of phase I reactions are oxidation, reduction, and hydrolysis. Oxidation is the most important type of phase I reaction. Phase I reactions are also called nonsynthetic because the original molecule undergoes degradation via electron loss. Oxygen serves as the electron acceptor. Phase I reactions are likely to yield molecules that are not significantly different from the original, and they commonly have pharmacologic activity. During this oxidative process, highly reactive, or even toxic, free radical compounds may be formed.

Phase II reactions involve the coupling, or conjugation, of the drug molecule with other compounds, such as an amino acid. These reactions are also known as synthetic reactions. Products of phase II reactions are often considerably different from the original and are usually inactive. Many drugs are metabolized sequentially, first by phase I, and then by phase II reactions. Some drugs are metabolized via only phase I or only phase II reactions.

Not all biotransformation reactions result in terminal, deactivated, nontoxic products. There are notable reactive, toxic compounds formed with many routinely used drugs. Examples are the hepatotoxicity seen with the common pain reliever acetaminophen, and nonsteroidal anti-inflammatory agents, such as ibuprofen, or isoniazid, which is used to treat tuberculosis.

The by-products of metabolism are called metabolites. Compared to the original drug, often called the parent compound, metabolites can be more active, less active, or inactive. As discussed in chapter 4, metabolites may possess similar activity to the original drug. These active metabolites may contribute to the intended effect of the medication. Metabolites can also demonstrate different properties than the parent drug. An example is seen in the substantially longer half-lives that metabolites of some benzodiazepines exhibit compared to the parent compounds, which can potentially lead to drug accumulation.

Metabolic Drug Interactions

The amount and activity of these enzymes are subject to change, especially when medications are co-administered. Significant drug interactions result from metabolic disruptions secondary to multiple medications. The fact that the particular enzymes involved in metabolizing many drugs have not been identified complicates the assessment and management of metabolic drug interactions. The two mechanisms by which enzyme activity is altered are enzyme induction and enzyme inhibition.

Induction takes place when the activity and amount of enzyme are increased. The result is usually a reduced serum concentration of the object drug by the precipitant drug. Another consequence of enzyme induction is the increased formation of toxic metabolites. Enzyme induction can result from a medication, such as carbamazepine (Tegretol), or a condition like smoking. Enzyme induction generally follows a gradual time course for both onset and dissipation. A two-to-three week time period is required for the production of new enzymes and for maximum effect to be achieved. Degradation and elimination of the increased enzymes require a similar, if not longer, period of time.

Inhibition occurs when there is a decrease in either production or activity of enzymes. The latter is usually secondary to enzyme competition at the binding site. This results in an increased serum concentration of the object drug. Such increases can be precipitous and, depending on the drugs involved, can lead to serious side effects and/or toxicity. Enzyme inhibition can result from a medication, such as cimetidine (Tagamet), or from a disease state, such as cirrhosis or hepatitis. Enzyme inhibition can be rapid, occurring within hours.

Anticipating, recognizing, and treating drug interactions present significant challenges in the use of medications, including psychotropics. Drug interactions may produce a range of outcomes, from toxicity to loss of desired effect. Drug interactions involving altered metabolism are the most common, the most widely researched, and present the greatest potential for undesirable medication effects. For example, recent attention has focused on drug interactions with SSRI and newer mixed-mechanism antidepressants. These antidepressants present potentially significant capacity to inhibit several key cytochrome P450 enzymes.

Another area of relevance in psychiatric practice are the drug-interactive effects of alcohol, which pose unique challenges. With acute ingestion, alcohol competitively blocks metabolic oxidation and, as such, is considered an enzyme inhibitor. Conversely, with chronic alcohol ingestion, enzyme induction occurs. Additionally, prescribers must take into account the physiological changes associated with chronic alcohol use, such as cirrhotic liver damage, which decreases drug-metabolizing capacity, or decreased serum albumin, which results in more "free" or active drug being available.

Throughout this book, key drug interactions are addressed. It is important to note, however, that there are real limitations in this field of study. The inherent research and interpretive challenges are described in detail by Greenblatt et al. (1998) and summarized below:

- Difficulty in identifying specific cytochrome P450 enzymes due to limitations of in vitro models

- Complexities involved in designing and conducting in vivo pharmacokinetic research studies

- Great interindividual variability in enzyme-metabolizing capabilities

- Assessing reliability of reported information

The study of drug interactions, especially those involving metabolism, is a highly complex, rapidly evolving field. Arriving at a clear understanding of clinical implications is greatly challenging to prescribers. Published information should be evaluated critically, especially if it is clearly promotional in nature.

There are several reliable, primary drug-interaction resources that physicians and pharmacists routinely consult.

Therapeutic Index

A critical pharmacokinetic parameter that directs safe and effective medication use is the *therapeutic index*. This parameter establishes a quantitative comparison between a drug's effective concentration and its toxic concentration. The closer these measurements are, the narrower the index, and therefore the more care that must be taken in prescribing. Lithium and anticonvulsants, for example, have narrow therapeutic indices.

Appendix B

Pharmacotherapy in Special Populations

Pregnancy

One of the most difficult dilemmas facing physicians is medication management in the psychiatric patient who is pregnant or considering pregnancy. Although therapists will not have to make ultimate prescribing decisions, they will undoubtedly remain involved in the patient's care. The information presented here summarizes general guidelines relevant to psychotropic medication use during pregnancy and nursing.[1]

It is important to remember that absolute data in this area is disturbingly incomplete. Experimental research obviously is limited by ethical restrictions. Animal studies are extensive but their results cannot be assumed to necessarily apply to humans. And, for infrequently prescribed medications, the available observational data are in some cases so limited that conclusions are impossible. Nevertheless, in some patients the risk of not medicating, especially in the presence of psychosis, mania, and severe depression, clearly outweighs the potential hazards to mother and child. The risk factors are these:

Risk factors associated with medications during pregnancy

- Teratogenesis (malformation of fetus or fetal organs)

---

1. Information from a variety of sources was compiled for this appendix: American Society of Health Systems Pharmacists (2012); *Facts and Comparisons* (2012); *Drug Information for the Health Care Professional* (USP-DI Drug Information for the Health Care Professional) (2007); Brown and Bryant (1992); Ereshefsky and Richards (1992); Jann (1992); Jinks and Fuerst (1992); Meyer (1992); Rubin (1992); Snodgrass (1992); Vestal, Montamat, and Nielson (1992); Briggs (2008).

- Drug effects on the growing and developing fetus

- Drug effects on labor and delivery

- Residual drug effects on the newborn (neonatal)

- Behavioral teratogenesis (long-term effects on the child resulting from drug exposure in utero)

- Pregnancy-induced changes in drug actions

- Drug effects on the breast-fed infant

Perhaps of most concern is the possibility of teratogenesis, with the risk being greatest during the period of organ formation (organogenesis) generally considered to be the first trimester. Avoiding medications as much as possible during this time can lower the risk of fetal malformation. However, since most drugs, with very few exceptions, cross the placenta, fetal medication exposure will continue throughout pregnancy. After the first trimester, safety concerns are related to effects on fetal growth and physiology, immediate and long-term effects on the child, and effects on breast-feeding. Figure B-1 provides guidelines for psychotropic medication use in pregnancy and nursing.

Psychotropic Medication Guidelines for Pregnancy and Lactation

Antidepressants:

- SSRIs and most TCAs not associated with teratogenesis, although extensive studies in humans have not been done. Animal studies with some agents indicate possible adverse effects.

- MAOIs, venlafaxine, and mirtazapine have not been studied extensively.

- Lack of adverse affects noted in animal studies with bupropion.

- Present in breast milk.

- Effects on neonate exposed to TCAs and SNRIs can include CNS depression and urinary retention.

- Inconclusive data on miscarriage rate.

- Effect on neonate exposed to SSRIs and SNRIs can include CNS depression or serotonin syndrome. There are reports of severe effects on neonates exposed to SSRIs or SNRIs during the third trimester requiring hospitalization and respiratory support.

Lithium:

- Established teratogen. First-trimester exposure strongly associated with fetal cardiac anomaly.

- For fetal lithium exposure in first trimester, consider cardiac ultrasound to detect presence or absence of malformation.

- If lithium is necessary after first trimester, dosage adjustments are necessary due to pregnancy-induced kidney function changes.

- Frequent lab monitoring is also required.

- Reductions in lithium dose are required several weeks prior to delivery.

Figure B-1

Psychotropic Medication Guidelines for Pregnancy and Lactation
(continued)

- Neonatal effects include impaired respiration, EKG and heart rate abnormalities, and renal impairment.
- Carbamazepine, clonazepam, and first-generation antipsychotics are *possible* alternatives to lithium.
- Significant concentrations in breast milk. Can cause decreased muscle tone, cyanosis, lethargy in infant. Nursing contraindicated.

Antipsychotics:

- High-potency agents may be preferred over low-potency agents.
- Establish lowest effective dose possible.
- Potential short-term abnormal neonatal motor activity.
- Possible alternative to lithium in mania.
- Present in breast milk.

Anticonvulsants:

- Carbamazepine is a probable teratogen (neural tube defects).
- Valproic acid is an established teratogen (neural tube defects).
- Lamotrigine is associated with neural tube defects.
- Carbamazapine and valproic acid both found in breast milk.

Benzodiazepines:

- Some benzodiazepines have established role in fetal abnormalities.
- Avoid use in first trimester. May need to taper dose.
- Switch to clonazepam if benzodiazepines absolutely indicated.
- Switch to tricyclic antidepressant for panic disorder if continued medication is required.
- Neonatal CNS depression, drug accumulation, and withdrawal symptoms possible.
- Excreted in breast milk. Produces drowsiness, failure to thrive in infant.

Sources: American Society of Health Systems Pharmacists (2008); *Facts and Comparisons* (2008); Drug Information for the Health Care Professional USP DI (2007); Cohen, Heller, and Rosenbaum (1989); Briggs (1992); Rubin (1992); Briggs (2008; 1992).

Figure B-1 *continued*

Geriatric Patients

Increasingly, our society is composed of greater numbers of elderly individuals, defined as sixty-five and older. Currently, the elderly constitute nearly 20 percent of the population. Consequently, psychotherapists are faced with diagnostic and treatment dilemmas specific to this population. Presented here are patterns and risks of medication use in the elderly (figure B-2) and age-specific factors contributing to adverse effects (figure B-3). Also discussed are recommended adjustments for use of psychotropics in the geriatric patient.

┌───┐

Medication Use and Risks in Geriatric Patients

■ Thirty percent of all prescription drugs are taken by people over sixty-five years of age.

■ Seventy percent of older adults self-medicate with over-the-counter products without physician or pharmacist consultation.

■ Fifty percent of accidental drug-related deaths occur in geriatric patients.

■ Adverse drug reactions occur at double the rate in geriatric patients than in other groups.

■ Common adverse drug-related effects are hip fractures, cognitive impairment, and neuroleptic-induced parkinsonism.

Figure B-2

Contributing Factors to Adverse Drug Reactions in the Elderly

■ Adverse drug reactions are proportional to the number of medications taken.

■ Elderly patients often have multiple prescribers without consolidated records.

■ Age-related factors increase the likelihood of adverse effects, such as the following:

    ■ Impaired organ function, especially decreased liver metabolism, leading to increased medication levels and effects

    ■ Multiple disease states

    ■ Exaggerated therapeutic response to medications

    ■ Increased sensitivity to side effects

■ Noncompliance in the elderly is common (usually underdosing) due to:

    ■ Complicated directions

    ■ Hearing and visual impairment

    ■ Cognitive and memory deficits

    ■ Child-resistant packaging

    ■ Cost

Figure B-3

Prescribing psychotropic medications in a population receiving numerous maintenance medications for medical conditions is inherently difficult. However, we present the following general recommendations to reduce the risk to this group.

Establish diagnosis and target symptoms

First-generation antipsychotics are frequently prescribed for geriatric patients, especially in long-term care facilities. However, these drugs may not be prescribed for psychotic symptoms but may merely be intended to control agitation and anxiety. An alternative to first-generation antipsychotics and benzodiazepines is buspirone (BuSpar).

Obtain complete medication history

Elderly people are at higher risk for developing drug-induced psychiatric symptoms from other prescribed medications, such as depression secondary to cardiovascular drugs or delirium and confusion secondary to CNS medications. Frequently, yet another medication is prescribed as a result, without the real cause of symptoms (the medication) having been identified. Also, additive drug effects are common in the elderly. For example, it is important to evaluate the total number of anticholinergic drugs before adding another one, since geriatric patients are especially prone to "anticholinergic delirium." Lastly, multiple medications (such as antihypertensives and diuretics) can increase the possibility of psychotropic-related falls.

Understand age-specific pharmacology

Some benzodiazepines, such as diazepam (Valium), chlordiazepoxide (Librium), and flurazepam (Dalmane), accumulate to a greater degree than others. Benzodiazepines considered to be safer are oxazepam (Serax), lorazepam (Ativan), and temazepam (Restoril). Additionally, the elderly in general are more likely to experience oversedation from benzodiazepines.

The most consistently predicable age-related change in drug response results from the normal decrease in kidney function that accompanies aging. This phenomenon probably contributes to the greatest number of adverse drug reactions in the elderly (Jinks and Fuerst 1992). Safe use of lithium, therefore, becomes particularly difficult. Aggressive serum-level monitoring and assessment of renal function are imperative.

Central nervous system changes are common with aging, including decreased cerebral blood flow, decreased cholinergic function, increased monoamine oxidase activity, and some brain atrophy. The result of these alterations can include the appearance of behavioral changes in the elderly and unpredictable medication response. Therefore, it is advisable to avoid frequent medication changes and not to experiment with medications in the elderly.

Adjust dosage

All psychotropics prescribed to elderly patients should begin with small doses and be titrated slowly. In addition, maintenance doses may sometimes be 30 to 50 percent lower than in younger patients. The aging person may demonstrate increased receptor or organ sensitivity to medications, and there is an age-associated decrease in albumin, resulting in more free (active) drug available.

In general, continuous attention should be paid to reducing the total number of drugs, eliminating duplicative agents, and simplifying the dosing schedule. Also, clearly instruct the patient and his or her spouse and family when medications are discontinued.

Use therapeutic monitoring

Liberally utilize laboratory monitoring capabilities.

Recognize and respond to side effects promptly

Psychotropic side effects that are more pronounced in the elderly are sedation, anticholinergic reactions, extrapyramidal symptoms, delirium, postural hypotension, cardiotoxicity, and cognitive impairments. Constipation is common and particularly troubling in the elderly. Therefore, add anticholinergic agents with caution, and recommend treatment at time of prescribing to prevent potentially serious gastrointestinal effects.

Pharmacogenetics

The rapidly developing field of pharmacogenetics examines variations in drug response attributable to genetic factors (Relling and Giacomini 2006). Advances in pharmacogenetics have accelerated since 2003, when the Human Genome Project was completed. The field of *pharmacogenomics* applies the knowledge of pharmacogenetics to broader goals, such as customizing drug therapy, enhancing patient safety, and guiding new drug development (Johnson 2003; Flowers and Veenstra 2004; Jin et. al. 2005; and Daly, King, and Leathart 2006). However, the two terms are used somewhat interchangeably in both professional and lay literature.

Genetic factors can affect drug response and side effects. For example, the genetic composition of one patient might result in inadequate drug response, while another patient might have an exaggerated response to the same drug and dose. Or one patient may experience severe side effects or toxicity from the same drug or dose that another patient tolerates quite well.

The dynamics and kinetics of drugs in the body are determined by genetically mediated patterns of protein structures, receptor sensitivities, and enzyme activity. Since protein synthesis is controlled by gene sequencing, there is a direct association between genetics and the proteins involved in drug absorption, metabolism, and receptor response.

We present current findings in this area, acknowledging that information is likely to expand in the future. Pharmacogenetics is extremely complex and definite conclusions and applications for clinical practice are elusive. Our intent is to summarize current concepts and knowledge that are of practical relevance to therapists.

Drug Metabolism

Genetically based individual variations in drug metabolism were first identified in the late 1950s. For the next several decades, through observation and clinical experience, it was discovered that some individuals are poor metabolizers of some drugs, while others are extensive metabolizers of drugs. Poor metabolizers may be at risk for exaggerated or unexpected side effects at normal dosages. Extensive metabolizers may experience a less-than-expected response to standard dosages of a given medication. Extensive metabolizers are also at risk for the buildup of intermediate toxic metabolites (see appendix A for a discussion of metabolic phases).

Beginning in the 1990s, paralleling the Human Genome Project, interest intensified to further refine the understanding of the genetic basis for alterations in drug metabolism. To date, over 50 cytochrome P450 (CYP) genes have been identified. The most widely studied genetic variations are linked to the specific enzymes CYP2D6, CYP2C19, and CYP2C9 (Katzung 2001; Zanger et al. 2008), all of which have significant drug metabolizing activity. CYP2D6 and CYP2C19 have been extensively studied for genetic variation. Among the drugs metabolized via CYP2D6 are antidepressants and antipsychotics.

There are distinct ethnic associations for metabolic enzyme variations. For example, nearly 7 percent of the Swedish population and 1 percent of Chinese are poor CYP2D6 metabolizers; whereas, for CYP2C19, 15 to 18 percent of Asians are poor metabolizers and 3 percent of Swedes and Caucasian Americans are poor metabolizers. In some instances, a genetic variation can result in multiple copies of the CYP2D6 gene, producing ultra-rapid metabolism of antidepressants (Ingelman-Sundberg et al. 2007). It is important to note that there are other drug metabolizing enzymes in addition to the cytochrome P450 system that are also subject to generic variation.

Membrane Transporters

Membrane transporters are proteins that transport ions and neurotransmitters across cell membranes. The serotonin transporter, for example, promotes serotonin reuptake and transports it to the presynaptic neuron. Genetic variations in the serotonin transporter have been implicated not only in altered drug response but also in the etiology of anxiety and depressive disorders. The dopamine transporter functions to transport dopamine from the synapse into neurons. Genetic variations in the dopamine transporter have been implicated in major depression, bipolar disorder, and ADHD (Zalsman et al. 2007; Contreras et al. 2009). At this time, individualized testing for altered membrane transporters is not near commercial application.

Clinical and Practical Implications

Despite the rapid growth of knowledge and significant research, there are few real-world applications for pharmacogenetics. There are, indeed, genetic tests available that determine altered drug metabolizing traits. For some cancer therapies and anticoagulants, genetic testing is highly recommended, if not routine. The FDA is increasingly including genetic information in drug product labeling. For example, carbamazepine products contain labeling advising genetic testing for patients with Asian ancestry who are at risk of a serious skin reaction, due to an altered genetically based immune response. Atomoxetine has labeling regarding poor metabolizers who may experience serious side effects and extensive metabolizers who may not respond as expected to the prescribed dosage.

There are, however, no expert guidelines or consensus decisions for most prescription medications about routine genetic testing to determine drug choice and dosage. Certainly, there is ample evidence to support increased emphasis on pharmacogenetics during medical training and heightened vigilance by health care providers for unusual medication effects that could signal a drug metabolism issue (Wilkinson 2005; de Leon 2009). Much of the pharmacogenetic research involves single or fixed dosages, usually with a single drug. Findings from these studies do not necessarily correlate with patients in clinical settings who are taking multiple medications, often changing dosages and combinations. Also, insurance companies do not routinely cover genetic testing and many patients cannot afford the out-of-pocket expense for commercially available tests. Nonetheless, pharmacogenetics and pharmacogenomics offer the future promise of personalized medications, safer drugs, and targeted therapies; realistically, however, widespread application is at least several years away.

Appendix C

Psychotropic Drug Interactions

This appendix provides a quick reference guide to frequent and significant drug interactions between psychotropic medications.[1] These tables are not absolute. Interactive effects will vary from person to person. In some instances an individual may experience the full range of symptoms presented here, while others may demonstrate only one or two symptoms from a range of possible effects.

Also note that the potential for an interaction between drugs does not preclude their concurrent use. Certain combinations are routinely prescribed without problems in many patients (as with lithium and antipsychotics), whereas others are contraindicated due to the severity of the interaction (for example, MAOIs and SSRIs). *However, whenever psychiatric medications are co-administered, the additive potential of central nervous system depression and anticholinergic effects must be considered.*

---

1. Information from a variety of sources was compiled for this appendix: American Society of Health Systems Pharmacists (2012); *Facts and Comparisons* (2012); *Drug Information for the Health Care Professional* (USP-DI Drug Information for the Health Care Professional) (2007); Hansten and Horn (2009).

Drug or Drug Category	Interacting Drug	Effect on TCA	Effect on Interacting Drug	Potential Result of Drug Interaction
Tricyclic Antidepressants (TCA)	**Monoamine Oxidase Inhibitors (MAOIs) contraindicated with TCAs include:** • **MAOI antidepressants,** phenelzine, isocarboxazid, and tranylcypromine • Other drugs with MAOI properties, such as selegeline, isoniazid, and linezolid	↑		Severe reaction causing excitation, dangerously high blood pressure, high body temperature, mania, seizures, coma, or **death**
	• Antiarrythmic drugs • Bupropion • Cimetidine • SSRI antidepressants	↑		Increased TCA levels, enhanced TCA response, increased TCA side effects or TCA toxicity
	• Amphetamines • Drugs used during surgery	↑	↑	Increased blood pressure, increased or irregular heart rate, very high fever
	Thyroid hormones	↑	↑	Increased or irregular heart rate, stimulation or excitation
	Quinolones		↑	Increased risk of serious, life-threatening cardiac arrhythmias
	Carbamazepine (CBZ)	↓	↑	• Decreased TCA levels, decreased TCA response • Increased CBZ levels, increased CBZ effects, increased CBZ side effects or CBZ toxicity
	Anticoagulants (blood thinners)		↑	Increased anticoagulant effect causing excessive bleeding or bruising
	Clonidine		→	Decreased antihypertensive effect of clonidine resulting in high blood pressure
	Antipsychotics		↑	Increased neurologic side effects

Figure C-1   Cyclic Antidepressants

Drug or Drug Category	Interacting Drug	Effect on SSRI	Effect on Interacting Drug	Potential Result of Drug Interaction
Serotonin Selective Reuptake Inhibitors (SSRI) *Certain interactions with SSRIs are assumed to occur with all medications in this category. For instance, all SSRIs should be avoided with MAOIs. However, interactions involving metabolic pathways, such as with anticonvulsants, may be more likely to occur with one SSRI than another. All SSRIs are not metabolized identically. Similarities and differences between SSRI antidepressants and all interacting drugs are beyond the scope of this reference.*	**Monoamine Oxidase Inhibitors (MAOIs) contraindicated with TCAs include:** • **MAOI antidepressants,** phenelzine, isocarboxazid, and tranylcypromine • Other drugs with MAOI properties, such as selegeline, isoniazid, and linezolid	↑		Severe serotonergic syndrome causing dangerously high blood pressure, high body temperature, tremor, muscle rigidity, seizures, coma, or **death**

	• Products containing L-tryptophan
	• Serotonin precursors and serotonin agonists include a wide range of drugs:
	  • "triptans" used to treat migraine headaches
	  • tramadol
	  • Saint-John's-wort
	  • Buspirone
	• Diet pills
		↑		Severe reaction causing headache, nausea, sweating, agitation, dangerously high blood pressure, high body temperature, seizures, or death (serotonergic syndrome)

	Amphetamines	↑	→	Increased blood pressure, increased or irregular heart rate, very high fever
	Anticonvulsants	→	↓↑	• Decreased SSRI levels, decreased SSRI response • Variable effect on anticonvulsants' levels depending on drug combination

Figure C-2 SSRI Antidepressants

Drug or Drug Category	Interacting Drug	Effect on SSRI	Effect on Interacting Drug	Potential Result of Drug Interaction
Serotonin Selective Reuptake Inhibitors (SSRI)	Beta blockers		↑	Increased effects of beta blockers, resulting in low blood pressure, low heart rate
	Antipsychotics		↑	• Increased neurologic side effects • Increased antipsychotic levels • SSRIs contraindicated with thioridazine due to risk of life-threatening cardiac arrhythmias
	TCA antidepressants		↑	Increased TCA levels (may be significant), enhanced TCA response, increased TCA side effects or TCA toxicity
	Benzodiazepines		↑	Increased BZ levels, enhanced BZ response, increased BZ side effects or BZ toxicity
	HIV protease inhibitors		↑	Increased levels of HIV protease inhibitors, increased serotonergic effects
	Lithium		↑ →	Increased or decreased lithium levels, increased serotonergic effects, neurotoxicity, confusion, dizziness, tremor muscle rigidity, incoordination
	• Anti-arrhythmic drugs • Nonsedating antihistamines		↑	Cardiotoxicity, arrhythmias
	• Anticoagulants • Aspirin • NSAIDs		↑	Increased anticoagulant effect causing excessive bleeding or bruising

Figure C-2 SSRI Antidepressants *Continued*

Drug or Drug Category	Interacting Drug	Effect on SNRI	Effect on Interacting Drug	Potential Result of Drug Interaction
Serotonin and Norepinephrine Reuptake Inhibitors (SNRI)	**Monoamine Oxidase Inhibitors (MAOIs) contraindicated with SNRIs include:** • **MAOI antidepressants,** phenelzine, isocarboxazid, and tranylcypromine • Other drugs with MAOI properties, such as selegeline, isoniazid, and linezolid	↑		Severe serotonergic syndrome causing dangerously high blood pressure, high body temperature, tremor, muscle rigidity, seizures, coma, or **death**

	• Products containing L-tryptophan
	• Serotonin precursors and serotonin agonists, include a wide range of drugs:
	   • triptans used to treat migraine headaches
	   • tramadol
	   • Saint-John's-wort
	   • buspirone
	• Diet pills
		↑		Severe reaction causing headache, nausea, sweating, agitation, dangerously high blood pressure, high body temperature, seizures, or death (serotonergic syndrome)

	• Cimetidine • Anti-arrythmics • Quinolones	↑		Increased SNRI levels, enhanced SNRI response, increased SNRI side effects or SNRI toxicity
	Antipsychotics		↑	• Increased neurologic side effects • Increased antipsychotic levels • SNRIs contraindicated with thioridazine due to risk of life-threatening cardiac arrythmias

Figure C-3 SNRI Antidepressants

Drug or Drug Category	Interacting Drug	Effect on SNRI	Effect on Interacting Drug	Potential Result of Drug Interaction
Serotonin and Norepinephrine Reuptake Inhibitors (SNRI)	TCA antidepressants		↑	Increased TCA levels (may be significant), enhanced TCA response, increased TCA side effects or TCA toxicity
	Lithium		↑	Increased serotonergic effects, neurotoxicity, confusion, dizziness, tremor, muscle rigidity, incoordination
	Anticoagulants		↑	Increased anticoagulant effect causing excessive bleeding or bruising

Figure C-3 SNRI Antidepressants *Continued*

Drug or Drug Category	Interacting Drug	Effect on Bupropion	Effect on Interacting Drug	Potential Result of Drug Interaction
Miscellaneous Antidepressants Buproprion (Wellbutrin)	**Monoamine Oxidase Inhibitors (MAOIs) contraindicated with bupropion include:** • **MAOI antidepressants**, phenelzine, isocarboxazid, and tranylcypromine • Other drugs with MAOI properties, such as selegeline, isoniazid, and linezolid	↑		Severe reaction causing excitation, dangerously high blood pressure, high body temperature, mania, seizures, coma, or **death**
	• Drugs that lower seizure threshold • Drug therapy changes that could lower seizure threshold (e.g., abrupt withdrawal of benzodiazepines)	↑	↑	Seizures
	• HIV protease inhibitors • Bupropion duplicative products (e.g., Zyban for smoking cessation)	↑		Increaesd bupropion levels, increased response, risk of toxicity
	L-dopa	↑		Excitability, restlessness, tremor, nausea, vomiting
	Carbamazepine (CBZ)	→		Decreased bupropion levels, decreased response
	• Anti-arrythmic drugs • Antipsychotics • Beta blockers • SSRI antidepressants • TCA antidepressants		↑	Bupropion inhibits metabolism of listed drugs resulting in increased levels of interacting drugs, increased response, and risk of toxicity. May require dosage reduction.

Figure C-4 Miscellaneous Antidepressants

Drug or Drug Category	Interacting Drug	Potential Result of Drug Interaction
Miscellaneous Antidepressants		
Monoamine Oxidase Inhibitors (MAOIs)	**Monoamine Oxidase Inhibitors (MAOIs) contraindicated with**	Severe reaction causing excitation, dangerously high blood pressure, high body temperature, mania, seizures, coma, or **death**
	• Antidiabetic agents	
	• Buproprion	MAOIs can adversely interact with numerous medications. These interactions are possible for up to two weeks even after the MAOI has been stopped. A washout period of up to five weeks after stopping some interacting medications may be necessary before starting an MAOI.
	• Buspirone (Buspar)	
	• Carbamazepine	
	• Cyclic antidepressants	
	• Dextromethorphan—found in prescription and over-the-counter cough syrups and lozenges	
	• Drugs used during surgery	
	• Ephedrine, pseudoephedrine—found in prescription and over-the-counter cough and cold or asthma medicines	See chapter 16 for a discussion of MAOI-food interactions and dietary restrictions
	• Levodopa	
	• L-tryptophan	
	• Meperidine (Demerol)	
	• Other drugs with MAOI properties, such as selegeline, isoniazid, linezolid, and triptans	
	• Phenylephrine, phenylpropanolamine—found in prescription and over-the-counter cough and cold or asthma medicines	
	• SSRI antidepressants	
	• Stimulants	

Figure C-4 Miscellaneous Antidepressants *Continued*

Drug or Drug Category	Interacting Drug	Effect on Mirtazapine	Effect on Interacting Drug	Potential Result of Drug Interaction
Miscellaneous Antidepressants **Mirtazapine (Remeron)** **(Note: drug interaction data for mirtazapine are limited)**	**Monoamine Oxidase Inhibitors (MAOIs) contraindicated with mirtazapine include:** • **MAOI antidepressants,** phenelzine, isocarboxazid, and tranylcypromine • Other drugs with MAOI properties, such as selegeline, isoniazid, and linezolid	↑		Severe reaction causing excitation, dangerously high blood pressure, high body temperature, mania, seizures, coma, or **death**

Figure C-4 Miscellaneous Antidepressants *Continued*

Drug or Drug Category	Interacting Drug	Effect on FGA	Effect on Interacting Drug	Potential Result of Drug Interaction
First-Generation Antipsychotics (FGA)	• HIV protease inhibitors • SSRI antidepressants	←		Increased FGA levels, enhanced FGA response, increased FGA side effects or FGA toxicity
	Beta blockers	←	←	• Increased effect of beta blocker • Thioridazine contraindicated with certain beta blockers due to risk of life-threatening cardiac arrhythmias
	Anticonvulsants	→	→	• Antipsychotic can lower seizure threshold, requiring dosage increase of anticonvulsant • Decreased FGA levels
	Tricyclic antidepressants (TCA)		←	Increased TCA levels, enhanced TCA response, increased TCA side effects or TCA toxicity
	Levodopa		→	Decreased effectiveness of levodopa in treating Parkinson's disease
	Amphetamines		←	Risk of psychosis
	Lithium		←	• Neurotoxicity (delirium, seizures, encephalopathy) • Increased EPS

Figure C-5 First-Generation Antipsychotics

Drug or Drug Category	Interacting Drug	Effect on SGA	Effect on Interacting Drug	Potential Result of Drug Interaction
Second-Generation Antipsychotics (SGA)	• HIV protease inhibitors • SSRI antidepressants • Oral antifungal agents • Macrolide antibiotics • Cimetidine • SSRI antidepressants • Caffeine	↑		Increased SGA levels, enhanced SGA response, increased SGA side effects or SGA toxicity
	Anticonvulsants	↓	↓	• Antipsychotic can lower seizure threshold requiring dosage increase of anticonvulsant • Decreased SGA levels
	Tricyclic antidepressants (TCA)		↑	Increased TCA levels, enhanced TCA response, increased TCA side effects or TCA toxicity
	Levodopa		↓	Decreased effectiveness of L-dopa in treating Parkinson's disease
	Lithium		↑	• Neurotoxicity (delirium, seizures, encephalopathy) • Increased EPS
	Amphetamines		↑	Risk of psychosis
	Anti-arrhythmic drugs		↑	Increased risk of cardiac arrhythmias

Figure C-6 Second-Generation Antipsychotics

Drug or Drug Category	Interacting Drug	Effect on Mood Stabilizer	Effect on Interacting Drug	Potential Result of Drug Interaction
Mood Stabilizers Carbamazepine (Tegretol)	**Monoamine Oxidase Inhibitors (MAOIs) contraindicated with carbamazepine** include: • **MAOI antidepressants,** phenelzine, isocarboxazid, and tranylcypromine • Other drugs with MAOI properties, such as selegeline, isoniazid, and linezolid	↑		Severe reaction causing excitation, dangerously high blood pressure, high body temperature, mania, seizures, coma or **death**
	• Calcium channel blockers • Cimetidine • Macrolide antibiotics • Oral antifungal agents	↑		Increased carbamazepine levels, increased side effects, risk of toxicity
	• TCA antidepressants • SSRI antidepressants	↑	↓	• Increased carbamazepine levels • Decreased TCA levels • Decreased SSRI levels
	Isoniazid	↑	↑	Increased carbamazepine levels, isoniazid toxicity, liver toxicity
	Anticonvulsants	↑ ↓	↑ ↓	Variable effect on anticonvulsants when used in combination
	HIV protease inhibitors	↑	↓	• Increased carbamazepine levels, increased side effects, risk of toxicity • Decreased levels of HIV protease inhibitors
	• Anticoagulants • Antipsychotics • Birth control pills • Buspirone		↓	Decreased levels or effectiveness of interacting drugs

Figure C-7 Mood Stabilizers

Drug or Drug Category	Interacting Drug	Effect on Mood Stabilizer	Effect on Interacting Drug	Potential Result of Drug Interaction
Mood Stabilizers Carbamazepine (Tegretol)	• Lithium		↑	Neurotoxicity (delirium, seizures, encephalopathy), or increased EPS
Divalproex (Depakote)	• Aspirin • NSAIDs	↑		• Increased divalproex levels • Increased risk of bleeding
	Anticonvulsants	↑	↓	Variable effect on anticonvulsants when used in combination
	Anticoagulants (blood thinners)	↓	↓↑	Risk of bleeding
Lamotrigine (Lamictal)	Birth control pills containing estrogen	↓		Adjust dose of lamotrigine when starting or stopping birth control pills
	Anticonvulsants	↓	↓	Variable effect on anticonvulsants when used in combination
Lithium	• ACE inhibitors • Calcium channel blockers • Diuretics • NSAIDs • Metronidazole	↓ ↑	↓	Increased lithium levels, lithium toxicity
	SSRI antidepressants	↑		Increased lithium levels, possible neurotoxicity (confusion, dizziness, tremor, muscle stiffness, incoordination)
	• Antipsychotics • Carbamazepine	↑		Neurotoxicity (delirium, seizures, encephalopathy) or increased EPS
	Theophylline	↓		Decreased lithium levels

Figure C-7 Mood Stabilizers *Continued*

Drug or Drug Category	Interacting Drug	Effect on Stimulant	Effect on Interacting Drug	Potential Result of Drug Interaction
Psychostimulants	**Monoamine Oxidase Inhibitors (MAOIs) contraindicated with stimulants include:** • **MAOI antidepressants,** phenelzine, isocarboxazid, and tranylcypromine • Other drugs with MAOI properties, such as selegeline, isoniazid, and linezolid	↑		Severe reaction causing excitation, dangerously high blood pressure, high body temperature, mania, seizures, coma, or **death**
	• SSRI antidepressants • TCA antidepressants		↑	• Increased risk of serotonin syndrome with SSRIs, increased SSRI levels. • Increased TCA levels • Increased side effects, especially nervousness, insomnia, and high blood pressure
	Thyroid hormones		↑	Increased or irregular heart rate, stimulation, or excitation
	Digoxin		↑	Additive effects on the heart resulting in cardiac arrhythmias
	Anticonvulsants		↑	Increased anticonvulsant levels
	Anticoagulants (blood thinners)		↑	Increased anticoagulant effect, causing excessive bleeding or bruising
	• Beta Blockers • Clonidine • Antihypertensive medications		↓	Decreased antihypertensive effect resulting in high blood pressure

Figure C-8 Stimulants

Handbook of Clinical Psychopharmacology for Therapists

Drug or Drug Category	Interacting Drug	Effect on Benzodiazepine	Effect on Interacting Drug	Potential Result of Drug Interaction
Benzodiazepines	• Beta blockers • Birth control pills • Calcium channel blockers • Cimetidine • Disulfiram • HIV protease inhibitors • Isoniazid • Macrolide antibiotics • Oral antifungal agents • Propoxyphene • SSRI antidepressants • Valproic acid	←		Increased BZ levels, increased BZ effects, increased BZ side effects or BZ toxicity
	Carbamazepine (CBZ)	→		Decreased benzodiazepine levels, decreased benzodiazepine effects
	Levodopa		→	Decreased effectiveness of levodopa
	Digoxin		←	Increased digoxin levels, risk of digoxin toxicity

Figure C-9   Benzodiazepines

Appendix D

Differentiating Psychotropic Side Effects from Psychiatric Symptoms

In this appendix we discuss a potentially problematic area: the identification of, and response to, psychotropic-induced side effects. The most obvious danger of failing to accurately differentiate medication side effects from a disease process is the possibility that one might increase the dose of the very medication responsible for the the side effects. Similarly, unwarranted diagnoses may be assigned or unnecessary medications added.

At times, making this distinction is nearly impossible. Not only is the clinician required to separate strikingly similar medication side effects and psychiatric symptomatology, but the patient may be only marginally able to give a useful subjective description.

Akathisia Versus Agitation Associated with Worsening Anxiety or Psychosis

Akathisia, the compulsion to be in motion, may present with a variety of associated symptoms. Patients often experience an inability to remain still and may pace, tap their feet while sitting, and shift their weight while standing. Along a continuum, mild akathisia may appear as increasing or emerging anxiety and, when more severe, may be mistaken for worsening psychosis.

Akathisia secondary to first-generation antipsychotics is more common in younger patients or with high-potency agents. The onset of akathisia can follow a variable course, appearing either early in treatment or up to several months later. Especially if the patient is not receiving anticholinergics, the possibility of medication-induced akathisia should be considered before more neuroleptic is administered. If symptoms diminish in response to anticholinergics, it is probably akathisia. If symptoms resolve with additional neuroleptic, it is more likely disease exacerbation. In some patients, response to anticholingerics is inadequate, requiring adding, or changing to, a benzodiazepine or beta blocker. In these cases, the patient will usually report a "physical" restlessness as opposed to "emotional" anxiety or agitation.

Akathisia has also been reported with the SSRIs, especially fluoxetine, and with the tricyclic antidepressants. Failure to recognize antidepressant-induced akathisia may lead to unnecessary prescribing of antianxiety agents or first-generation antipsychotics.

Excessive Anticholinergic Effects Versus Psychosis

An acute onset of primary organic symptoms may signal anticholinergic delirium, with associated mental status changes of confusion, disorientation, and tactile or visual hallucinations. Physiologic indicators include dry mucous membranes, increased heart rate, and dilated pupils. Recovery usually occurs within several days following discontinuation of the suspected anticholinergic drug, but occasionally this syndrome may last up to two weeks. Elderly people are especially prone to anticholinergic overload.

Drug treatment of anticholinergic delirium is typically not recommended, although benzodiazepines can be used to treat severe agitation. First-generation antipsychotics, with their anticholinergic properties, are relatively contraindicated.

Parkinsonian Side Effects Versus Depression

Neuroleptic-induced Parkinsonian side effects are characterized by the triad of tremor, muscle stiffness, and slowness of motion. For the most part, these physical indicators are relatively easy to identify. The tremor, which is somewhat coarse and may include classic "pill-rolling," is worse at rest and is distinguishable from the fine, intention tremor of lithium. Muscle stiffness or rigidity is notable for the increased resistance to passive movement ("cogwheeling").

The absence of movement (akinesia) does not occur as frequently as slowed movement (bradykinesia). Moderate to severe bradykinesia includes postural abnormalities of shuffling gait, stooped appearance, and feeling off balance. Drooling and slowed, nonexpressive speech are also common. It is the mildly bradykinetic patient, without noticeable tremor or rigidity, whose presentation can mimic a depressive mood disorder. Overall, the slowed motion, lack of facial expression, apathy, and social withdrawal present markedly similar to depression. A careful evaluation should be made to determine the presence of associated Parkinsonian characteristics before revising a diagnosis or initiating an antidepressant.

Acute Dystonia Versus Tardive Dyskinesia

Dystonic reactions occur within hours or days of initiating treatment with (or increasing the dose of) a neuroleptic. Tardive dyskinesia (TD) presents with a more insidious onset and is associated with long-term neuroleptic treatment. Figure D-1 summarizes the characteristics of acute dystonia and TD.

Not only is there no effective treatment for TD, but administration of anticholinergics is likely to worsen the symptoms. Therefore, the differential diagnosis of these two syndromes is critically important.

Acute Dystonia Versus Tardive Dyskinesia

Acute Dystonia

Fixed upward gaze
(oculogyric crisis)
Neck twisting (torticollis)
Arching of the head
backward (opisthotonos)
Clenched jaw or "lockjaw"
(trismus)
Facial grimacing due to
involuntary muscle contraction
Difficulty swallowing
Difficulty breathing
(larynogospasm)

Tardive Dyskinesia

Abnormal, involuntary, rhythmic movements
of the mouth, tongue, and lips, including
protruding tongue, wormlike tongue
movements, mouth puckering,
lip smacking, and chewing motions
Irregular, purposeless, involuntary quick
movements of the extremities, flailing, or
jerky in appearance
Continuous writhing movements of
extremities, including trunk or pelvis

Figure D-1

Antidepressant Toxicity Versus Worsening or Reemerging Depression

Symptoms of depression that reappear, or are slow to resolve with antidepressant treatment, may be explained by several factors, including noncompliance and poor therapeutic response requiring a medication change. Consideration should also be given to medication-related CNS toxicity. The most obvious of these symptoms that are also diagnostic of depression are irritability, confusion, memory impairment, anxiety, agitation, and lethargy. In determining a differential diagnosis, the clinician can assess for the physiologic symptoms of antidepressant toxicity (as described in chapters 16 and 20) and utilize laboratory monitoring for antidepressant blood levels.

A small percentage of patients treated with SSRIs for more than six months will report a reemergence of what are experienced as depressive symptoms. A close review of the clinical status will reveal that many of the previously reported depressive symptoms continue, in fact, to be well controlled by the antidepressant. However, what can develop are symptoms of apathy, low motivation, and emotional blunting (e.g., an inability to cry). One hypothesis is that the chronic effect of increased serotonin action in the CNS is to gradually inhibit dopamine neurons in the frontal cortex (inhibitory serotonin receptors are found on dopamine cell bodies). This dopaminergic hypometabolic state has been demonstrated on metabolic brain scans (Hoehn-Saric et al. 1990). This phenomenon also may be responsible for the rare occurrence of emotional disinhibition, sometimes seen with chronic SSRI treatment.

This condition, which should be distinguished from primary depressive illness, can be eliminated by the discontinuation of the SSRI, or oftentimes it is resolved by the co-administration of a dopamine agonist (e.g., bupropion).

Appendix E

Neurocognitive Mental Status Exam

Figure E-1 is a short exam that can be administered to patients as an aid in making a diagnosis. Notes on each question appear below. For a more comprehensive review of a neurologically based mental status exam, the reader is referred to an excellent text: *The Mental Status Examination in Neurology* (Strub and Black 2000).

Notes on the Use of the Brief Neurocognitive Mental Status Exam

1. *Behavioral observations*

    a. Look for signs of drowsiness or fluctuating degrees of alertness.

    b. This may be formally tested by administering a digit span test or by careful observation during the interview.

    c. Make note of slurred speech or word-finding problems.

    d. Watch for unsteady gait and poor gross motor coordination.

2. *Orientation*—Ask: "What is the date (month, day, year), and what time of day is it now?" "Can you tell me where you are right now? Please be specific." Ask the patient to identify relatives who have accompanied him or her.

3. *Recent memory*—Present three items and ask for immediate recall. Then after a period of five minutes, ask the patient to again recall the three items. Most

normal adults should be able to recall three items. Inability to do so may suggest recent memory problems. A second trial may be conducted later in the interview.

4.   *Calculations*—Ask the patient to begin with the number 100 and subtract 7 from this number, then subtract 7 again, and so forth. This test provides a rough measure of concentration.

5.   *Reproduction of cross and cube*—Present stimulus illustrations shown below. You can copy them onto a 3-by-5-inch, unlined, white index card. Allow the patient to copy the designs one at a time onto a blank sheet of paper. Drawing performance can be compared to samples (see figure E-2) to derive rough estimates of the patient's constructional ability.

Cross   **Cube**

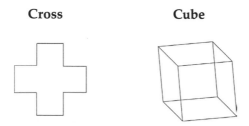

6.   *Thinking/Speech*—Note the presence of incoherent or irrelevant speech.

Brief Neurocognitive Mental Status Exam

Name _____ Age _____ Date _____

Level of education _____ Occupation _____

Onset of symptoms _____

Medications _____

1. Behavioral observations

   a. Level of awakeness/alertness _____

   b. Signs of impaired attention or distractibility _____

   c. Quality of speech _____

   d. Gait _____

2. Orientation: Time _____ Place _____ Person _____

3. Recent memory (three-item recall with five-minute delay)

   Trial A: House, Orange, Robert _____

   Trial B: Petunia, Buick, Wind _____

4. Calculations: 100 – 93 – 86 – 79 – 72 – 65 – 58 – 51

5. Reproduction of cross _____ cube _____

6. Thinking/Speech: Coherent? _____ Relevant? _____

Figure E-1

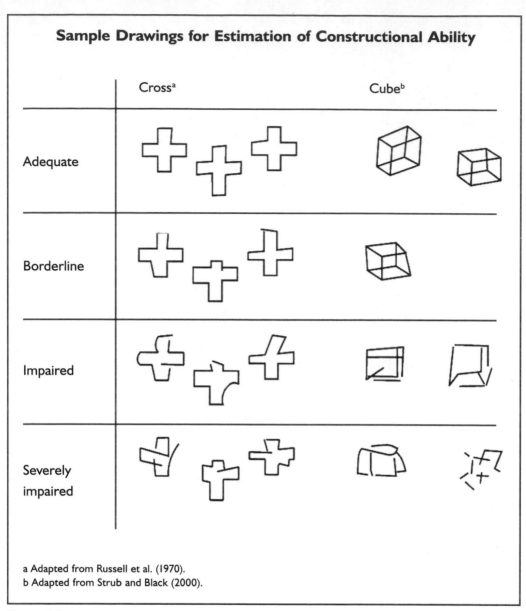

Sample Drawings for Estimation of Constructional Ability

	Cross[a]	Cube[b]
Adequate		
Borderline		
Impaired		
Severely impaired		

a Adapted from Russell et al. (1970).
b Adapted from Strub and Black (2000).

Figure E-2

Appendix F

Trade Versus Generic Drug Names: A Quick Reference

The following tables will enable you to quickly find the corresponding generic or trade name of a medication when you know only one of its names.

Trade to Generic

Trade Name	Generic Name	Trade Name	Generic Name
Abilify	Aripiprazole	Metadate ER	Methylphenidate extended release
Adderall	Amphetamine combination	Nardil	Phenelzine
Akineton	Biperiden	Navane	Thiothixene
Ambien	Zolpidem	Neurontin	Gabapentin
Anafranil	Clomipramine	Norpramin	Desipramine
Artane	Trihexyphenidyl	Orap	Pimozide
Asendin	Amoxapine	Pamelor	Nortriptyline
Atarax	Hydroxyzine HCl	Parnate	Tranylcypromine
Ativan	Lorazepam	Paxil	Paroxetine
Aventyl	Nortriptyline	Paxipam	Halazepam
Benadryl	Diphenhydramine	Permitil	Fluphenazine
BuSpar	Buspirone	Pristiq	Desvenlafaxine
Catapres	Clonidine	Prolixin	Fluphenazine
Celexa	Citalopram	ProSom	Estazolam
Clozaril	Clozapine	Prozac	Fluoxetine
Cogentin	Benztropine	Remeron	Mirtazapine
Concerta	Methylphenidate sustained release	Restoril	Temazepam
		Risperdal	Risperidone
Cymbalta	Duloxetine	Ritalin	Methylphenidate
Dalmane	Flurazepam	Rozerem	Ramelteon
Depakene	Valproic acid	Saphris	Asenapine
Depakote	Divalproex	Sarafem	Fluoxetine
Desyrel	Trazodone	Serax	Oxazepam
Dexedrine	Dextroamphetaìmine	Seroquel	Quetiapine
Doral	Quazepam	Serzone	Nefazodone
Effexor XR	Venlafaxine extended release	Sinequan	Doxepin
		Sonata	Zaleplon
Elavil	Amitriptyline	Stelazine	Trifluoperazine
Eldepryl	Selegiline (deprenyl)	Strattera	Atomoxetine
Emsam	Selegiline	Surmontil	Trimipramine
Equetro	Carbamazepine	Symbyax	Fluoxetine/Olanzapine
Eskalith	Lithium carbonate		
Eskalith CR	Lithium carbonate controlled release	Symmetrel	Amantadine
		Tegretol	Carbamazepine
Fanapt	Iloperidone	Tegretol XR	Carbamazepine extended release
Focalin	Dexmethylphenidate		
Gabitril	Tiagabine	Tenex	Guanfacine
Geodon	Ziprasidone	Tenormin	Atenolol
Halcion	Triazolam	Thorazine	Chlorpromazine
Haldol	Haloperidol	Tindal	Acetophenazine
Inderal	Propranolol	Tofranil	Imipramine
Invega	Paliperidone	Topamax	Topiramate
Klonopin	Clonazepam	Tranxene	Clorazepate
Lamictal	Lamotrigine	Trilafon	Perphenazine
Lexipro	Escitalopram	Trileptal	Oxcarbazepine
Librium	Chlordiazepoxide	Valium	Diazepam
Lithobid	Lithium carbonate slow release	Versed	Midazolam
		Vestra	Reboxetine
Lithonate	Lithium carbonate	Vistaril	Hydroxyzine pamoate
Lithotabs	Lithium carbonate	Vivactil	Protriptyline
Loxitane	Loxapine	Wellbutrin	Bupropion
Ludiomil	Maprotiline	Wellbutrin SR	Bupropion sustained release
Lunesta	Eszopiclone		
Luvox	Fluvoxamine	Xanax	Alprazolam
Marplan	Isocarboxazid	Zoloft	Sertraline
Mellaril	Thioridazine	Zyprex	Olanzapine

Generic to Trade

Generic Name	Trade Name	Generic Name	Trade Name
Acetophenazine	Tindal	Imipramine	Tofranil
Alprazolam	Xanax	Isocarboxazid	Marplan
Amantadine	Symmetrel	Lamotrigine	Lamictal
Amitriptyline	Elavil	Lithium carbonate	Lithotabs,
Amoxapine	Asendin		Lithonate,
Amphetamine	Adderall		Eskalith
combination		Lithium carbonate,	Eskalith CR,
Aripiprazole	Abilify	long acting	Lithobid
Asenapine	Saphris	Lorazepam	Ativan
Atenolol	Tenormin	Loxapine	Loxitane
Atomoxetine	Strattera	Maprotiline	Ludiomil
Benztropine	Cogentin	Methylphenidate	Concerta
Biperiden	Akineton	sustained release	
Bupropion	Wellbutrin	Methylphenidate	Metadate ER
Bupropion	Wellbutrin SR	extended release	
sustained release		Midazolam	Versed
Buspirone	BuSpar	Mirtazpine	Remeron
Carbamazepine	Tegretol	Nefazodone	Serzone
Carbamazepine	Equetro	Nortriptyline	Pamelor, Aventyl
Chlordiazepoxide	Librium	Olanzapine	Zyprexa
Chlorpromazine	Thorazine	Oxazepam	Serax
Citalopram	Celexa	Oxcarbazepine	Trileptal
Clomipramine	Anafranil	Paliperidone	Invega
Clonazepam	Klonopin	Paroxetine	Paxil
Clonidine	Catapres	Perphenazine	Trilafon
Clorazepate	Tranxene	Phenelzine	Nardil
Clozapine	Clozaril	Pimozide	Orap
d- and	Adderall	Propranolol	Inderal
l-amphetamine		Protriptyline	Vivactil
Desipramine	Norpramin	Quazepam	Doral
Desvenlafaxine	Pristiq	Quetiapine	Seroquel
Dexmethylphenidate	Focalin	Ramelteon	Rozerem
Dextroamphetamine	Dexedrine	Reboxetine	Vestra
Diazepam	Valium	Risperidone	Risperdal
Diphenhydramine	Benadryl	Selegeline	Eldepryl
Divalproex	Depakote	(deprenyl)	
Doxepin	Sinequan	Selegiline	Emsam
Duloxetine	Cymbalta	Sertraline	Zoloft
Escitalopram	Lexipro	Temazepam	Restoril
Estazolam	ProSom	Thioridazine	Mellaril
Eszopiclone	Lunesta	Thiothixene	Navane
Fluoxetine	Serafem	Tiagabine	Gabitril
Fluoxetine/	Symbyax	Topiramate	Topamax
Olanzapine		Tranylcypromine	Parnate
Fluphenazine	Prolixin, Permitil	Trazodone	Desyrel
Flurazepam	Dalmane	Triazolam	Halcion
Fluoxetine	Prozac	Trifluoperazine	Stelazine
Fluvoxamine	Luvox	Trihexyphenidyl	Artane
Gabapentin	Neurontin	Trimipramine	Surmontil
Guanfacine	Tenex	Valproic acid	Depakene
Haloperidol	Haldol	Venlafaxine	Effexor
Hydroxyzine HCl	Atarax	Venlafaxine	Effexor XR
Hydroxyzine	Vistaril	extended release	
pamoate		Zaleplon	Sonata
Iloperidone	Fanapt	Ziprasidone	Geodon
		Zolpidem	Ambien

Appendix G

Medication Safety

The Joint Commission (formerly known as the Joint Commission on Accreditation of Health Care Organizations [JCAHO]) has established a National Patient Safety Goal to reduce medication errors. Included in this initiative are several lists of dangerous abbreviations, symbols, or acronyms that should be eliminated from handwritten, patient-specific communications. In addition, the Institute of Safe Medication Practices (ISMP) provides practitioners and patients with education to promote safe medication use. While the *Handbook* is not governed by the Joint Commission standards, many of our readers practice in settings that are subject to its regulations. The authors support all efforts to promote medication safety for our patients and provide the following information to raise awareness about this extremely important issue.

Problems Associated with Drug Names

Look-alike, sound-alike drugs can be problematic for practitioners and patients, especially in cases of unclear handwriting. Readers are cautioned about the following examples:

- Celexa and Cerebryx have been confused on handwritten orders.

- Lexipro and Loxitane have similar names and strengths (10 mg).

- Medication errors related to the similarity in spelling between Lamictal, Lamisil, Lomotil, labetolol, and lamivudine have been reported.

- Plavix and Paxil have been associated with medication errors.

- Drug name suffixes can be confusing to prescribers and patients, and lead to inappropriate dosing. Examples include XL, XR, SR, CD, ER, and LA for products such as Depakote, Wellbutrin, Effexor, Ritalin, and Metadate.

Potential Problems with Abbreviations, Symbols and Dose Designations

While not all-inclusive, listed below are examples taken from comprehensive lists issued by ISMP (2003) and Joint Commission (2004) of error-prone abbreviations, symbols, and dose designations. These examples might be of particular relevance to therapists for handwritten, patient-specific documentation.

Abbreviation/Dose Designation/Symbol	Intended Action or Meaning	Potential Misinterpretation	Correct Term
qhs	At bedtime	Mistaken as qhr (every hour)	Write "at bedtime"
qd or q.d.	Every day	Mistaken as qid (four times daily)	Write "daily"
qod or q.o.d.	Every other day	Mistaken as "qd" (daily) or qid (four times daily)	Write "every other day"
IU or U	International unit or unit	IU mistaken as IV (intravenous) or 10 (ten); U mistaken as zero, four, or cc	Write "international units" or "units"
SSRI	Sliding scale regular insulin	Selective serotonin reuptake inhibitor	Write "sliding scale regular insulin"
Trailing zero after decimal point (e.g., 10.0 mg)	10 mg	Mistaken as 100 mg if decimal point not seen	Do not write a zero after a decimal point
No leading zero before a decimal dose (e.g., .5 mg)	0.5 mg	Mistaken as 5 mg if decimal point not seen	Always use a zero before decimal point
Drug name and dose run together, especially for drugs ending in "L" (e.g., Tegretol300 mg)	Tegretol 300 mg	Mistaken as Tegretol 1300 mg	Place adequate space between the drug name, dose, and unit of measure
Numerical dose and unit of measure run together (e.g., 10mg)	10 mg	The "m" is sometimes mistaken as a zero or two zeros, leading to a 10- to 100-fold overdose	Place adequate space between the dose and unit of measure
cc	cubic centimeter	Mistaken for units	Write "ml"
μg	mcg	Mistaken for "mg" resulting in 1000-fold overdose	Write "mcg"
@	At	Mistaken as "2"	Write "at"
&	And	Mistaken as "2"	Write "and"
+	Plus or and	Mistaken as "4"	Write "and"
°	Hour	Mistaken as a zero (e.g., q2° seen as q 20)	Write "hr" or "h" or "hour"

Patient Education

We can promote the safe use of medications by encouraging our patients and caregivers to be as informed as possible and to never be afraid to ask questions of prescribers, therapists, nurses, and pharmacists. We can encourage patients to obtain accurate and organized information about medications using the structured discussion points listed below:

1. Be familiar with the brand and generic names of the medications. Write them down and always compare to the labeling on the prescription bottle.

2. Know what the medication looks like. For refills, if the product looks different than before, insist upon an explanation.

3. Ask your prescriber why you are taking the medicine. You can request that your doctor include the reason for use on the prescription.

4. Know the dose, how often it should be taken, and at what times of the day.

5. When starting a new medication, ask how long you will need to take it. Ask your doctor to periodically evaluate all your medications.

6. Be informed about the possible side effects and what to do if you experience a side effect. Know what to do if you miss a dose.

7. Make sure you have received information about interactions with other medications or any foods.

8. When being started on a new medicine, ask if it replaces anything else you are taking.

9. Know what the storage requirements are for the prescription.

Appendix H

Books for Patients About Medication Treatment

General Information

Consumer's Guide to Psychiatric Drugs, by John Preston, John O'Neal, and Mary Talaga. New York: Pocket Books, 2009.

Depression

You Can Beat Depression: A Guide To Recovery, fourth edition, by J. Preston. San Luis Obispo, CA: Impact Publishers, 2004.

The Depression Workbook, by Mary Ellen Copeland. Oakland, CA: New Harbinger Publications, 2002.

Getting Things Done When You're Depressed, by J. Fast and J. Preston. New York: Penguin Books, 2008.

Bipolar Disorder

Loving Someone with Bipolar Disorder: How to Help and Understand Your Partner, second edition, by J. Fast and J. Preston. Oakland, CA: New Harbinger Publications, 2012.

An Unquiet Mind, by Kay Redfield Jamison. New York: Alfred A. Knopf, 1995.

Bipolar Disorder: A Guide for Patients and Families, second edition, by Francis Mark Mondimore. Baltimore, MD: Johns Hopkins University Press, 2006.

Take Charge of Bipolar Disorder, by J. Fast and J. Preston. New York: Warner Books, 2006.

Anxiety

The Anxiety and Phobia Workbook, fourth edition, by Edmund Bourne. Oakland, CA: New Harbinger Publications, 2005.

Psychosis

Surviving Schizophrenia: A Manual for Families, Patients, and Providers, by E. F. Torrey. New York: HarperCollins, 2006.

Alzheimer's Disease

The 36-Hour Day, third edition, by N. L. Mace and P. V. Rabins. New York: Warner Books, 2006.

Obsessive-Compulsive Disorder

Brain Lock: Free Yourself from Obsessive-Compulsive Behavior, by J. Schwartz. New York: Harper Perennial, 1997.

Obsessive-Compulsive Disorder: A Complete Guide to Getting Well and Staying Well, by Fred Penzel. UK: Oxford University Press, 2000.

Attention-Deficit Disorder

Taking Charge of ADHD: The Complete Authoritative Guide for Parents, second edition, by Russell Barkley. New York: Guilford Press, 2000.

Borderline Personality Disorder

I Hate You—Don't Leave Me, by J. Kreisman and H. Kraus. Los Angeles: Price Stern Publishers, 1991.

Stop Walking on Eggshells: Taking Your Life Back When Someone You Care About Has Borderline Personality Disorder, by Paul T. Mason and Randi Kreger. Oakland, CA: New Harbinger Publications, 1998.

Medications and Psychotherapy

Make Every Session Count, by J. Preston, N. Varzos, and D. Liebert. Oakland, CA: New Harbinger Publications, 1998.

Complete Idiot's Guide to Managing Your Mood, by J. Preston. New York: Penguin Books, 2007.

Appendix I

Patient Information Sheets on Psychiatric Medications

Patient Information on Antidepressants

The name of your medication is: _____

IMPORTANT NOTE: The following information is intended to supplement, not substitute for, the expertise and judgment of your physician, pharmacist, or other health care professional. It is not intended to imply that use of the drug is safe, appropriate, or effective for you. This information contains limited and general information about these medications, and it is not all-inclusive. Not all uses, side effects, precautions, or drug interactions are listed. Your doctor or pharmacist will provide you with official patient information that is more complete and detailed. Consult your health care professional before using this drug.

Uses

SSRI antidepressants and other, more recently developed, antidepressants such as Effexor, Remeron, and Cymbalta are used in the treatment of a number of disorders, including major depressive disorder, depression associated with manic depressive illness (bipolar disorder), obsessive-compulsive disorder, panic disorder, generalized anxiety disorder, eating disorders, social phobia, post-traumatic stress disorder, and premenstrual changes in mood. The antidepressant Wellbutrin is an effective antidepressant, but is generally not used to treat anxiety or eating disorders. These drugs have also been found to be effective in the treatment of several other disorders, including mild depression, separation anxiety disorder, and impulsive or aggressive behavior, although they are not currently approved for these indications.

The doctor may choose to prescribe this medication for a reason not listed here. If you are not sure why this medication is being prescribed, please ask the doctor.

How To Use

Take as directed, usually once a day by mouth. Some side effects, such as nausea, may be reduced by taking the medication with food. It is best to take it at about the same time each day. The dosage is based on your medical condition and response to therapy.

Missed Dose

If you miss a dose, take it as soon as you remember. However, if it is near the time of the next dose, or the next day, skip the missed dose and resume your usual dosing schedule. *Do not double the dose in order to catch up.*

Side Effects

Side effects occur, to some degree, with all medications. They are usually not serious and do not occur in all individuals. They may sometimes occur before beneficial effects of the medication are noticed. Most side effects will decrease or disappear with time. If a side effect persists, speak to the doctor about appropriate treatment.

Common side effects that should be reported to the doctor at the next appointment include drowsiness and fatigue; anxiety or nervousness, including problems sleeping; headache; nausea or heartburn; muscle tremor; twitching; changes in sex drive or sexual performance; blurred vision; dry mouth; nightmares; and loss of appetite.

Tell your doctor immediately if any of the following unlikely but serious side effects occur: soreness of the mouth, gums, or throat; skin rash or itching; swelling of the face; any unusual bruising or bleeding; nausea; vomiting; loss of appetite; fatigue; weakness; fever or flu-like symptoms; yellow tinge of the eyes or skin; dark-colored urine; inability to pass urine; tingling in the hands and feet; severe muscle twitching; severe agitation or restlessness; *a switch in mood to an unusual state of happiness, excitement, or irritability, or a marked disturbance in sleep*; or thoughts of suicide or hostility (in rare instances this medication has been associated with some suicidal or hostile thoughts; although these thoughts may be seen as a part of the disorder, you should definitely discuss these kinds of thoughts with your doctor).

Report any other side effects not listed above to your physician.

Drug Interactions

Because SSRI antidepressant drugs can change the effects of other medication or may be affected by other medication, always check with the doctor or pharmacist before taking any other drugs, including over-the-counter medications such as cold remedies. Inform all doctors and dentists who examine or treat you that you are taking an antidepressant drug.

PRECAUTIONS

■ Before taking this medication, tell your doctor or pharmacist if you are allergic to it (if known) or if you have any other allergies.

■ Do not increase or decrease your dose without consulting your doctor.

■ This drug may make you dizzy or drowsy; use caution engaging in activities requiring alertness, such as riding a bike, driving, or using machinery.

■ Avoid alcoholic beverages.

■ Avoid excessive amounts of caffeine.

■ Do not stop your drug suddenly, as this may result in withdrawal symptoms such as muscle aches, chills, tingling in your hands or feet, nausea, vomiting, and dizziness.

■ All antidepressants can increase the likelihood of seizures. Because of this risk, bupropion (Wellbutrin), in particular, should not be used by persons with bulimia.

■ Antidepressant medicines may increase suicidal thoughts or actions in some children, teenagers, and young adults when the medicine is first started.

■ *If you have any questions regarding this medication, do not hesitate to contact the doctor, pharmacist, or nurse.*

Patient Information on Antianxiety Medications

The name of your medication is: _____

IMPORTANT NOTE: The following information is intended to supplement, not substitute for, the expertise and judgment of your physician, pharmacist, or other health care professional. It is not intended to imply that use of the drug is safe, appropriate, or effective for you. This information contains limited and general information about these medications, and it is not all-inclusive. Not all uses, side effects, precautions, or drug interactions are listed. Your doctor or pharmacist will provide you with official patient information that is more complete and detailed. Consult your health care professional before using this drug.

Uses

Antianxiety medications can help relieve the symptoms of anxiety but will not alter its cause. In usually prescribed doses, they help to calm and sedate the individual; in higher doses these drugs may be used to induce sleep. These medications, known as benzodiazepines, may also be used as a muscle relaxant, to treat agitation, to suppress seizures, and prior to some diagnostic procedures or surgery.

The doctor may choose to use this medication for a reason not listed here. If you are not sure why this medication is being prescribed, please ask the doctor.

How To Use

Anxiolytic drugs can reduce agitation and induce calm or sedation usually within an hour. Depending on the medication, they may be taken up to three or four times per day.

Missed Dose

Often this type of medication is taken on a PRN, or as needed, basis. However, if you have been instructed to take the medication on a regular basis, you may wait until the next scheduled time if you miss a dose. *Do not double the dose in order to catch up.*

Side Effects

Side effects occur, to some degree, with all medications. They are usually not serious and do not occur in all individuals. They may sometimes occur before beneficial effects of the medication are noticed. Most side effects will decrease or disappear with time. If a side effect persists, speak to the doctor about appropriate treatment.

Common side effects that should be reported to the doctor at the next appointment include drowsiness and fatigue, loss of coordination, weakness or dizziness, forgetfulness, memory lapses, slurred speech, nausea, and heartburn.

Tell your doctor immediately if any of the following unlikely but serious side effects occur: disorientation; confusion; worsening of memory; difficulty learning new things; blackouts; amnesia; nervousness, restlessness, excitement, or any other behavior changes; loss of coordination leading to falls; or skin rash.

This type of medication may impair the mental and physical abilities required for driving a car or riding a bike. Avoid these activities if you feel drowsy or slowed down.

Do not stop taking the drug suddenly, especially if you have been on the medication for a number of months or have been taking high doses. Benzodiazepines need to be reduced gradually in order to prevent withdrawal reactions.

Report any other side effects not listed above to your physician.

Drug Interactions

Because antianxiety medications may be affected by other medication, always check with the doctor or pharmacist before taking any other drugs, including over-the-counter medication such as cold remedies, especially those that are sedating. Inform all doctors and dentists who examine or treat you that you are taking an antianxiety medication.

PRECAUTIONS

- Before taking this medication, tell your doctor or pharmacist if you are allergic to it (if known) or if you have any other allergies.

- Do not increase or decrease your dose without consulting your doctor.

- *If you have any questions regarding this medication, do not hesitate to contact the doctor, pharmacist, or nurse.*

Patient Information on Anticonvulsant Mood Stabilizers

The name of your medication is: _____

IMPORTANT NOTE: The following information is intended to supplement, not substitute for, the expertise and judgment of your physician, pharmacist, or other health care professional. It is not intended to imply that use of the drug is safe, appropriate, or effective for you. This information contains limited and general information about these medications, and it is not all-inclusive. Not all uses, side effects, precautions, or drug interactions are listed. Your doctor or pharmacist will provide you with official patient information that is more complete and detailed. Consult your health care professional before using this drug.

Common Drug Names

(Brand and generic)

Depakote	(divalproex)
Depakene	(valproic acid)
Lamictal	(lamotrigine)
Tegretol, Equetro	(carbamazepine)

Uses

These medications can be used to treat bipolar disorder, but they are primarily used to treat seizure disorders.

How To Use

A variety of products are available in different strengths; some are short acting and some are long acting. A lower starting dose is prescribed, followed by slowly increasing dosages. Your doctor will determine the best dosing schedule for you. You will need to have regular blood tests to check the amount of medication in your system. After the medication is started, some improvement may be noted within the first week, followed by continued lessening of symptoms over the next several weeks or months. Treatment with the medication is considered long term.

Missed Dose

If you miss a dose, take it as soon as you remember. However, if it is near the time of the next dose, or the next day, skip the missed dose and resume your usual dosing schedule. *Do not double the dose in order to catch up.*

Side Effects

Side effects occur, to some degree, with all medications. They are usually not serious and do not occur in all individuals. They may sometimes occur before beneficial effects of the medication are noticed. Most side effects will decrease or disappear with time. If a side effect persists, speak to the doctor about appropriate treatment.

You should seek immediate medical attention if you experience rash, blistering, or crusting of the skin; itching; swelling; difficulty breathing; mouth sores; lethargy; weakness; confusion; blurred vision; unusual eye movements; lack of coordination; tremor; fever or flu-like symptoms; unusual bruising; bleeding or skin blotching; yellow discoloration of the skin or yellow tinge in the eyes; nausea; vomiting; extreme loss of appetite; difficulty urinating; or dark-colored urine.

Although rare, severe liver problems may occur with these medications. Contact your doctor immediately if you experience vomiting, unusual tiredness, or swelling of the face.

A rare and serious side effect of divalproex is pancreatitis. Tell your doctor immediately if you develop stomach pain, nausea, vomiting, or loss of appetite.

Common side effects that should be reported to the doctor as soon as possible include drowsiness, dizziness, dry mouth, nausea, hair loss (valproate), changes in the menstrual cycle (valproate), and weight change.

Report any other side effects not listed above to your physician.

Drug Interactions

Check with the doctor or pharmacist before starting, stopping, or changing the dose of any other medicines, including over-the-counter and herbal products.

Certain antibiotics may cause carbamazepine levels to increase. Carbamazepine may cause birth controls pills to be less effective.

PRECAUTIONS

- Before taking this medication, tell your doctor or pharmacist if you are allergic to it (if known) or if you have any other allergies.

- Take exactly as prescribed. Do not increase your dose unless instructed by your doctor. Taking too much medication can result in serious side effects.

- Follow your doctor's instructions regarding getting your blood levels checked.

- Do not chew or crush the tablets or capsules unless directed to do so by your doctor or pharmacist.

- Take with food or milk to prevent stomach upset.

- This medicine may cause fatigue, light-headedness, or blurred vision. Use caution when operating machinery, driving, or performing tasks that require alertness or clear vision.

- Carbamazepine may cause increased sensitivity to sunlight.

- Do not stop taking your medication suddenly unless told to do so by your doctor. Abruptly stopping the medicine may cause your bipolar symptoms to return.

- Make sure that your doctor knows about all your medical conditions.

- Inform your doctor or pharmacist about all other medicines you are taking, including over-the-counter products.

- Avoid drinking grapefruit juice while taking carbamazepine, since it can affect the level of carbamazepine in your body.

- Do not drink alcohol while taking this medication.

- Tell your doctor if the medicine does not seem to be working or if your condition gets worse.

- Consult with your doctor if you think you might be pregnant.

- Check with your doctor before breastfeeding.

- Anticonvulsants may cause suicidal thoughts. Notify your doctor immediately if you notice changes in mood, behavior, or actions, or if you have thoughts of harming yourself.

- *If you have any questions regarding this medication, do not hesitate to contact the doctor, pharmacist, or nurse.*

Patient Information on Lithium

The name of your medication is: _____

IMPORTANT NOTE: The following information is intended to supplement, not substitute for, the expertise and judgment of your physician, pharmacist, or other health care professional. It is not intended to imply that use of the drug is safe, appropriate, or effective for you. This information contains limited and general information about these medications, and it is not all-inclusive. Not all uses, side effects, precautions, or drug interactions are listed. Your doctor or pharmacist will provide you with official patient information that is more complete and detailed. Consult your health care professional before using this drug.

Common Brand Names

Eskalith, Lithonate, Lithobid

Use

Lithium is primarily used to treat bipolar disorder.

How To Use

A variety of products are available in different strengths; some are short acting, and some are long acting. A lower starting dose is prescribed, followed by slowly increasing dosages. Your doctor will determine the best dosing schedule for you. You will need to have regular blood tests to check the amount of lithium in your system. After the medication is started, some improvement may be noted within the first week, followed by continued lessening of symptoms over the next several weeks or months. Treatment with the medication is considered long term.

Missed Dose

If you miss a dose, take it as soon as you remember. However, if it is near the time of the next dose, or the next day, skip the missed dose and resume your usual dosing schedule. *Do not double the dose in order to catch up.*

Side Effects

Side effects occur, to some degree, with all medications. They are usually not serious and do not occur in all individuals. They may sometimes occur before beneficial effects of the medication are noticed. Most side effects will decrease or disappear with time. If a side effect persists, speak to the doctor about appropriate treatment.

Although rare, rash, itching, swelling, or difficulty breathing sometimes occurs with lithium. Contact your doctor immediately if you experience vomiting, unusual tiredness, or swelling of the face while taking lithium.

Some side effects might mean that you have too much lithium in your system, which could be very serious. You should report the following side effects to the doctor *immediately*: clumsiness, loss of balance, feeling of intoxication, slurred speech, double vision, vomiting or diarrhea, tremors or shakiness of the hands, and change in mood or behavior.

Common side effects that should be reported to the doctor as soon as possible include difficulty concentrating, mild nausea, weight change, increased thirst and urination, and acne or skin problems.

Report any other side effects not listed above to your physician.

Drug Interactions

Check with the doctor or pharmacist before starting, stopping, or changing the dose of any other medicines, including over-the-counter and herbal products.

Potentially serious drug interactions can occur with diuretic medications (water pills) and nonsteroidal anti-inflammatory medications by causing lithium levels to rise.

PRECAUTIONS

- Before taking this medication, tell your doctor or pharmacist if you are allergic to it (if known) or if you have any other allergies.

- Take exactly as prescribed. Do not increase your dose unless instructed by your doctor. Taking too much lithium can result in serious side effects.

- Follow your doctor's instructions regarding getting your blood levels checked.

- Do not chew or crush the tablets or capsules unless directed to do so by your doctor or pharmacist.

- Take with food or milk to prevent stomach upset.

- Drink eight to twelve glasses of water or fluid every day.

- Maintain your normal diet and do not change the amount of salt in your diet unless instructed by your doctor.

- Limit caffeine intake.

- This medicine may cause fatigue, light-headedness, or blurred vision. Use caution when operating machinery, driving, or performing tasks that require alertness or clear vision.

- Do not stop taking your medication suddenly unless told to do so by your doctor. Abruptly stopping the medicine may cause your bipolar symptoms to return.

- Make sure that your doctor knows about all your medical conditions.

- If you become sick with any flu-like virus or have a fever, check with your doctor to see if any changes in your lithium dose are necessary.

- Be careful not to become dehydrated when exercising, during hot weather, or any time you sweat excessively (for example, in saunas and hot tubs). Losing water and salt from your body may cause your blood lithium level to increase.

- Inform your doctor or pharmacist about all other medicines you are taking, including over-the-counter products.

- Do not drink alcohol while taking this medication.

- Tell your doctor if the medicine does not seem to be working or if your condition gets worse.

- Consult with your doctor if you think you might be pregnant.

- Check with your doctor before breastfeeding.

- *If you have any questions regarding this medication, do not hesitate to contact the doctor, pharmacist, or nurse.*

Patient Information on Psychostimulants

The name of your medication is: _____

IMPORTANT NOTE: The following information is intended to supplement, not substitute for, the expertise and judgment of your physician, pharmacist, or other health care professional. It is not intended to imply that use of the drug is safe, appropriate, or effective for you. This information contains limited and general information about these medications, and it is not all-inclusive. Not all uses, side effects, precautions, or drug interactions are listed. Your doctor or pharmacist will provide you with official patient information that is more complete and detailed. Consult your health care professional before using this drug.

Uses

Psychostimulants are used primarily in the treatment of attention-deficit/hyperactivity disorder (ADHD) in children and adults. These drugs are also approved for use in the treatment of narcolepsy.

Although they are not currently approved for this indication, psychostimulants have been found useful in the treatment of refractory depression.

The doctor may choose to use this medication for a reason not listed here. If you are not sure why this medication is being prescribed, please ask the doctor.

How To Use

Take as directed, usually starting in the morning, up to three times per day by mouth. Some side effects may be reduced by taking the medication with food. It is best to take it at about the same time each day. The dosage is based on your medical condition and response to therapy.

Missed Dose

If you miss a dose, take it as soon as you remember. However, if it is near the time of the next dose, or the next day, skip the missed dose and resume your usual dosing schedule. *Do not double the dose in order to catch up.*

Side Effects

Side effects occur, to some degree, with all medications. They are usually not serious and do not occur in all individuals. They may sometimes occur before beneficial effects of the medication are noticed. Most side effects will decrease or disappear with time. If a side effect persists, speak to the doctor about appropriate treatment.

Common side effects that should be reported to the doctor at the next appointment include difficulty sleeping, nervousness, excitability, loss of appetite, weight loss, increased heart rate and blood pressure, headache, nausea or heartburn, dry mouth, and dizziness.

Tell your doctor immediately if any of the following unlikely but serious side effects occur: muscle twitches or tics; fast or irregular heartbeat; persistent throbbing headache; soreness of mouth, gums, or throat; rash; unusual bruising or bleeding;

nausea and vomiting; yellow tinge of eyes or skin; severe agitation or restlessness; *a switch in mood to an unusual state of happiness or irritability; or other fluctuations in mood.*

Report any other side effects not listed above to your physician.

Drug Interactions

Because psychostimulants can change the effects of other medication, or may be affected by other medication, always check with the doctor or pharmacist before taking other drugs, including over-the-counter medication such as cold remedies. Inform all doctors and dentists who treat or examine you that you are taking a psychostimulant drug.

PRECAUTIONS

- Before taking this medication, tell your doctor or pharmacist if you are allergic to it (if known) or if you have any other allergies.

- Do not increase or decrease your dose without consulting your doctor.

- *If you have any questions regarding this medication, do not hesitate to contact the doctor, pharmacist, or nurse.*

Patient Information on Antipsychotics

The name of your medication is: _____

IMPORTANT NOTE: The following information is intended to supplement, not substitute for, the expertise and judgment of your physician, pharmacist, or other health care professional. It is not intended to imply that use of the drug is safe, appropriate, or effective for you. This information contains limited and general information about these medications, and it is not all-inclusive. Not all uses, side effects, precautions, or drug interactions are listed. Your doctor or pharmacist will provide you with official patient information that is more complete and detailed. Consult your health care professional before using this drug.

Uses

This medication is used to treat certain mental or mood conditions, such as schizophrenia and bipolar mania. It works by helping to restore the balance of certain natural chemicals in the brain (neurotransmitters). Some of the benefits of continued use of this medication include reduced nervousness, better concentration, and reduced episodes of confusion.

How To Use

Take as directed, usually once a day by mouth, with or without food. Stand up slowly, especially when starting this medication, to avoid dizziness. The dosage is based on your medical condition and response to therapy. Use this medication regularly in order to get the most benefit from it. Remember to use it at the same time each day.

Missed Dose

If you miss a dose, take it as soon as you remember. However, if it is near the time of the next dose, or the next day, skip the missed dose and resume your usual dosing schedule. *Do not double the dose in order to catch up.*

Side Effects

Side effects occur, to some degree, with all medications. They are usually not serious and do not occur in all individuals. They may sometimes occur before beneficial effects of the medication are noticed. Most side effects will decrease or disappear with time. If a side effect persists, speak to the doctor about appropriate treatment.

Common side effects that should be reported to the doctor at the next appointment include dizziness, stomach pain, dry mouth, constipation, weight gain, and drowsiness. If any of these effects persist or worsen, notify your doctor or pharmacist promptly.

To minimize dizziness or fainting, stand up slowly when rising from a seated or lying position, especially when you first start using this medication.

Tell your doctor immediately if any of the following unlikely but serious side effects occur: fast heartbeat, ankle or leg swelling, agitation, confusion, restlessness, weakness, difficulty speaking, numbness or tingling of hands or feet, trouble walking (abnormal gait), painful menstrual periods, pink urine, tremor, muscle spasm or rigidity, chest pain, yellowing of the eyes or skin, one-sided weakness, sudden vision changes or other eye problems, headache, painful urination, seizures, or difficulty swallowing.

This drug infrequently causes blood sugar levels to rise, which can cause or worsen diabetes. High blood sugar can in rare cases cause serious (sometimes fatal) conditions, such as diabetic coma. Tell your doctor immediately if you develop symptoms of high blood sugar, such as unusual increased thirst and urination. If you already have diabetes, be sure to check your blood sugars regularly.

This drug may also cause significant weight gain and a rise in your blood cholesterol (or triglyceride) levels. These effects, along with diabetes, may increase your risk for developing heart disease. Discuss the risks and benefits of treatment with your doctor.

This medication can, in rare cases, cause a serious condition called neuroleptic malignant syndrome (NMS). Tell your doctor immediately if you develop any of the following symptoms: fever, muscle stiffness, severe confusion, sweating, or fast or irregular heartbeat.

In rare cases antipsychotics cause a condition known as tardive dyskinesia. In some cases, this condition may be permanent. Tell your doctor immediately if you develop any unusual or uncontrolled movements (especially of the face or tongue).

Report any other side effects not listed above to your physician.

Drug Interactions

Before using this medication, tell your doctor or pharmacist about all prescription medications and over-the-counter or herbal products you are using, especially carbamazepine, fluvoxamine, omeprazole, rifampin, drugs for high blood pressure, and drugs for Parkinson's disease.

Report drugs that cause drowsiness, because this effect will be increased by taking them in combination with this medication.

Do not start or stop any medicine without doctor or pharmacist approval.

PRECAUTIONS

- Before taking this medication, tell your doctor or pharmacist if you are allergic to it (if known) or if you have any other allergies.

- Do not increase or decrease your dose without consulting your doctor.

- This drug may make you dizzy or drowsy; use caution when engaging in activities requiring alertness, such as riding a bike, driving, or using machinery.

- Avoid alcoholic beverages.

- Avoid excessive amounts of caffeine.

- This medication can make you prone to heat stroke. Avoid activities that might cause you to overheat (such as doing strenuous work, exercising in hot weather, and using hot tubs).

- Do not share this medication with others.

- Laboratory and/or medical tests (such as fasting blood sugar, weight, blood pressure, blood cholesterol/triglyceride levels, and liver function tests) should be performed periodically to monitor your progress and check for side effects. Consult your doctor for more details.

- Go for regular eye exams as part of your regular health care regimen, and to check for any unlikely, but possible, eye problems.

- *If you have any questions regarding this medication, do not hesitate to contact the doctor, pharmacist, or nurse.*

References

Agras, S. 1985. *Panic: Facing Fears, Phobias, and Anxiety*. New York: W. H. Freeman.

Ahearn, E. P., A. Krohn, K. M. Connor, et al. 2003. Pharmacologic treatment of PTSD: A focus on antipsychotic use. *Annals of Clinical Psychiatry* 15 (3-4):193-201.

Ahearn, E. P., E. Winston, M. Mussey, and J. R. T. Davidson. 2003. Atypical antipsychotics, improved intrusive symptoms in patients with PTSD. *Military Medicine* 168(9):x–xi.

Akiskal, H. S. 1996. The prevalent clinical spectrum of bipolar disorders: Beyond DSM-IV. *Journal of Clinical Psychopharmacology* 16(Suppl):4S–14S.

Akiskal, H. S., M. L. Bourgeios, J. Angst, R. Post, H. J. Möller, and R. Hirshfeld. 2000. Re-evaluating the prevalence of and diagnostic composition within the broad clinical spectrum of bipolar disorders. *Journal of Affective Disorders* 59(Suppl):S5–530.

Akiskal, H. S., and C. L. Bowden. 2000. The spectrum of bipolarity. Symposium conducted at the American Psychiatric Association 153rd Annual Meeting, Chicago, IL, May.

Akiskal, H. S., and G. B. Cassano, eds. 1997. *Dysthymia and the Spectrum of Chronic Depression*. New York: Guilford Press.

Akiskal, H. S., and R. E. Weise. 1992. The clinical spectrum of so-called "minor" depressions. *American Journal of Psychotherapy* 46:9–22.

American Academy of Child and Adolescent Psychiatry. 2001. Practice parameters for the assessment and treatment of children and adolescents with schizophrenia (American Academy of Child and Adolescent Psychiatry). *Journal of the American Academy of Child and Adolescent Psychiatry* 40:4S–23S.

American Psychiatric Association. 2000. *Diagnostic and Statistical Manual of Mental Disorders, Fourth Edition: Text Revision*. Washington DC: American Psychiatric Association.

———. 2002. Practice Guideline for the Treatment of Patients with Bipolar Disorder (Revision). *American Journal of Psychiatry* 159(Suppl 4):1–50.

American Society of Health Systems Pharmacists. 2004. *American Hospital Formulary Service Drug Information*. Bethesda, MD: American Society of Health Systems Pharmacists.

———. 2008. *American Hospital Formulary Service Drug Information*. Bethesda, MD: American Society of Health Systems Pharmacists.

———. 2012. *American Hospital Formulary Service Drug Information*. Bethesda, MD: American Society of Health Systems Pharmacists.

Arndt, S., R. J. Alliger, and N. C. Andreasen. 1991. The distinction of positive and negative symptoms: The failure of a two-dimensional model. *British Journal of Psychiatry* 158:340–45.

Atshuler, L. L., R. M. Post, G. S. Leverich, K. Mikalauskas, A. Rosoff, and L. Ackerman. 1995. Antidepressant-induced mania and cycle acceleration: A controversy revisited. *American Journal of Psychiatry* 152:1130–1138.

Aursnes, I., I. F. Tvete, J. Gaasemyr, and B. Natvig. 2005. Suicide attempts in clinical trials with paroxetine randomized against placebo. *BMC Medicine* 3:14 (electronic journal) Standard number: 1741–7015. Journal identifier: 101190723.

Avis, H. 1998. *Drugs and Life*. New York: McGraw-Hill Higher Education.

Ayd, F. J. 2000. Evaluating interactions between herbal and psychoactive medications. *Psychiatric Times*, December, 45-47.

Ballenger, J. C., and R. M. Post. 1980. Carbamazepine in manic-depressive illness: A new treatment. *American Journal of Psychiatry* 137:782–90.

Barkley, R. A. 2000. *Taking Charge of ADHD*. New York: Guilford Press.

Baron, M., N. Risch, R. Hamburger, B. Mandel, S. Kushner, M. Newman, et al. 1987. Genetic linkage between X-chromosome markers and bipolar affective illness. *Nature* 326:289–292.

Baroni, A., J. R. Lunsford, D. A. Luckenbaugh, K. E Towbin, and E. Leibenluft. 2009. Practitioner review: The assessment of bipolar disorder in children and adolescents. *Journal of Child Psychology and Psychiatry* 50:203–15.

Barnes, N. M., and T. Sharp. 1999. A review of central 5-HT receptors and their function. *Neuropharmacology* 38:1083–1152.

Barnhart, W. J., E. H. Makela, and M. J. Latocha. 2004. SSRI-induced apathy syndrome: A clinical review. *Journal of Psychiatric Practice* 10(3):196–99.

Bauer, M. S., A. M. Callahan, C. Jampala, F. Petty, M. Sajatovic, V. Schaefer, et al. 1999. Clinical practice guidelines for bipolar disorder from the Department of Veterans Affairs. *Journal of Clinical Psychiatry* 60:9–21.

Baxter, L. R. 1991. PET studies of cerebral function in major depression and obsessive-compulsive disorder: The emerging profrontal cortex consensus. *Annals of Clinical Psychiatry* 3:103–09.

Baxter, L. R., J. M. Schwartz, K. S. Bergman, M. P. Szuba, B. H. Guze, J. C. Marriotta, et al. 1992. Caudate glucose metabolic rate changes with both drug and behavior therapy for obsessive-compulsive disorder. *Archives of General Psychiatry* 49:681–89.

Beasley, C. M., and B. E. Dornseif. 1991. Fluoxetine and suicide: A meta-analysis of controlled trials of treatment of depression. *British Medical Journal* 303:685–92.

Beaubrun, G., and G. E. Gray. 2000. A review of herbal medicines for psychiatric disorders. *Psychiatric Services* 51(9):1130–34

Beck, A. T. 1976. *Cognitive Therapy and the Emotional Disorders*. New York: International Universities Press.

Beitman, B. D., and G. L. Klerman, eds. 1991. *Integrating Pharmacotherapy and Psychotherapy*. Washington, DC: American Psychiatric Press.

Bender, K. J., ed. 1993. Narcotic antagonist for alcoholism. *Psychotropics* 13:6–8.

Benet, L. Z., D. L. Kroetz, and L. B. Sheiner. 1996. Pharmacokinetics: The dynamics of drug absorption, distribution, and elimination. In *Goodman and Gilman's: The Pharmacological Basis of Therapeutics*. J. G. Hardman, L. E. Limbird, P. B. Molinoff, R. W. Ruddon, and A. G. Gilman, eds. New York: McGraw-Hill.

Benet, L. Z., J. R. Mitchell, and L. B. Sherner. 1990a. General principles. In *Goodman & Gilman's: The Pharmacological Basis of Therapeutics*. A. G. Gilman, T. W. Rall, A. S. Nies, and P. Taylor, eds. New York: Pergamon Press.

———. 1990b. Pharmacokinetics: The dynamics of drug absorption, distribution, and elimination. In *Goodman & Gilman's: The Pharmacological Basis of Therapeutics*, A. G. Gilman, T. W. Rall, A. S. Nies, and P. Taylor, eds. New York: Pergamon Press.

Berigan, T. R., and A. Holzgang. 1995. Valproate as an alternative in post-traumatic stress disorder: A case report. *Military Medicine* 160(6):318.

Bhalla, U. S., and R. Iyengar. 1999. Emergent properties of networks of biological signaling pathways. *Science* 283:381–87.

Biederman, J., T. Wilens, T. J. Spencer, M. Harding, D. O'Donnell, and S. Griffin. 1999. Pharmacotherapy for ADD reduces risk for substance abuse disorder. *Pediatrics* 104(2):20.

Bieck, P. R., and K. Antonin. 1988. Oral tyramine pressor test and the safety of monoamine oxidase inhibitor drugs: Comparison of brofaromine and tranylcypromine in healthy subjects. *Journal of Clinical Psychopharmacology* 8:237–45.

Bleuler, M. 1968. Prognosis of schizophrenic psychoses: A summary of personal research. In *The Schizophrenias*. F. Flach, ed. New York: Norton.

Bly, R. 1990. *Iron John*. Reading, MA: Addison-Wesley Publishing.

Bochus, S. E., and J. E. Kleinman. 1996. The neuropathology of schizophrenia. *Journal of Clinical Psychiatry* 57(Suppl):72–83.

Bogenschutz, M. P., and G. H. Nurnberg. 2004. Olanzapine versus placebo in the treatment of borderline personality disorder. *Journal of Clinical Psychiatry* 65(1):104–09.

Boullata, J. I., and A. M. Nace. 2000. Safety issues with herbal medicine. *Pharmacotherapy* 20:257–69.

Bourne, H. R., and M. von Zastrow. 2001. Drug receptors and pharmacodynamics. In *Basic and Clinical Pharmacology*. B. G. Katzung, ed. New York: McGraw-Hill.

Bowden, C. L. 1996. Role of newer medications for bipolar disorder. Journal of Clinical Psychopharmacology 16(Suppl):48S–55S.

———. 2003. Rapid cycling disorder. *Medscape Psychiatry and Mental Health* 8(1), www.medscape.com.

Bowden, C. L., A. M. Brugger, A. C. Swann, J. R. Calabrese, P. G. Janicak, F. Petty, et al. 1994. Efficacy of divalproex vs. lithium, placebo in the treatment of mania. *Journal of the American Medical Association* 271:918–24.

Bowes, M. 2001. OCD: Will immunotherapy succeed where other approaches have failed? *Neuropsychiatry Reviews* 2:1–25.

Bowlby, J. 1986. *Attachment and Loss*. New York: Basic Books.

Brady, K., T. Pearlstein, G. M. Asnis, D. Baker, B. Rothbaum, C. R. Sikes, et al. 2000. Efficacy and safety of sertraline treatment of post-traumatic stress disorder: A randomized controlled trial. *Journal of the American Medical Association* 283:1837–44.

Brenner, R., et al. 2000. Comparison of an extract of hypericum (LI-160) and sertraline in the treatment of depression: A double-blind randomized pilot study. *Clinical Therapeutics* 22:411-419.

Briggs, G. G., R. K. Freeman, and S. J. Yaffe. 2008. *Drugs in Pregnancy and Lactation*. Philadelphia, PA: Lippincott Williams & Wilkins.

Briggs, G. G. 1992. Drugs in pregnancy and lactation. In *Applied Therapeutics: The Clinical Use of Drugs*, 5th ed. M. A. Koda-Kimble, L. Y. Young, W. A. Kradjan, and B. J. Guglielmo, eds. Vancouver, WA: Applied Therapeutics.

Brotman, A. 1992. *Practical Reviews in Psychiatry* (audiotape). Birmingham, AL: Educational Reviews.

Brown, C. S., and S. G. Bryant. 1992. Major depressive disorders. In *Applied Therapeutics: The Clinical Use of Drugs*, 5th ed. M. A. Koda-Kimble, L. Y. Young, W. A. Kradjan, and B. J. Guglielmo, eds. Vancouver, WA: Applied Therapeutics.

Brown, S. A., and M. A. Schuckit. 1988. Changes in depression among abstinent alcoholics. *Journal of the Study of Alcoholism* 49:412–17.

Brown University. 2004. Experts, parents weigh in at FDA's public hearing on SSRI safety. *Child and Adolescent Psychopharmacology Update* 6(3):1–3.

Burton, T. M. 1991. Antidepression drug of Eli Lilly loses sales after attack by sect. *Wall Street Journal*, April 19, A1–A2.

Calabrese, J. R., S. H. Fatemi, M. Kujawa, and M. J. Woyshville. 1996. Predictors of response to mood stabilizers. *Journal of Clinical Psychopharmacology* 16(Suppl):24S–31S.

Calabrese, J. R., P. E. Keck, W. Macfadden, M. Minkwitz, et al. 2005. A randomized, double-blind, placebo-controlled trial of quetiapine in the treatment of bipolar I or II depression. *American Journal of Psychiatry* 162:1351-1360.

Calabrese, J. R., and M. Woyshville. 1995. A medication algorithm for treatment of bipolar rapid cycling? *Journal of Clinical Psychiatry* 56(Suppl):11–18.

Carlson, G. A., and F. K. Goodwin. 1973. The stages of mania. *Archives of General Psychiatry* 28:221–28.

Carpenter, W. T., T. E. Hanlon, D. W. Heinrichs, A. T. Summerfelt, B. Kirkpatrick. J. Levine, et al. 1990. Continuous versus targeted medication in schizophrenic outpatients: Outcome results. *American Journal of Psychiatry* 147:1138–48.

Castellanos, F. X., P. P. Lee, W. Sharp, N. O. Jeffries, D. K. Greenstein, L. S. Clasen, et al. 2002. Developmental trajectories of brain volume abnormalities in children and adolescents with attention-deficit/hyperactivity disorder. *Journal of the American Medical Association* 288(14):1740–48.

Cauffield, J. S. 2000. The psychosocial aspects of complementary and alternative medicine. *Pharmacotherapy* 20:1289–94.

Chang, D. M. 2000. Lithium as a neuroprotective drug in vivo and in vitro: Mechanisms and implications. *International Journal of Neuropsychopharmacology* 3(Suppl):S11.

Clayton, A. H., J. F. Pradko, H. A. Montano, C. B. Ledbetter, et al. 2002. Prevalence of sexual dysfunction among newer antidepressants. *Journal of Clinical Psychiatry* 63:357–66.

Clerc, G. E., P. Ruimy, and J. Verdeau-Palles. 1994. A double-blind comparison of venlafaxine and fluoxetine in patients hospitalized for major depression and melancholia. *International Journal of Clinical Psychopharmacology* 9:139–43.

Clothier, J., A. C. Swann, and T. Freeman. 1992. Dysphoric mania. *Journal of Clinical Psychopharmacology* 12(Suppl):13S–22S.

Coccaro, E. F. 1998. Clinical outcome of psychopharmacologic treatment of borderline and schizotypal personality disordered subjects. *Journal of Clinical Psychiatry* 59(Suppl):130–35.

———. 2004. Borderline personality disorder therapy with Omega-3 fatty acids. Current Psychiatry Reports 6(1):42.

Coghill, D. 2003. Current issues in child and adolescent psychopharmacology. Part 2: Anxiety and obsessive-compulsive disorders, autism, Tourette's and schizophrenia. *Advances in Psychiatric Treatment* 9:289–99.

Cohen, L. S., V. L. Heller, and J. F. Rosenbaum. 1989. Treatment guidelines for psychotropic drug use in pregnancy. *Psychosomatics* 30:25–33.

Connor, K. M., S. M. Sutherland, L. A. Tupler, M. L. Malik, and J. R. Davidson. 1999. Fluoxetine in post-traumatic stress disorder: Randomized, double-blind study. *British Journal of Psychiatry* 175:17–22.

Consumer Reports. 2000. Emotional aspirin? December, 60–62.

Contreras, J., L. Hare, B. Camarena, D. Glahn, A. Dassori, R. Medina, et al. 2009. The serotonin transporter 5-HTTPR polymorphism is associated with current and lifetime depression in persons with chronic psychotic disorders. *Acta Psychiatrica Scandinavica* 119:117–27.

Cook, E. H., K. D. Wagner, J. S. March, J. Biederman, P. Landau, R. Wolkow, and M. Messig. 2001. Long-term sertraline treatment of children and adolescents with obsessive-compulsive disorder. *Journal of the American Academy of Child and Adolescent Psychiatry* 40:1175–81.

Cornelius, J. R., P. H. Soloff, J. M. Perel, and R. F. Ulrich. 1991. A preliminary trial of fluoxetine in refractory borderline patients. *Journal of Clinical Psychopharmacology* 11:116–20.

Cowdry, R. W., and D. L. Gardner. 1988. Pharmacotherapy of borderline personality disorder. *Archives of General Psychiatry* 45:111–19.

Cowley, G., K. Springer, E. A. Leonard, K. Robins, and J. Gorden. 1990. The promise of Prozac. *Newsweek*, March 26, 38–41.

Crutchfield, J. P., J. Farmer, N. H. Packard, and R. Shaw. 1986. Chaos. *Scientific American* 255:46–57.

Daly, A. K., B.P. King, and J. B. Leathart. 2006. Genotyping for cytochrome P450 polymorphisms. *Methods in molecular biology* 320:193–207.

Davidson, J., H. Kudler, R. Smith, S. L. Mahorney, et al. 1990. Treatment of PTSD with amitriptyline and placebo. *Archives of General Psychiatry* 47:259–66.

Davidson, J., S. Roth, and E. Newman. 1991. Fluoxetine in post-traumatic stress disorder. *Journal of Traumatic Stress* 4:419–23.

Davidson, J. R. T., and K. M. Connor. 2000. *Herbs for the Mind: What Science Tells Us About Nature's Remedies for Depression, Stress, Memory Loss and Insomnia*. New York: Guilford Press.

Davidson, S. R. 2003. Treatment of PTSD: The impact of paroxetine. *Psychopharmacology Bulletin* 37(Suppl 1):76–88.

Davis, K., R. Kahn, G. Ko, and M. Davidson. 1991. Dopamine in schizophrenia: A review and reconceptualization. *American Journal of Psychiatry*. 148:1474–1484.

Davis, K. L., M. S. Buchsbaum, L. Shihabuddin, J. Spiegel-Cohen, et al. 1998. Ventricular enlargement in poor-outcome schizophrenia. *Biological Psychiatry* 43:783–93.

DeBattista, C., K. Doghramji, M. A. Menza, M. H. Rosenthal, et al. 2003. Adjunct Modafinil for the short-term treatment of fatigue and sleepiness in patients with major depressive disorder: A preliminary double-blind, placebo-controlled study. *Journal of Clinical Psychiatry* 64(9):1057-1064.

Deckert, G. 1985. Advances in neuro-biology. Paper presented at Continuing Education Advanced Psychiatric Update, San Francisco, CA.

De La Cancela, V. 2000. Diversity in psychopharmacology. *Public Service Psychology* 25(3):11–12, 28.

de Leon, J. 2009. The future (or lack of future) of personalized prescription in psychiatry. *Phamacological Research* 59:81–89.

Deltito, J. A. 1993. The effect of valproate on bipolar spectrum temperamental disorders. *Journal of Clinical Psychiatry* 54:301–04.

DerMarderosian, A., and J. A. Beutler. 2008. *The Review of Natural Products*. St. Louis, MO: Wolters Kluwer Health.

Devlin, M. J., S. Z. Yanovski, and G. T. Wilson. 2000. Obesity: What mental health professionals need to know. *American Journal of Psychiatry* 157:854–66.

Dilsaver, S. C., A. C. Swann, A. M. Shoaib, T. C. Bowers, et al. 1993. Depressive mania associated with non-response to antimanic agents. *American Journal of Psychiatry* 150:1548–51.

Donnelly, C. L. 2003. Pharmacologic treatment approaches for children and adolescents with posttraumatic stress disorder. *Child and Adolescent Psychiatric Clinics of North America* 12(2):251–69.

Drent, M. L., and E. A. van der Veen. 1993. Lipase inhibition: A novel concept in the treatment of obesity. *International Journal of Obesity and Related Metabolic Disorders* 17:241–44.

Drug Information for the Health Care Professional. 2007. USP DI vol. I: Drug Information for the Health Care Professional. Greenwood Village, CO: Thomson Micromedex.

Eisenberg, D. M., R. B. Davis, S. L. Ettner, S. Appel, et al. 1998. Trends in alternative medicine use in the United States, 1990–1997. *Journal of the American Medical Association* 280:1569–75.

Emslie, G. J., and T. C. Mayes. 2001. Mood disorders in children and adolescents: Psychopharmacological treatment. *Biological Psychiatry* 49:1082–90.

Emslie, G. J., A. J. Rush, W. A. Weinberg, R. A. Kowatch, C. W. Hughes, T. Carmody, et al. 1997. A double-blind randomized, placebo-controlled trial of fluoxetine in children and adolescents with depression. *Archives of General Psychiatry* 54:1031–37.

Ereshefsky, L., and A. L. Richards. 1992. Psychoses. In *Applied Therapeutics: The Clinical Use of Drugs,* 5th ed. M. A. Koda-Kimble, L. Y. Young, W. A. Kradjan, B. J. Guglielmo, eds. Vancouver, WA: Applied Therapeutics.

Evans, D. L., M. J. Byerly, and R. A. Greer. 1995. Secondary mania: Diagnosis and treatment. *Journal of Clinical Psychiatry* 56(Suppl):31–37.

Eysenck, H. J. 1965. The effects of psychotherapy: An evaluation. *Journal of Consulting Psychology* 16:319–24.

Facts and Comparisons. 2012. St. Louis, MO: Facts and Comparisons.

Fava, M., K. I. Anderson, and J. Rusenbaum. 1993. Are thymoleptic-responsive "anger attacks" a discrete clinical syndrome? *Psychosouratics* 34(4):350–55.

Fava, M., and J. F. Rosenbaum. 1991. Suicidality and fluoxetine: Is there a relationship? *Journal of Clinical Psychiatry* 52:108–11.

Fava, M., M. E. Schmidt, S. Zhang, J. Gonzales, N. J. Raute, and R. Judge. 2002. Treatment approaches to major depressive disorder relapse. Part 2: Reinitiation of antidepressant treatment. *Psychotherapy and Psychosomatics* 71(4):195–199.

Fesler, F. A. 1991. Valporate in combat-related post-traumatic stress disorder. *Journal of Clinical Psychiatry* 52:361–64.

Flowers, C. R., and D. Veenstra. 2004. The role of cost-effectiveness analysis in the era of pharmacogenomics. *Pharmacogenomics* 22:481–93.

Flockhart, D. A. 1996. Drug interactions, cardiac toxicity and terfenadine: From bench to clinic? *Journal of Clinical Psychopharmacology* 16:101–02.

Forster, P. L., F. B. Schoenfeld, C. R. Marmar, and A. J. Lang. 1995. Lithium for irritability in post-traumatic stress disorder. *Journal of Traumatic Stress* 8:143–49.

Frances, A. J. 1989. *Borderline Personality Disorder* (audiotape). New York: Guilford Publications.

Frances, A. J., D. A. Kahn, D. Carpenter, J. P. Docherty, and S. L. Donovan. 1998. The expert consensus guidelines for treating depression in bipolar disorder. *Canadian Journal of Psychiatry* 59(Suppl): 73-79.

Frances, A. J., and P. H. Soloff. 1988. Treating the borderline patient with low-dose neuroleptics. *Hospital and Community Psychiatry* 39:246–48.

Frank, J. D. 1991. *Persuasion and Healing,* 3rd ed. Baltimore: Johns Hopkins University Press.

Freud, S. 1895. Project for a scientific psychology. In vol. 1 of *The Standard Edition of the Complete Psychological Works of Sigmund Freud,* J. Strachey, ed. London: Hogarth Press, 1953.

———. 1917. Mourning and melancholia. In vol. 14 of *The Standard Edition of the Complete Psychological Works of Sigmund Freud*. London: Hogarth Press, 1957.

Fugh-Berman, A. 2000. Herb-drug interactions. *Lancet* 355:134.

Gabbard, G. O. 2000. A neurobiologically informed perspective on psychotherapy. *British Journal of Psychiatry* 177:117–22.

Gardner, D. L., and R. W. Cowdry. 1986. Positive effects of carbamazepine on behavioral dyscontrol in borderline personality disorder. *American Journal of Psychiatry* 143:519–22.

Garlow, S. J., D. L. Musselman, and C. B. Nemeroff. 1999. The neurochemistry of mood disorders clinical studies. In *Neurobiology of Mental Illness*. D. S. Charney, E. J. Nester, and B. S. Bunney, eds. New York: Oxford University Press.

Gelenberg, A. J., and S. C. Schoonover. 1991. Bipolar disorder. In *The Practitioner's Guide to Psychoactive Drugs*, 3rd ed. A. J. Gelenberg, E. L. Bassuk, and S. C. Schoonover, eds. New York: Plenum.

Geller, B., J. L. Craney, K. Bolhofner, M. J. Nickelsburg, et al. 2002. Two-year prospective follow-up of children with a prepubertal and early adolescent bipolar disorder phenotype. *American Journal of Psychiatry* 159:927–33.

Geller, B., J. L. Craney, K. Bolhofner, M. P. DelBello, et al. 2003. Phenomenology and longitudinal course of children with a prepubertal and early adolescent bipolar disorder phenotype. In *Bipolar Disorder in Childhood and Early Adolescence*. B. Geller, and M. P. DelBello, eds. New York: Guilford Press.

Geller, B., and M. P. DelBello, eds. 2003. *Bipolar Disorder in Childhood and Early Adolescence*. New York: Guilford Press.

Geller, D. A., J. Biederman, B. Mullin, A. Martin, et al. 2003. Which SSRI? A meta-analysis of pharmacotherapy trials in pediatric obsessive-compulsive disorder. *American Journal of Psychiatry* 160:1919–28.

Gelpin, E., O. Bonne, D. Brandes, and A. Y. Shalev. 1996. Treatment of recent trauma survivors with benzodiazepines: A prospective study. *Journal of Clinical Psychiatry*. 57(9):390–94.

Gennaro, A. R. 1980. Inorganic pharmaceutical chemistry. In *Remington's Pharmaceutical Sciences*, 16th ed. A. Osol, ed. Easton, PA: Mack.

George, A., and P. H. Soloff. 1986. Schizotypal symptoms in patients with borderline personality disorder. *American Journal of Psychiatry* 143:212–215.

Ghaemi, S. N. 2000. New treatments for bipolar disorder: The role of atypical neuroleptic agents. *Journal of Clinical Psychiatry* 61(Suppl):33–42.

Gilbert, D. A., K. Z. Altshuler, W. V. Rago, S. P. Shon, et al. 1998. Texas medication algorithm project: Definitions, rationale, and methods to develop medication algorithms. *Journal of Clinical Psychiatry* 59:345–351.

Gitlin, M. 1993. Pharmacotherapy of personality disorders: Conceptual framework and lineal strategies. *Journal of Clinical Psychopharmacology* 13(5):343–53.

———. 1999. Lithium and the kidney: An updated review. *Drug Safety* 20:2331–43.

———. 2002. *Depression Myths and Contrary Realities*. Continuing Education Series, Department of Psychiatry, UCLA.

Glass, R. M. 2004. Treatment of adolescents with major depression: Contributions of a major trial. *Journal of the American Medical Association* 292(7):861–63.

Glazener, F. S. 1992. Adverse drug reactions. In *Melmon and Morrelli's Clinical Pharmacology: Basic Principles in Therapeutics*, 3rd ed. D. W. Nierenberg, ed. New York: McGraw-Hill.

Goff, D. C., and J. T. Coyle. 2001. The emerging role of glutamate in the pathophysiology and treatment of schizophrenia. *American Journal of Psychiatry* 158(9):1367–77.

Goldberg, J. F. 2000. Treatment guidelines: Current and future management of bipolar disorder. *Journal of Clinical Psychiatry* 61(Suppl):12–18.

Goldberg, J. F., M. Harrow, and L. S. Grossman. 1995. Course and outcome in bipolar affective disorder: A longitudinal follow-up study. *American Journal of Psychiatry* 152:379–84.

Goldberg, S. C., S. C. Schulz, P. M. Schulz, R. J. Resnick, et al. 1986. Borderline and schizotypal personality disorders treated with low dose thiothixene vs. placebo. *Archives of General Psychiatry* 43:680–86.

Goodman, A. 1991. Organic unit theory: The mind-body problem revisited. *American Journal of Psychiatry* 148:553–63.

Goodwin, F. K., and K. R. Jamison. 1990. *Manic Depressive Illness*. New York: Oxford University Press.

Gordon, B. 1990. *I'm Dancing As Fast As I Can*. New York: Bantam.

Gottschalk, A., M. S. Bauer, and P. C. Whybrow. 1995. Evidence of chaotic mood variation in bipolar disorder. *Archives of General Psychiatry* 52:947–59.

Greenblatt, D. J., L. L. von Moltke, J. S. Harmatz, and R. I. Shader. 1998. Drug interactions with newer antidepressants: Role of human cytochromes P450. *Journal of Clinical Psychiatry* 1998(Suppl):19–27.

Gur, R. E., P. Cowell, B. I. Turetsky, N. Gallacher, et al. 1998. A follow-up magnetic resonance imaging study of schizophrenia: Relationship of neuroanatomical changes to clinical and neurobehavioral measures. *Archives of General Psychiatry* 55:145–52.

Hall, R., M. K. Popkin, R. Devaul, L. Fairlace, and S. K. Stickney. 1978. Physical illness presenting as psychiatric disease. *Archives of General Psychiatry* 35.1315–20.

Hamner, M. B., S. E. Deitsch, S. P. Brodrick, et al. 2003. Quetiapine treatment with patients with PTSD: An open trial of adjunctive therapy. *Journal of Clinical Psychopharmacology* 23(1):15–20.

Hammer, M., H. Ulmer, and D. Horne. 1997. Buspirone potential of antidepressants in the treatment of PTSD. *Depression and Anxiety* 5:137–39.

Hanotin, C., F. Thomas, S. P. Jones, E. Leutenegger, et al. 1998. A comparison of sibutramine and dexfenfluramine in the treatment of obesity. *Obesity Research* 6:285–91.

Hansten, P. D., and J. R. Horn. 2009. *Drug Interactions Analysis and Management.* St. Louis, MO: Wolters Kluwer Health.

———. 1993. *Drug Interactions and Updates.* Vancouver, WA: Applied Therapeutics.

Hardan, A., K. Johnson, C. Johnson, and B. Hrecznyj. 1996. Case study: Risperidone treatment of children and adolescents with developmental disorders. *Journal of the American Academy of Child and Adolescent Psychiatry* 35:1551–56.

Harlow, H. F., and M. K. Harlow. 1971. Psychopathology in monkeys. In *Experimental Psychopathology.* H. D. Kimmal, ed. New York: Academic Press.

Harvey, P. D., and R. S. E. Keefe. 2001. Studies of cognitive changes in patients with schizophrenia following novel antipsychotic treatment. *American Journal of Psychiatry* 158:176–84.

Harris, I. M. 2000. Regulatory and ethical issues with dietary suppements. *Pharmacotherapy* 20:1295–02.

Heim, C., D. J. Newport, S. Heit, and Y. P. Graham. 2000. Pituitary-adrenal and autonomic responses to stress in women after sexual and physical abuse in childhood. *Journal of the American Medical Association* 284(5):592–97.

Heim, C., and C. P. Nemeroff. 2002. Neurobiology of early life stress: Clinical studies. *Seminars in Clinical Neuropsychiatry* 7(2):147–59.

Henderson, D. C. 1995. Psychopharmacological issues in the treatment of African Americans. Proceedings of the Second Symposium for Mental Health Professionals of Color, College of the Holy Cross. Worcester: MA. 97–106.

Hidalgo, R. B., and J. R. Davidson. 2000. Selective serotonin reuptake inhibitors in PTSD. *Journal of Psychopharmacology* 14(1):70–76.

Hidalgo, R. B., et al. 1999. Nefazodore in PTSD: Results from six open-label trials. *International Clinical Psychopharmacology* 14(2):61–68.

Hilger, E., C. Barnas, and S. Kasper. 2003. Quetiapine in the treatment of borderline personality disorder. *World Journal of Biological Psychiatry* 4(1):42–44.

Hirschfeld, R. M., and F. K. Goodwin. 1988. Mood disorders. In *The American Psychiatric Press Textbook of Psychiatry.* J. A. Talbott, R. E. Hales, and S. C. Yudofsky, eds. Washington, DC: American Psychiatric Press.

Hoehn-Saric, R., J. R. Lipsey, and D. R. McCloud. 1990. Apathy and indifference in patients on fluvoxamine and fluoxetine. *Journal of Clinical Psychopharmacology* 10:343–45.

Hoffman, R. E., and T. H. McGlashan. 1997. Synaptic elimination, neurodevelopment, and the mechanism of hallucinated "voices" in schizophrenia. *American Journal of Psychiatry* 154:1683–89.

Hollander. E., J. Bartz, W. Chaplin, A. Phillip, J. Sumner, L. Soorya, et al. 2007. Oxytocin increases retention of social cognition in autism. *Biological Psychiatry* 61(4):498–503.

Hollander, E., and J. Rosen. 2000. Impulsivity. *Journal of Psychopharmcology* 14:S39–S44.

Hollister, L. E. 1992. Psychiatric disorders. In *Melmon and Morrelli's Clinical Pharmacology: Basic Principles in Therapeutics,* 3rd ed. K. L. Melmon, H. F. Morrelli, B. B. Hoffman, and D. W. Nierenberg, eds. New York: McGraw-Hill.

Hori, A. 1998. Pharmacotherapy for personality disorders. *Clinical Neuroscience* 52(1):13–19.

Horowitz, M. J. 1976. *Stress Response Syndromes.* New York: Jason Aronson.

Hyman, S. E., and E. J. Nestler. 1996. Initiation and adaptation: A paradigm for understanding psychotropic drug action. *American Journal of Psychiatry* 153(2):151–62.

Ingelman-Sundberg, M., S. C. Sim, A. Gomez, and C. Rodriguez-Antona. 2007. Influence of cytochrome P450 polymorphisms on drug therapies: Pharmacogenetic, pharmacoepigenetic, and clinical aspects. *Pharmacology & Therapeutics* 116:496–526.

Institute of Safe Medication Practices List of Error-Prone Abbreviations, Symbols, and Dose Designations. 2003. *ISMP MedicationSafetyAlert!* November, vol. 8, issue 24. Huntingdon Valley, PA.

Jacobsen, F. M. 1993. Low-dose valproate: A new treatment for cyclothymia, mild rapid cycling disorders, and premenstrual syndrome. *Journal of Clinical Psychiatry* 54:229–34.

Jann, M. W. 1992. Anxiety. In *Applied Therapeutics: The Clinical Use of Drugs*, 5th ed. M. A. Koda-Kimble, L. Y. Young, W. A. Kradjan, and B. J. Guglielmo, eds. Vancouver, WA: Applied Therapeutics.

Jaskiw, G. E., and D. R. Weinberger. 1992. Dopamine and schizophrenia—A cortically corrective perspective. *Seminars in the Neurosciences* 4:179–88.

Javitt, D., and S. Zukin. 1991. Recent advances in the phencyclidine model of schizophrenia. *American Journal of Psychiatry* 148:1301–07.

Jin, Y., Z. Desta, V. Stearns, B. Ward, et al. 2005. CYP2D6 genotype, antidepressant use, and tamoxifen metabolism during adjuvant breast cancer treatment. *Journal of the National Cancer Institute* 97:30–39.

Jinks, M. J., and R. H. Fuerst. 1992. Geriatric therapy. In *Applied Therapeutics: The Clinical Use of Drugs*, 5th ed. M. A. Koda-Kimble, L. Y. Young, W. A. Kradjan, and B. J. Guglielmo, eds. Vancouver, WA: Applied Therapeutics.

Johnson, G. 1998. Lithium: Early development, toxicity, and renal function. *Neuropsychopharmacology* 19:200–05.

Johnson, J. A. 2003. Pharmacogenetics: Potential for individualized drug therapy through genetics. *Trends in Genetics* 19:660–66.

Johnston, A. M., and J. M. Eagles. 1999. Lithium associated clinical hypothyroidism: Prevalence and risk factors. *British Journal of Psychiatry* 175:336–39.

Joint Commission on the Accreditation of Health Care Organizations. 2004. National Patient Safety Goal #2 (Communication). Oakbrook Terrace, IL.

Joseph, S. 1997. *Personality Disorders: New Symptom-Focused Only Therapy*. New York: Haworth Press.

Journal of Clinical Psychiatry. 2004. Consensus development conference on antipsychotic drugs and obesity and diabetes. *Journal of Clinical Psychiatry* 65:267–72.

Jureidini, J., C. J. Doecke, P. R. Mansfield, M. M. Haby, et al. 2004. Efficacy and safety of antidepressants for children and adolescents. *British Medical Journal* 328:879–83.

Kagan, J. 1998. *Galen's Prophecy: Temperament in Human Nature*. New York: Basic Books.

Kane, J. M. 1990. Treatment programme and long-term outcome in chronic schizophrenia. *Acta Psychiatrica Scandinavica* 82(Suppl):358:151–57.

Kapfhamner, H. P., and H. Hippius. 1998. Pharmacotherapy in personality disorders. *Journal of Personality Disorders* 12(3):277–88.

Katzung, B. G. 2001. Basic principles. In *Basic and Clinical Pharmacology*, B. G. Katzung, ed. New York: McGraw-Hill.

Keck, P. E., and S. L. McElroy. 1996. Outcome in the pharmacologic treatment of bipolar disorder. *Journal of Clinical Psychopharmacology* 16(Suppl):15S–23S.

Keck, P. E., S. L. McElroy, K. C. Tugrul, and J. A. Bennett. 1993. Valproate oral loading in the treatment of acute mania. *Journal of Clinical Psychiatry* 54:305–08.

Keck, P. E., R. H. Perlis, M. W. Otto, D. Carpenter, et al. 2004. The Expert Consensus Guideline Series: Treatment of Bipolar Disorder 2004. *Postgraduate Medicine Special Report:* 1-120.

Keller, M. B., P. Lavori, W. Coryell, J. Endicott, et al. 1993. Bipolar I: A five-year prospective follow-up. *Journal of Nervous and Mental Disease* 181:238–45.

Kelsoe, J. R., M. A. Spence, E. Loetscher, M. Foguet, et al. 2001. A genome survey indicates a possible susceptibility locus for bipolar disorder on chromosome 22. *Proceedings of the National Academy of Science USA* 98:585–90.

Ketter, T. A., H. K. Manji, and R. M. Post. 2003. Potential mechanisms of action of lamotrigine in the treatment of bipolar disorder. *Journal of Clinical Psychopharmacology* 23(5):484–95.

Kety, S. S. 1975. Progress toward an understanding of the biological substrates of schizophrenia. In *Genetic Research in Psychiatry*, R. R. Fieve, ed. Baltimore: Johns Hopkins University Press.

Kety, S. S., D. Rosenthal, T. H. Wender, and F. Schulsinger. 1971. Mental illness in the biological and adoptive families of adopted schizophrenics. *American Journal of Psychiatry* 128:302–06.

Kleiner, J., L. Altshuler, V. Hendrick, and J. M. Hershman. 1999. Lithium-induced subclinical hypothyroidism: Review of the literature and guidelines for treatment. *Journal of Clinical Psychiatry* 60:249–55.

Klerman, G. L., M. M. Weissman, B. J. Rounsaville, and E. Chevron. 1984. *Interpersonal Psychotherapy of Depression*. New York: Basic Books.

Knipling, R., and J. Wang. 1994. Crashes and fatalities related to driver drowsiness/fatigue. Research Note from the Office of Crash Avoidance Research, Nov.: 1–8. Washington, DC: National Highway Traffic Safety Administration.

Koran, L., H. Sox, K. Marton, S. Moltzen, et al. 1989. Medical evaluation of psychiatric patients: I. Results in a state mental health system. *Archives of General Psychiatry* 46:733–40.

Kosfeld, M., M. Heinrichs, P. J. Zak, U. Fischbacher, and E. Fehr. 2005. Oxytocin increases trust in humans. *Nature* 435(7042):673–76.

Kowatch, R. A., T. Suppes, T. J. Carmody, J. P. Bucci, et al. 2000. Effect size of lithium, divalproex sodium, and carbamazepine in children and adolescents with bipolar disorder. *Journal of American Academy of Children and Adolescent Psychiatry* 39:713–20.

Knoll, J. L., IV, D. L. Garver, J. E. Ramberg, S. J. Kingsbury, et al. 1998. Heterogeneity of the psychoses: Is there a neurodegenerative psychosis? *Schizophrenia Bulletin* 24:365–79.

Korn, M. 2000. Developments in the treatment of bipolar disorder. Symposium conducted at the 23rd Annual Congress of the Collegium Internationale Neuro-Psychopharmacologicum, July.

Kraemer, G. W., M. H. Ebert, and S. R. Lake. 1984. Hypersensitivity to d-amphetamine several years after early social deprivation in rhesus monkeys. *Psychopharmacology* 82:266–71.

Kraepelin, E. 1921. *Textbook of Psychiatry*, 7th ed. (abstracted). Trans. Diefendorf. London: MacMillan, 1907.

Kramer, A. M. 2000. New advances in the use of lithium. Symposium conducted at the 23rd Annual Congress of the Collegium Internationale Neuro-Psychopharmacologicum, 23–27, 2000. Montreal, Canada. July.

Kramer, P. D. 1993. *Listening to Prozac*. New York: Viking.

Krashin, D., and E. W. Oates 1999. Risperidone as an adjunct therapy for post-traumatic stress disorder. *Military Medicine* 164(8):605–06.

Krystal, J. H., A. Anand, and B. Moghaddam. 2002. Effects of NMDA receptor antagonists: Implications for the pathophysiology of schizophrenia. *Archives of General Psychiatry* 59(7):663–64.

Kuczenski, R., et al. 2002. Exposure of adolescent rats to oral methylphenidate. *Journal of Neuroscience* 22:264–71.

Kupfer, D. J., L. L. Carpenter, and E. Frank. 1988. Possible role of antidepressants in precipitating mania and hypomania in recurrent depression. *American Journal of Psychiatry* 145:804–08.

LaFrance, W. C., E. C., Lauterbach, E. C. Coffey, C. E. Salloway, et al. 2000. The use of herbal alternative medicines in neuropsychiatry. *Journal of Neuropsychiatry and Clinical Neurosciences* 12:177–92.

Langtry, H. D., and P. Benfield. 1990. Zolpidem: A review of its pharmacodynamic and pharmacokinetic properties and therapeutic potential. *Drug* 40:291–13.

Le Doux, J. 1996. *The Emotional Brain*. New York: Simon and Schuster.

Lee, S., Y. K. Wing, and K. C. Wong. 1992. Knowledge and compliance towards lithium therapy among Chinese psychiatric patients in Hong Kong. *Australia and New Zealand Journal of Psychiatry* 26:444–49.

Letterman, L, and J. S. Markowitz. 1999. Gabapentin: A review of published experience in the treatment of bipolar disorder and other psychiatric conditions. *Pharmacotherapy* 19:565–72.

Leucht, S., K. Komossa, C. Rummel-Kluge, C. Corves, H. Hunger, F. Schmid, C. A. Lobos, et al. 2009. A meta-analysis of head-to-head comparisons of second-generation antipsychotics in the treatment of schizophrenia. *American Journal of Psychiatry* 166:152–63.

Lewis, T., F. Amini, and R. Lennon. 2000. *A General Theory of Love*. New York: Random House.

Li, X., T. A. Ketter, and M. A. Frye. 2002. Synaptic, intracellular, and neuroprotective mechanisms of anticonvulsants: Are they relevant for the treatment and course of bipolar disorders? *Journal of Affective Disorders* 69(1–3):1–14.

Liddle, P. F., T. R. E. Barnes, D. Morris, and S. Haque. 1989. Three syndromes in chronic schizophrenia. *British Journal of Psychiatry* 155(Suppl 7):119–22.

Lieberman J., and D. Shore. 1995. Clinical implications of clozapine discontinuation: Report of an NIMH workshop. *Schizophrenia Bulletin* 21(2): 333-338.

Lieberman, J. A. 1999. Is schizophrenia a neurodegenerative disorder? A clinical and neurobiological perspective. *Biological Psychiatry* 46:729–39A

Lieberman, J. A., J. M. Alvir, A. Koreen, S. Geisler, M. Chakos, B. Sheitman, and M. Woerner. 1996. Psychobiologic correlates of treatment response in schizophrenia. *Neuropsychopharmacology* 14:13S–21S.

Lieberman, J. A., T. S. Stroup, J. P. McEvoy, M. S. Swartz, R. A. Rosenheck, D. O. Perkins et al. 2005. Effectiveness of antipsychotic drugs in patients with chronic schizophrenia. *New England Journal of Medicine* 353:1209–23.

Liebowitz, M. R., and D. F. Klein. 1979. Hysteroid-dysphoria. *Psychiatric Clinics of North America* 2:555–75.

———. 1981. Interrelationships of hysteroid-dysphoria and borderline personality disorder. *Psychiatric Clinics of North America* 4:67–87.

Lindenmayer, J. P., P. Czobor, J. Volavka, L. Citrome, et al. 2003. Changes in glucose and cholesterol levels in patients with schizophrenia treated with typical or atypical antipsychotics. *American Journal of Psychiatry* 160(2):290–96.

Links, P. S., A. Boggild, and N. Sarin. 2001. Psychopharmacology of personality disorders: Review and emerging issues. *Current Psychiatry Reports* 3(1):70–76.

Loebel, A. D., J. A. Lieberman, J. M. J. Alvir, D. I. Mayerhoff, et al. 1992. Duration of psychosis and outcome in first episode schizophrenia. *American Journal of Psychiatry* 149:1183–88.

Luby, E. D., J. S. Gottlieb, B. D. Cohen, G. Rosenbaum, et al. 1962. Model psychoses and schizophrenia. *American Journal of Psychiatry* 119:61–67.

Luby, E. D., M. A. Marrazzi, and J. Kinzie 1987. Letter to the editor. *Journal of Clinical Psychopharmacology* 7:52–53.

Luby, J. L., A. Hefflinger, C. Mrakotsky, M. Hessler, et al. 2002. Preschool major depressive disorder: Preliminary validation for developmentally modified DSM-IV criteria. *Journal of the American Academy of Child and Adolescent Psychiatry* 41(8):928–37.

Mahler, J. 2004. The antidepressant dilemma. *New York Times Magazine.* November 21, 2000.

Mahler, M., F. Pine, and A. Berman. 1975. *The Psychological Birth of the Human Infant: Symbiosis and Individuation.* New York: Basic Books.

Malaspina, O., H. M. Quitkin, and C. A. Kaufmann. 1992. Epidemiology and genetics of neuropsychiatric disorders. In *The American Psychiatric Press Textbook of Neuropsychiatry.* S. C. Yudofsky and R. E. Hales, eds. Washington, DC: American Psychiatric Press.

MacQueen, G. M., and L. Trevor Young. 2001. Bipolar II disorder: Symptoms, course, and response to treatment. *Psychiatric Services* 52:358–61.

Manji, H. K. 2001. The neurobiology of bipolar disorder. *The Economics of Neuroscience* 3:37–44.

Manji, H. K., and R. H. Lennox. 2000. The nature of bipolar disorder. *Journal of Clinical Psychiatry* 61(Suppl):42–57.

Manji, H. K., G. J. Moore, G. Rajkowska, and G. Chen. 2000. Neuroplasticity and cellular resilience in mood disorders. *Molecular Psychiatry* 5:578–93.

Manji, H. K., and W. Z. Potter. 1997. Monoaminergic systems. In *Bipolar Disorder: Biological Models and Their Clinical Application.* L. T. Young and R. T. Joffe, eds. New York: Marcel Dekker.

March, J., J. Silva, S. Petrycki, J. Curry, et al. 2004 Fluoxetine, cognitive-behavioral therapy, and their combination for adolescents with depression. *Journal of the American Medical Association* 292:807–20.

March, J. S., J. Biederman, R. Wolkow, A. Safferman, J. Mardekian, et al. 1998. Sertraline in children and adolescents with obsessive-compulsive disorder. *Journal of the American Medical Association* 280(20):1752–56.

Markovitz, P. J., J. R. Calabrese, S. C. Schulz, and H. Y. Meltzer. 1991. Fluoxetine in the treatment of borderline and schizotypal personality disorders. *American Journal of Psychiatry* 148(8):1064–67.

Marneros, A. 2001. Expanding the group of bipolar disorders. *Journal of Affective Disorders* 62:39–44.

Mayberg, H. S. 1997. Limbic-cortical dysregulation. *The Neuropsychiatry of Limbic and Subcortial Disorders.* Washington, DC: American Psychiatric Press, 167–77.

McCann, U. G. Hatzidimitriou, A. Ridenour, C. Fischer, et al. 1994. Dexfenfluramine and serotonin neurotoxicity: Further preclinical evidence that clinical caution is indicated. *Pharmacological Experimental Therapy* 269(2):792–98.

McCracken, J. T., J. McGough, B. Shah, P. Cronin, et al. 2002. Risperidone in children with autism and serious behavioral problems. *New England Journal of Medicine* 347:314–21.

McCullough, J. P. 2000. *Treatment for Chronic Depression*. New York: Guilford Press.

McDougle, C. J., S. T. Naylor, D. J. Cohen, F. R. Volkmar, et al. 1996. A double-blind, placebo-controlled study of fluvoxamine in adults with autistic disorder. *Archives of General Psychiatry* 53:1001–08.

McElroy, S. L., P. E. Keck, H. G. Pope, J. I. Hudson, et al. 1992. Clinical and research implications of the diagnosis of dysphoric or mixed mania or hypomania. *American Journal of Psychiatry* 149:1633–44.

Menninger, K. 1963. *The Vital Balance*. New York: Viking.

Metzner, R. J. 2000. Neurotransmitters and depression: New possibilities. Annual Meeting: American Psychiatric Association.

Meyer, U. A. 1992. Drugs in special patient groups: Clinical importance of genetics in drug effects. In *Melmon and Morrelli's Clinical Pharmacology: Basic Principles in Therapeutics*, 3rd ed. K. L. Melmon, H. F. Morrelli, B. B. Hoffman, and D. W. Nierenberg, eds. New York: McGraw-Hill.

Michaels, R. 1992. Principles of psychodynamic psychotherapy. *Audio Digest Psychiatry* 20:13.

Michalets, E. L. 1998. Update: Clinically significant cytochrome P-450 drug interactions. *Pharmacotherpy* 18:84–112.

Miklowitz, D. J. 1996. Psychotherapy in combination with drug treatment for bipolar disorder. *Journal of Clinical Psychopharmacology* 16(Suppl):56S–66S.

Mischoulon, D., M. Fava, and J. F. Rosenbaum. 1999. Strategies for augmentation of SSRI treatment: A survey of an academic psychopharmacology practice. *Harvard Review of Psychiatry* 6:322–26.

Moleman, P., K. van Dam, and V. Dings. 1999. Psychopharmacological treatment of personality disorders: A review. In *Treatment of Personality Disorders*, 207. New York and Heidelberg: Kluwer Academic/Plenum Publishers.

Mooallem, J. 2007. The sleep-industrial complex. *The New York Times Magazine*. November 18, 2007.

Musselman, D. L., C. DeBattista, K. I. Nathan, C. D. Kilts, et al. 1998. Biology of mood disorders. In *Textbook of Psychopharmacology*, 2nd ed., 549–88. A. F. Schatzberg and C. B. Nemeroff eds. Arlington, VA: American Psychiatric Publishing, Inc.

Nagy, L. M., C. A. Morgan, S. M. Southwick, and D. S. Charney. 1993. Open prospective trial of fluoxetine for post-traumatic stress disorder. *Journal of Clinical Psychopharmacology* 13:107–13.

National Institutes of Health. 2008. Barnes, P. M., B. Bloom, and R. Nahin. 2008. Complementary and alternative medicine use among adults and children: United States, 2007. *National Health Statistics Report* No. 12.

National Sleep Foundation. 2005. Sleep in America Poll. Washington, DC. National Sleep Foundation: www.sleepfoundation.org.

Nemeroff, C. B., C. L. DeVane, and B. G. Pollock. 1996. Newer antidepressants and the cytochrome P450 system. *American Journal of Psychiatry* 153:311–20.

Nemeroff, C. B. 1997. The role of early adverse life events in the etiology of depression and post-traumatic stress disorder: Focus on CRF. *Annals of the New York Academy of Sciences* 821:194–207.

Nemets, B., Z. Stahl, and R. H. Belmaker. 2002. Addition of omega-3 fatty acid to maintenance medication treatment for recurrent unipolar depressive disorder. *American Journal of Psychiatry* 159(3):477–79.

Ness, J., F. T. Sherman, and C. X. Pan. 1999. Alternative medicine: What data says about common herbal therapies. *Geriatrics* 54(10):33–38.

Nester, P. G., M. E. Shenton, and R. W. McCarley. 1993. Neuropsychological correlates of MRI temporal lobe abnormalities in schizophrenia. *American Journal of Psychiatry* 150:1849–55.

Nicolson, R., G. Awad, and L. Sloman. 1998. An open trial of risperidone in young autistic children. *Journal of the American Academy of Child and Adolescent Psychiatry* 37:372–76.

Nishino, S., E. Mignot, and W. C. Dement. 1998. Sedative-hypnotics. In *Textbook of Psychopharmacology*, 2nd ed. A. F. Schatzberg and C. B. Nemeroff, eds. Arlington, VA: American Psychiatric Publishing, Inc. 487–502.

Norden, M. J. 1989a. Fluoxetine in borderline personality disorder. *Progress in Neuropsychopharmacological Biological Psychiatry* 13:885–93.

———. 1989b. Is there an effective drug treatment for borderline personality disorder? *Harvard Mental Health Letter* 6:8.

Nurnberger, J. I., and T. Foroud. 2000. Genetics of bipolar affective disorder. *Current Psychiatry Reports* 2:147–57.

Otte, C., K. Wiedermann, A. Yassouridis, and M. Kellner. 2004. Valproate monotherapy in the treatment of civilian patients with non-combat-related PTSD: An open label study. *Journal of Clinical Psychopharmacology* 24(1):106–108.

Pande, A. C., J. G. Crockatt, C. A. Janney, J. L. Werth, et al. 2000. Gabapentin in bipolar disorder: A placebo-controlled trial of adjunctive therapy. Gabapentin bipolar disorder study group. *Bipolar Disorder* 2:249–255.

Papolos, D., and J. Papolos. 2007. *The Bi-Polar Child*. 3rd ed. New York: Broadway Books.

Pazzaglia, P. J., R. M. Post, T. A. Ketter, M. S. George, et al. 1993. Preliminary controlled trial of nimopidine in ultra-rapid cycling affective dysregulation. *Psychiatry Research* 49:257–73.

PDR. 1998. *PDR for Herbal Medicines*, 6. Montvale, NJ: Medical Economics.

Peet, M., and D. F. Horrobin. 2002. A dose-ranging study of the effects of ethyleicosapentaenoate in patients with on-going depression despite apparently adequate treatment with standardized drugs. *Archives of General Psychiatry* 59:913–19.

Perlis, R. H. 2007. Treatment of bipolar disorder: The evolving role of atypical antipsychotics. *American Journal of Managed Care*. 13:S178–88.

Petrovic, P., R. Kalisch, T. Singer, and R. J. Dolan. 2008. Oxytocin attenuates affective evaluations of conditioned faces and amygdala activity. *Journal of Neuroscience* 28(26):6607–15.

Petty, F., L. L. Davis, A. L. Nugent, et al. 2002. Valproate therapy for chronic, combat-induced PTSD. *Journal of Clinical Psychopharmacology* 22(1):100–01.

Perugi, G., C. Toni, F. Frare, G. Ruffolo, L. Moretti, C. Torti, and H. S. Akiskal. 2002. Effectiveness of adjunctive gabapentin in resistant bipolar disorder: Is it due to anxious alcohol abuse comorbidity? *Journal of Clinical Psychopharmacology* 22(6):584–91.

Pies, R. 2002. The "softer" end of the bipolar spectrum. *Journal of Psychiatric Practice* 8:189–95.

Pine, D., P. Cohen, D. Gurley, J. Brook, and Y. Ma. 1998. The risk for early-adulthood anxiety and depressive disorders in adolescents with anxiety and depressive disorders. *Archives of General Psychiatry* 55:56–64.

Pinsker, H., I. Kupfermann, V. Castellucci, and E. Kandel. 1970. Habituation and dishabituation of the gill-withdrawal reflex in Aplysia. *Science* 167:1740–42.

Pollock, V. E. 1992. Meta-analysis of subjective sensitivity to alcohol in sons of alcoholics. *American Journal of Psychiatry* 149:1534–38.

Pomerantz, J. M., S. N. Finklestein, E. R. Berndt, A. W. Poret, L. E. Walker, R. C. Alber, V. Kadiyam, M. Das, et al. 2004. Prescriber intent, off-label usage, and early discontinuation of antidepressants: A retrospective physician survey and data analysis. *Journal of Clinical Psychiatry* 65(3): 395–404.

Popper, C. 2004. Bipolar disorder in children and adolescents. *Audio Digest Psychiatry* 33(2).

Post, R. M. 2011. Acquired lithium resistance revisited: Discontinuation-induced refractoriness versus tolerance. *Journal of Affective Disorders*, December 7. Epub ahead of print retrieved April 13, 2012, from http://dx.doi.org/10.1016/j.jad.2011.09.021

Post, R. M., and S. R. B. Weiss. 1997. Emergent properties of neural systems: How focal molecular neurobiological alterations can affect behavior. *Development and Psychopathology* 9:907–29.

Post, R. M., S. R. B. Weiss, and O. Chuang. 1992. Mechanisms of action of anticonvulsants in affective disorders: Comparisons with lithium. *Journal of Clinical Psychopharmacology* 12:23S–35S.

Post, R. M., S. R. B. Weiss, and G. S. Leverich. 1994. Recurrent affective disorder: Roots in developmental neurobiology and illness progression based on changes in gene expression. *Development and Psychopathology* 6:781–813.

Potash, J. B., and J. R. DePaulo. 2000. Searching high and low: A review of the genetics of bipolar disorder. *Bipolar Disorder* 2:8–26

Preston, J. D. 1993. *Depression and Anxiety Management* (audiotape). Oakland, CA: New Harbinger Publications.

———. 2006. *Integrative Treatment for Borderline Personality Disorder*. Oakland, CA: New Harbinger Publications.

Quintana, H., B. Birmaher, D. Stedge, S. Lennon, et al. 1995. Use of methylphenidate in the treatment of children with autistic disorder. *Journal of Autism and Developmental Disorders* 25:283–94.

Rabkin, J. G., F. M. Quitkin, P. McGrath, W. Harrison, et al. 1985. Adverse reactions to monoamine oxidase inhibitors, part II: Treatment correlates and clinical management. *Journal of Clinical Psychopharmacology* 5:2–9.

Rapoport, J. L. 1991. Recent advances in obsessive-compulsive disorder. *Neuropsychopharmacology* 5:1–10.

Raskin, J., D. J. Goldstein, C. H. Mallinckrodt, and M. B. Ferguson. 2003. Duloxetine in the long-term treatment of major depressive disorder. *Journal of Clinical Psychiatry* 64(10):1237–44.

Relling, M. V., and K. M. Giacomini. 2006. Pharmacogenetics. In Goodman & Gilman's: *The Pharmacological Basis of Therapeutics*. L. L. Brunton, J. S. Lazo, and K. L. Parker, eds. New York: McGraw-Hill.

Ricaurte, G. A., M. E. Molliver, M. B. Martello, J. L. Katx, M. A. Wilson, et al. 1991. Dexfenfluvamine neurotoxicity in brains of non-human primates. *Lancet* 338:1487–88.

Rizvi, S. T. 2002. Lamotrigine and borderline personality disorder. *Journal of Child and Adolescent Psychopharmacology* 12(4):365–66.

Rocca, P, L. Marchiaro, E. Cocuzza, and F. Bogetto. 2002. Treatment of borderline personality disorder with risperidone. *Journal of Clinical Psychiatry* 63(3):241–44.

Robertson, M. M., and J. S. Stern. 1997. The Gilles de la Tourette syndrome. *Critical Reviews in Neurobiology* 11:1–19.

Rosenthal, J., A. Strauss, L. Minkoff, and A. Winston. 1986. Identifying lithium-responsive bipolar depressed patients using nuclear magnetic resonance. *American Journal of Psychiatry* 143:779–80.

Rosenthal, M. 2003. Tiagabine for the treatment of generalized anxiety disorder: A randomized, open-label, clinical trial with paroxetine as a positive control. *Journal of Clinical Psychiatry* 64(10):1245–49.

Rosenthal, N. E. 2006. *Winter Blues*. New York: Guilford Press.

Rubin, P. C. 1992. Drugs in special patient groups: Pregnancy and nursing. In *Melmon and Morrelli's Clinical Pharmacology: Basic Principles in Therapeutics*, 3rd ed. K. L. Melmon, H. F. Morrelli, B. B. Hoffman, and D. W. Nierenberg, eds. New York: McGraw-Hill.

Russell, E. W., C. Neuringer, and G. Goldstein. 1970. *Assessment of Brain Damage: A Neuropsychological Key Approach*. New York: Wiley.

Sachs, G. S. 1996. Bipolar mood disorder: Practical strategies for acute and maintenance phase treatment. *Journal of Clinical Psychopharmacology* 16(Suppl):32S–47S.

Sachs, G. S., D. J. Printz, D. A. Kahn, D. Carpenter, and J. P. Doherty. 2000. The expert consensus guideline series: Medication treatment of bipolar disorder. *Postgraduate Medicine* 4(Special):1–104.

Sachs, G. S., A. A. Nierenberg, J. R. Calabrese, L. B. Marangell, S. R. Wisniewski, L. Gyulai, et al. 2007. Effectiveness of adjunctive antidepressant treatment for bipolar depression. *New England Journal of Medicine* 356:1711–22.

Sackett, G. P. 1965. Effects of rearing conditions on the behavior of the rhesus monkey. *Child Development* 36:855–68.

Safer, D. J., and J. M. Krager. 1992. Effect of a media blitz and a threatened lawsuit on stimulant treatment. *Journal of the American Medical Association* 268:1004–07.

Salzman, C., A. N. Wolfson, A. Schatzberg, A. Looper, et al. 1995. Effect of fluoxetine on anger in asymptomatic volunteers with borderline personality disorder. *Journal of Clinical Psychopharmacology* 15(1):23–29.

Sapolsky, R. M. 1994. *Why Zebras Don't Get Ulcers*. New York: W. H. Freeman & Company.

———. 1996. Glucocorticoids and atrophy of the human hippocampus. *Science* 273:749–75.

Sato, T., R. Bottlender, N. Kleindiendst, and H. J. Moller. 2002. Syndromes and phenomenological subtypes underlying acute mania: A factor analytic study of 576 manic patients. *American Journal of Psychiatry* 159(6):968–74.

Schatzberg, A. F., and J. J. Schildkraut. 1995. Recent studies on norepinephrine systems in mood disorders. In *Psychopharmacology: The Fourth Generation of Progress*. F. E. Bloom and D. J. Kupfer, eds. New York: Raven Press.

Schou, M. 1997. Forty years of lithium treatment. *Archives of General Psychiatry* 54:9–13.

Schuckit, M. A., E. Gold, and C. Risch. 1987. Serum prolactin levels in sons of alcoholics and control subjects. *American Journal of Psychiatry* 144:854–59.

Schuckit, M. A., M. Irwin, and S. A. Brown. 1990. The history of anxiety symptoms among 171 primary alcoholics. *Journal of the Study of Alcoholism* 51:34–41.

Schulz, S. C., K. L. Camlin, S. A. Berry, and J. A. Jesburger. 1999. Olanzapine safety and efficacy in patients with borderline personality disorder and comorbid dysthymia. *Biological Psychiatry* 46(10):1429–35.

Schwartz, J., and S. Begley. 2003. *The Mind and the Brain*. New York: Harper Perennial.

Seedat, S., D. J. Stein, C. Ziervogel, T. Middleton, et al. 2002. Comparison of response to an SSRI in children, adolescents, and adults with posttraumatic stress disorder. *Journal of Child and Adolescent Psychopharmacology* 12(1):37-46.

Seligman, M. E. P. 1990. *Learned Optimism*. New York: Pocket Books.

Sharma, V., L. N. Yatham, D. R. Haslam, P. H. Silverstone, et al. 1997. Continuation and prophylactic treatment of bipolar disorder. *Canadian Journal of Psychiatry* 42(Suppl):92S–100S.

Shea, S. C. 2006 *Improving medication adherence: How to talk with patients about their medications* (1st ed.). Philadelphia: Lippincott, Williams and Wilkins.

Shelton, R. C., and A. J. Tomarken. 2001. Can recovery from depression be achieved? *Psychiatric Services* 52(11):1469–78.

Shimoda, K., T. Minowada, T. Noguchi, and S. Takahashi. 1993. Interindividual variations of desmethylation and hydroxylation of clomipramine in an Oriental psychiatric population. *Journal of Clinical Psychopharmacology* 13:181–88.

Shinba, T., T. Shinozaki, and G. Mugishima. 2001. Clonidine immediately after immobilization stress prevents long-lasting locomotion reduction in the rat. *Progress in Neuro-Psychopharmacology and Biological Psychiatry* 25:1629–40.

Shore, D., S. Matthews, J. Cott, and J. A. Lieberman. 1995. Clinical implications of clozapine discontinuation: Report of an NIMH workshop. *Schizophrenia Bulletin* 21(2):333–338.

Shulman, K. I., S. E. Walker, S. MacKenzie, and S. Knowles. 1989. Dietary restriction, tyramine, and the use of monoamine oxidase inhibitors. *Journal of Clinical Psychopharmacology* 9:397–402.

Smith, D. E., and D. R. Wesson. 1983. Benzodiazepine dependency syndromes. *Journal of Psychoactive Drugs* 15:85–95.

Smith, S. S., B. F. O'Hara, A. M. Persico, D. A. Gorelick, et al. 1992. Genetic vulnerability to drug abuse. *Archives of General Psychiatry* 49:723–27.

Snodgrass, W. R. 1992. Drugs in special patient groups: Neonates and children. In *Melmon and Morrelli's Clinical Pharmacology: Basic Principles in Therapeutics*, 3rd ed. K. L. Melmon, H. F. Morrelli, B. B. Hoffman, and D. W. Nierenberg, eds. New York: McGraw-Hill.

Snyder, S. H., and C. D. Ferris. 2000. Novel neurotransmitters and their neuropsychiatric relevance. *American Journal of Psychiatry* 157:1738–51.

Soares, J. C. 2000. Recent advances in the treatment of bipolar mania, depression and mixed states, and rapid cycling. *International Clinical Psychopharmacology* 15:183–96.

Soares, J. C., and J. J. Mann. 1997. The anatomy of mood disorders: Review of structural neuroimaging studies. *Biological Psychiatry* 41:86–106.

Soloff, P. H., A. George, R. S. Nathan, P. M. Schulz, et al. 1986. Progress in psychopharmacology of borderline disorders. *Archives of General Psychiatry* 43:691–97.

Solomon, D. A., G. J. Keitner, J. W. Miller, M. T. Shea, et al. 1995. Course of illness and maintenance treatments for patients with bipolar disorder. *Journal of Clinical Psychiatry* 56:5–13.

Southwick, S. M., J. D. Bremner, A. Rasmusson, C. A. Morganhill, A. Arnstein, and D. S. Charney. 1999. Role of norepinephrine in the pathophysiology and treatment of PTSD. *Biological Psychiatry* 46:1192–1203.

Spiegel, R., and H. J. Aebi. 1989. *Psychopharmacology: An Introduction.* Chichester, U.K.: John Wiley and Sons.

Stein, D. J., et al. 2000. Selective serotonin reuptake inhibitors in the treatment of post-traumatic stress disorder: A meta-analysis of randomized controlled trials. *International Journal of Clinical Psychopharmacology* 15:S31–S39.

Stein, M. B., N. A. Kline, and J. L. Matloff. 2002. Adjunctive olanzapine for SSRI-resistant combat-related PTSD: A double-blind, placebo-controlled study. *American Journal of Psychiatry* 159(10):1777–79.

Stern, E., D. A. Silbersweig, K. Chee, A. Holmes, et al. 2000. A functional neuroanatomy of tics in Tourette Syndrome. *Archives of General Psychiatry* 57:741–48.

Stoll, A. L., P. V. Mayer, M. Kolbrener, E. Goldstein, B. Suplit, J. Lucier, B. M. Cohen, and M. Tohen. 1994. Antidepressant-associated mania: A controlled comparison with spontaneous mania. *American Journal of Psychiatry* 151:1642–45.

Stoll, A. L., W. E. Severus, M. P. Freeman, S. Reuter, et al. 1999. Omega 3 fatty acids in bipolar disorder. A preliminary double-blind, placebo-controlled trial. *Archives of General Psychiatry* 56:407–12.

Stone, M. H. 1988. Toward a psychobiological theory of borderline disorder. *Dissociation* 1:2–15.

Stoudemire, A., R. Frank, N. Hedemark, M. Kamlet, and D. Blazer. 1986. The economic burden of depression. *General Hospital Psychiatry* 8:387–94.

Strub, R. L., and F. W. Black. 2000. *The Mental Status Examination in Neurology*, 4th ed. Philadelphia: F. A. Davis.

Suppes, T. E., B. Dennehy, R. M. Hirschfeld, L. L. Althsuler, et al. 2004. The Texas Implementation of Medication Algorithms: Update to the algorithms for treatment of bipolar I disorder. *Journal of Clinical Psychiatry.* 66: 870–86.

Sutherland, S. M., and J. R. Davidson. 1994. Pharmacotherapy for PTSD. *Psychiatric Clinics of North America* 17:409–23.

Svanborg, C., A. A. Wistedt, and P. Svanborg. 2008. Long-term outcome of patients with dysthymia and panic disorder: A naturalistic 9-year follow-up study. *Nordic Journal of Psychiatry* 62(1):17-24.

Swann, A. C. 1995. Mixed or dysphoric manic states: Psychopathology and treatment. *Journal of Clinical Psychiatry* 56(Suppl):6–10.

Tailor, S. A., K. I. Shulman, S. E. Walker, J. Moss, and D. Gardner. 1994. Hypertensive episide associated with Phenelzine and tap beer—An analysis of the role of pressor aminos in beer. *Journal of Clinical Psychopharmacology* 14:5–14.

Taylor, F. B. 2003. Tiagabine for posttraumatic stress disorder: A case series of 7 women. *Journal of Clinical Psychiatry* 64(12):1421–25.

Taylor, R. L. 1990. *Distinguishing Psychological from Organic Disorders.* New York: Springer Publishing.

Teicher, M. H., C. Glod, and J. O. Cole. 1990. Emergence of intense suicidal preoccupation during fluoxetine treatment. *American Journal of Psychiatry* 147:207–210.

Terr, L. C. 1991. Childhood traumas: An outline and overview. *American Journal of Psychiatry* 148:10–20.

Thoenen, H. 1995. Neurotropins and neural plasticity. *Science* 270:593–98.

Thomsen, P. H., C. Ebbesen, and C. Persson. 2001. Long-term experience with citalopram in the treatment of adolescent OCD. *Journal of the American Academy of Child and Adolescent Psychiatry* 40:895-902.

Tindle, H. A., R. B. Davis, R. S. Phillips, and D. M.Eisenberg. 2005. Trends in use of complementary and alternative medicine by U.S. adults: 1997–2002. *Alternative Therapies in Health and Medicine* 11:42–9.

Townsend, M. H., K. M. Cambre, and J. G. Barber. 2001. Treatment of borderline personality disorder with mood instability with divalproex sodium: Series of ten cases. *Journal of Clinical Psychopharmacology.* 21(2):249–51.

Tsuang, M. T., and S. V. Faraone. 1990. *The Genetics of Mood Disorders.* Baltimore: Johns Hopkins University Press.

Tsuang, M. T., W. Stone, and S. V. Faraone. 2000. Toward reformulating the diagnosis of schizophrenia. *Journal of Psychiatry* 157:1041–50.

Tucker, P., R. Potter-Kimball, D. B. Wyatt, D. E. Parker, et al. 2003. Can physiologic assessment and side effects team out differences in PTSD trials? A double-blind comparison of citalopram, sertraline, and placebo. *Psychopharmacology Bulletin* 37(3):135–49.

Turnbull, G. J. 1998. A review of post-traumatic stress disorder: Part II. *Treatment Injury* 29:169–75.

Turner, S. 1999. Place of pharmacotherapy in post-traumatic stress disorder. *Lancet* 354:1404–05.

Ulenhuth, E. H., H. DeWit, M. B. Balter, C. E. Johanson, and G. D. Mellinger. 1988. Risks and benefits of long-term benzodiazepine use. *Journal of Clinical Psychopharmacology* 8:161–67.

van der Kolk, B. A. 1987. *Psychological Trauma.* Washington, DC: American Psychiatric Press.

van der Kolk, B. A., D. Dreyfuss, M. Michaels, M. Shera, et al. 1994. Fluoxetine in post-traumatic stress disorder. *Journal of Clinical Psychiatry* 55:517–22.

Vandel, P., E. Haffen, S. Vandel, B. Bonin, et al. 1999. Pharmacokinetics and disposition: Drug extrapyramidal side effects. CYP2D6 genotypes and phenotypes. *European Journal of Clinical Pharmacology* 55:659–65.

Vestal, R. E., S. C. Montamat, and C. P. Nielson. 1992. Drugs in special patient groups: The elderly. In *Melmon and Morrelli's Clinical Pharmacology: Basic Principles in Therapeutics,* 3rd ed. K. L. Melmon, H. F. Morrelli, B. B. Hoffman, and D. W. Nierenberg, eds. New York: McGraw-Hill.

Vestergaard, P., A. Amdisen, and M. Schow. 1980. Clinically significant side effects of lithium treatment. *Acta Psychiatrica Scandinavica* 62:193–200.

von Moltke, L. L., D. J. Greenblatt, J. S. Harmatz, and R. I. Shader. 1994. Cytochromes in psychopharmacology. *Journal of Clinical Psychopharmacology* 14:1–4.

Wagner, K. D., P. Ambrosini, M. Ryann, C. Wohlberg, et al. 2003. Efficacy of sertraline in the treatment of children and adolescents with major depression disorder: Two randomized, controlled trials. *Journal of the American Medical Association* 290:1033–41.

Walkup, J. T. 2002. What's new in pediatric psychopharmacology: Anxiety disorders. *U.S. Psychiatric Congress,* Las Vegas, NV.

———. 2003. What's new in pediatric psychopharmacology? *U.S. Psychiatric and Mental Health Congress,* Orlando, FL.

————. 2004. Child and adolescent psychopharmacology: What's new? *U.S. Psychiatric and Mental Health Congress,* San Diego, CA.

Walkup, J. T., J. J. Labellante, M. A. Riddle, D. S. Pine, et al. 2001. Fluvoxamine for the treatment of anxiety disorders in children and adolescents. *New England Journal of Medicine* 344(17):1279–85.

Ward, N. 1992. Psychopharmacology update. Pharmaceutical company presentation, Sacramento, CA.

Watsky, E. J., and C. Salzman. 1991. Psychotropic drug interactions. *Hospital and Community Psychiatry* 42:247–56.

Weber, S. S., S. R. Saklad, and K. V. Kastenholz. 1992. Bipolar affective disorders. In *Applied Therapeutics: The Clinical Use of Drugs,* 5th ed. M. A. Koda-Kimble, L. Y. Young, W. A. Kradjan, and B. J. Guglielmo, eds. Vancouver, WA: Applied Therapeutics.

Weinberger, D. R. 1996. On the plausibility of "the neurodevelopmental hypothesis" of schizophrenia. *Neuropsychopharmacology* 14:15–115.

Weinberger, D. R., K. F. Berman, R. Suddath, and E. F. Torrey. 1992. Evidence of dysfunction of a prefrontal-limbic network in schizophrenia: A magnetic resonance imaging and regional cerebral blood flow study of discordant monozygotic twins. *American Journal of Psychiatry* 149:890–97.

Weiss, J., H. I. Glazer, and L. A. Pohorecky. 1976. Coping behavior and neurochemical changes in rats: An alternative explanation for the original "learned helplessness" experiments. In *Animal Models in Human Psychobiology,* G. Servan and A. Kling, eds. New York: Plenum Press.

Wells, G. B., C. C. Chu, R. Johson, C. Nasdahl, et al. 1991. Buspirone in the treatment of post-traumatic stress disorder. *Pharmacotherapy* 11: 340–43.

Weng, G., U. S. Bhalla, and R. Iyengar. 1999. Complexity in biological signaling systems. *Science* 284:92–96.

Wheatley, D. P., M. van Moffaert, L. Timmerman, and C. M. E. Kremer. 1998. Mirtazapine: Efficacy and tolerability in comparison with fluoxetine in patients with moderate to severe major depressive disorder. *Journal of Clinical Psychiatry* 59:306–12.

Whittington, C. J., T. Kendall, P. Fonagy, D. Cottrell, et al. 2004. SSRIs in childhood depression: Systematic review of published versus unpublished data. *Lancet* 363(9418):1341–45.

Wilkinson, G. R. 2005. Drug metabolism and variability among patients in drug response. *New England Journal of Medicine* 352:2211–21.

Willner, P. 1995. Dopaminergic mechanisms in depression and mania. In *Psychopharmacology: The Fourth Generation of Progress.* F. E. Bloom and D. J. Kupfer, eds. New York: Raven Press.

Winchel, R. M., and M. Stanley. 1991. Self-injurious behavior: A review of the behavior and biology of self-mutilation. *American Journal of Psychiatry* 148:306–17.

Winter, M. E. 1988. *Basic Clinical Pharmacokinetics.* Vancouver, WA: Applied Therapeutics.

Wirshing, D. A., J. A. Boyd, L. R. Meng, J. S. Ballon, et al. 2002. The effects of novel antipsychotics on glucose and lipid levels. *Journal of Clinical Psychiatry* 63(10):856–65.

Yamazaki, H. 2000. Roles of human cytochrome P450 enzymes involved in drug metabolism and toxicological studies. *Yakugaku Zasshi* 120:1347–57.

Yager, J., M. J. Devlin, K. A. Halmi, D. B. Herzog, et al. 2006. American Psychiatric Association Practice Guidelines: Treatment of patients with eating disorders, 3rd edition. *American Journal of Psychiatry* 163(7 Suppl):5–54.

Yatham, L. N., V. Kusumakar, J. R. Calabrese, R. Rao, et al. 2002. Third generation anticonvulsants in bipolar disorder: A review of efficacy and summary of clinical recommendations. *Journal of Clinical Psychiatry* 63(4):275–83.

Young, J. Z. 1987. *Philosophy and the Brain.* Oxford: Oxford University Press.

Zalsman, G., Y. Y. Huang., M. A. Oquendo, A. K. Burke, X. Z. Hu, D. A. Brent, S. P. Ellis, D. Goldman, and J. J. Mann. 2007. Association of a triallelic serotonin transporter gene promoter region (5-HTTLPR) polymorphism with stressful life events and severity of depression. *American Journal of Psychiatry* 164:829–30. www

Zanger, U. M., M. Turpeinen, K. Klein, and M. Scwab. 2008. Functional pharmacogenetics/genomics of human cytochromes P450 involved in drug biotransformation. *Analytical and Bioanalytical Chemistry* 392:1093–108.

Zisook, S., Y. Chentsova-Dutton, and S. R. Shuchter. 1999. PTSD following bereavement. *Annals of Clinical Psychiatry* 10(4):157–63.

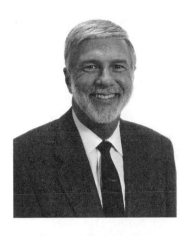

John D. Preston, PsyD, ABPP, is a licensed psychologist and the author or coauthor of twenty books. He is a professor of psychology at Alliant International University, and has also served on the faculty of the University of California, Davis, School of Medicine. He has lectured widely in the United States and abroad. He is the recipient of the Mental Health Association's President's Award for contributions to the mental health professions, and is a fellow of the American Psychological Association.

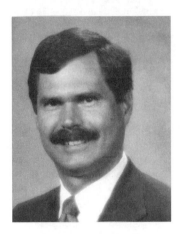

John H. O'Neal, MD, is a board-certified psychiatrist who has been in private practice since 1977. He is past chief of the department of psychiatry at Sutter Community Hospital in Sacramento, CA. He is an associate clinical professor of psychiatry at the University of California, Davis, School of Medicine and a fellow of the American Psychiatric Association. He lectures on depression and psychopharmacology to mental health professionals, employee assistance programs, and the public. Dr. O'Neal received his MS in clinical psychology from Harvard University.

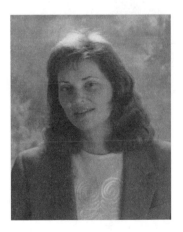

Mary Talaga, RPh, PhD, is administrative services leader for Kaiser Permanente Pharmacy Operations in the Northern California region. She has been a pharmacist for more than thirty years, and specializes in psychiatric pharmacy. Talaga has extensive experience in health care and has practiced in a variety of clinical settings. She is particularly interested in promoting collaborative care models and developing best-practice guidelines. She provides training and mentoring to health care professionals and general education to patients and consumers.

Index

A

abbreviation errors, 318
abnormal involuntary movements, 230, 231
absorption of medications, 46–47, 275–276
acamprosate, 154–155
acetylcholine, 42
action potential, 30
activation, 57, 185
acute dystonia, 306–307
acute organic brain syndromes, 70
acute stress disorder, 106
acute treatment phase, 184
addiction issues, 58, 60, 253–254
adenosine, 33
adenosine triphosphate (ATP), 35
adequate trials, 243
ADHD. *See* attention-deficit/hyperactivity
    disorder
adolescents. *See* child and adolescent
    psychopharmacology
adrenergic neurons, 42
adverse effects. *See* side effects
affect regulation, 141, 142
affective disorders. *See* depressive disorders
age-specific pharmacology, 285
aggression, 168–169
agitation, 305–306
agonist, 53, 64
agoraphobia, 107–108, 113, 118
agranulocytosis, 226, 228
AIMS scale, 230, 231
akathisia, 135, 224, 227, 231, 305–306
akinesia, 231
Alcoholics Anonymous (AA), 119
alcoholism, 153–155; biological basis for,
    153–154; depression and, 78, 79; diagnosis
    of, 67–68; disorders associated with, 154;

quick reference on, 158; treatment of,
    154–155; unexplained relapse and, 244. *See
    also* substance abuse
Alexander, Franz, 17
allergic reactions, 51
alpha-2 adrenergic agonists, 142, 257–258
alprazolam, 115, 119
Alzheimer's disease, 322
amantadine, 155
American Psychiatric Association (APA), 10,
    197
amino acids, 33
amitriptyline, 173
amphetamines, 155, 256
amygdala, 40, 111
angry-impulsive borderline personality, 147,
    148, 149
anhedonia, 76, 77, 79
anorexia nervosa, 122, 160, 161
antagonist, 53, 64
anterograde amnesia, 213
antiadrenergic side effects, 224
antianxiety medications, 213–221; anxiety
    disorders and, 117–119; borderline
    personality disorders and, 148; child and
    adolescent use of, 268–269; discontinuation
    of, 241; dosages of, 216; educating
    patients about, 220; half-lives of, 213, 214;
    indications for, 218; length of treatment
    with, 218; mechanism of action for, 214,
    215; patient information sheet on, 326–327;
    quick reference to, 221; side effects of,
    213, 247; signs of toxicity or overdose,
    248; types of, 214–215, 217; withdrawal
    symptoms from, 218–219. *See also* anxiety
    disorders
anticholinergic side effects, 224, 226, 306

anticonvulsants, 203–206; aggressive behavior and, 169; bipolar disorder and, 265, 266; blood level monitoring of, 204–205; child and adolescent use of, 265, 266; discontinuation symptoms, 241; dosage guidelines for, 205; eating disorders and, 160, 161; less commonly used, 205–206; patient information sheet on, 328–330; pregnancy/lactation guidelines for, 283; side effects of, 204–205, 247, 266; signs of toxicity or overdose, 248

antidepressant medications, 173–196; ADHD and, 258–259; aggressive behavior and, 168; anxiety disorders and, 117, 119, 269; atypical, 177; bipolar disorder and, 265; blood levels of, 183; borderline personality disorders and, 148; child and adolescent use of, 258–259, 260–263, 269; choosing, 181, 183–184; chronic pain and, 169; comparison of, 180; cyclic, 174, 175; depressive disorders and, 88–89; development of, 6–7, 173; discontinuation of, 239–240; dosages of, 181, 182; eating disorders and, 160, 161; educating patients about, 187, 189; mechanism of action for, 179, 181; monoamine oxidase inhibitors, 173, 177, 179; noncompliance issues with, 58–59; norepinephrine reuptake inhibitors, 173, 177; obsessive-compulsive disorder and, 123, 124, 125; over-the-counter options as, 189; patient information sheet on, 323–325; phases of treatment with, 184–185; post-traumatic stress disorder and, 141; pregnancy/lactation guidelines for, 282; quick reference to, 192–196; schizophrenia and, 135; selective action of, 90, 188; selective serotonin reuptake inhibitors, 173, 175–176; serotonin and norepinephrine reuptake inhibitors, 173, 176; side effects of, 174–175, 176, 177, 179, 181, 183, 185–186, 246; signs of toxicity or overdose, 248; stimulants as, 179; suicidality and, 261–263; toxicity effects from, 307; treatment-resistant depression and, 186–187, 191; tricyclic, 174–175; types of, 89, 174–179. *See also* depressive disorders

antihistamines, 217, 247
antipanic medications, 119
antiparkinsonian medications, 135, 225, 227
antipsychotic medications, 223–233; aggressive behavior and, 169; child and adolescent use of, 265, 270; considerations for choosing, 229–230; discontinuation

of, 241; dopamine receptors and, 132, 133, 223; dosages of, 225; drug interactions with, 298–299; educating patients about, 231; first-generation, 224, 225, 226–227, 232, 298; length of treatment with, 230–231; managing side effects from, 227; mechanism of action of, 223; patient information sheet on, 336–338; post-traumatic stress disorder and, 144; pregnancy/lactation guidelines for, 283; psychotic depressions and, 81; quick reference to, 232–233; reassessing prescriptions for, 227; schizophrenia and, 135–136; second-generation, 206, 225, 227–229, 233, 299; self-injurious behavior and, 162; side effects of, 224, 226–229, 247; signs of toxicity or overdose, 248. *See also* psychotic disorders

anxiety: akathisia and, 305–306; book for patients about, 322; drugs that can cause, 114; medical disorders and, 108, 113–114, 118; panic vs., 105–106; stress reactions and, 107, 117

anxiety disorders, 105–120; agoraphobia, 107–108, 113, 118; biologic theories of, 109–116; childhood and adolescent, 266–269; diagnosis of, 105–108, 267–268; educating patients about, 220; etiology of, 108–116; facts about, 107; generalized anxiety disorder, 107, 112, 116–117; length of treatment for, 218; medications for, 117–119, 213–221, 268–269; neurotic anxiety, 108, 115, 118; over-the-counter products for, 238; panic disorder, 108, 115–116, 118–119; patients medicated for, 24; phobias, 107, 113, 117–118; psychotherapy for, 116, 117, 118, 119; quick reference to, 120; symptoms of, 106; treatments for, 116–119, 213–221, 268–269; types of, 106–108. *See also* antianxiety medications

Aplysia study, 18
appetite disturbance, 80
aripiprazole, 228, 229
asenapine, 228
Asian patients, 26
aspartate, 33
Asperger's syndrome, 270
atenolol, 217
atomoxetine, 177, 180, 287
attachment compulsion, 140–141
attachment theories, 85
attention-deficit/hyperactivity disorder (ADHD), 254–259; alpha-2 adrenergic agonists and, 257–258; antidepressants

and, 258–259; bipolar disorder and, 263–264, 266; book for patients about, 322; diagnosis of, 254–255; medications for, 8–9, 256–259; neurobiology of, 255; residual, 161; Ritalin controversy and, 8–9; stimulants and, 256–257; symptoms of, 254–255, 264; Tourette syndrome and, 159; treatment of, 256–259

atypical antidepressants, 177; dosages of, 182; side effects of, 176, 177

atypical antipsychotics. *See* second-generation antipsychotics

atypical benzodiazepines, 215, 216

atypical depressions, 80, 83

atypical neurotransmitters, 33

atypical side effects, 226

augmentation, 187

autism spectrum disorders, 270

autonomic nervous system, 41–42

Axis I and II disorders (DSM-IV), 63–66, 67

axons, 29

B

barbiturates, 213

basal ganglia, 123

behavioral treatments, 19; for obsessive-compulsive disorder, 124; for phobias, 117

benign side effects, 245, 246–247

benzodiazepines, 213, 214–215; anxiety disorders and, 111, 117, 118, 119, 213, 269; atypical, 215, 216; bipolar disorders and, 265; borderline personality disorders and, 148; child and adolescent use of, 253, 269; discontinuation of, 240, 241; dosages of, 216; drug interactions with, 303; GABA receptor interactions, 214, 215; half-lives of, 213, 214; length of treatment with, 218; mechanism of action of, 214, 215; post-traumatic stress disorder and, 144; pregnancy/lactation guidelines for, 283; quick reference to, 221; schizophrenia and, 135; side effects of, 213, 247; sleep disorders and, 167; withdrawal symptoms from, 218–219, 240

beta blockers: aggressive behavior and, 169; akathisia and, 227; anxiety disorders and, 118, 217

binge-eating disorder, 160–161

bioavailability, 275

biogenic amines, 32

biological factors: alcoholism and, 153–154; anxiety disorders and, 109–116; bipolar disorders and, 100–103; borderline personality disorders and, 147–148;

depressive disorders and, 77, 79–80; personality traits and, 66, 67; psychiatric disorders and, 43; psychological functioning and, 16–20; schizophrenia and, 132–134; stress and, 140–142

biological psychiatry: cultural context of, 26–27; history of, 4–13; managed care dilemma and, 11–12; psychodynamics of, 21–25; reasons for learning about, 13–14

biotransformation, 48–49, 277

bipolar disorders, 93–104; ADHD and, 263–264, 266; bipolar I disorder, 95–97; bipolar II disorder, 97–98; books for patients about, 321–322; childhood-onset, 263–266; clinical depression and, 76; course specifiers for, 99; cyclothymia, 98–99; depression and, 84–85, 95; diagnosis of, 93–95, 263–265; drugs inducing mania in, 97; educating patients about, 207–208; episode specifiers for, 99; etiology of, 100–103; facts about, 95; length of treatment for, 207, 249; medical conditions associated with, 95; medications for, 103, 197–211, 265–266; model for expanded spectrum of, 100; psychotherapy for, 103, 208; quick reference to, 104; rapid cycling, 100; stages of acute mania, 94; symptoms of, 94, 104, 263, 264; treatments for, 103, 197–211, 265–266; unspecified, 99

bipolar medications, 197–211; anticonvulsants, 203–206; bipolar disorders and, 197–198, 265–266; blood level monitoring of, 202, 204–205; child and adolescent use of, 265–266; combinations of, 206–207; discontinuation of, 241; dosage guidelines for, 199, 205; drug interactions with, 300–301; educating patients about, 207–208; length of treatment with, 207; lithium, 199–203, 331–333; mechanism of action for, 202–203; psychotherapy used with, 208; quick reference to, 209–211; second-generation antipsychotics, 206; side effects of, 200–202, 203, 204–205, 247, 266; treatment guidelines for, 198–199; trends in using, 197

blocking, 53

blood level monitoring: of anticonvulsants, 204–205; of lithium, 202

blood-brain barrier, 46, 53

books for patients, 321–322

borderline personality disorders, 145–149; books for patients about, 322; diagnosis of, 145–147; discontinuing treatment for, 249; etiology of, 147–148; facts about,

146; medications for, 148–149; patients medicated for, 24; quick reference to, 149; symptoms of, 146; treatments for, 148–149

brain: acute organic syndromes of, 70; biological functioning of, 16–17; chronic organic syndromes of, 71; information processing by, 40; psychological functions of, 39; psychopathology and, 39, 43; schizophrenia and, 132; structures of, 37–42; traumatic experiences and, 140–142

brain imaging techniques, 11–12, 18–19, 36

brain-derived neurotropic factor (BDNF), 87, 88, 173

breakthrough symptoms, 244

brief psychotic disorder, 129

brief therapy, 118

bromocriptine, 155

Brotman, Andrew, 8, 9, 10

bulimia nervosa, 160, 161

bupropion, 177, 180; anxiety disorders and, 119n; borderline personality disorders and, 148; depressive disorders and, 177; drug interactions with, 295; eating disorders and, 160; nicotine dependence and, 157; quick reference to, 195

buspirone, 215, 217; aggressive behavior and, 169; anxiety disorders and, 117, 215, 217; depressive disorders and, 177; educating patients about, 220; side effects of, 247

C

caffeine: content in common substances, 69; diagnosing use of, 68; overuse of, 157

calcium signaling theory, 102

carbamazepine, 203–205, 209, 219, 287, 300–301

carbon dioxide, 33

cardiovascular effects, 201

catatonic schizophrenia, 130

catecholamine theory, 101–102

CATIE study, 229

cellular resiliency, 102

central nervous system, 41, 46

cerebral cortex, 40

chaotic attractor theory, 101

Charcot, Jean-Martin, 4

child abuse and neglect: anxiety disorders and, 112; post-traumatic stress disorder and, 140–141

child and adolescent psychopharmacology, 251–271; addiction issues in, 253–254; ADHD and, 254–259; anxiety disorders and, 266–269; autism spectrum disorders and, 270; bipolar disorder and, 263–266;

clinical considerations in, 251–252; depression and, 259–263; diagnostic issues in, 254–255, 259–260, 263–265, 267–268; metabolism issues in, 253; obsessive-compulsive disorder and, 267, 268; post-traumatic stress disorder and, 267–268, 269; psychotic disorders and, 269–270; quick reference to, 271; research studies on, 253; suicidality and, 261–263; treatment issues in, 256–259, 260–263, 268–269

chlordiazepoxide, 7, 213

chloride ion channels, 110, 111

chlorpromazine, 6, 223

chronic organic brain syndromes, 71

chronic pain, 169

Church of Scientology, 8, 9, 10

citalopram, 175, 180

clinical depression, 76

clonazepam, 115, 119

clonidine, 142, 156, 169, 217, 257, 258

clozapine, 133, 227–228, 229

clozaril, 270

cocaine, 155

cognitive behavioral psychotherapy, 12

cognitive functioning: medical disorders and, 70–71; mental status exam of, 309–312

cognitive model, 85

complementary and alternative medicine (CAM), 235

compliance issues, 11, 57–60, 231, 244

compounding pharmacies, 58

conduction, 31

continuation treatment phase, 184–185

corticotropin releasing factor (CRF), 32, 86, 173

cortisol, 87, 88, 142

countertransference issues, 25

CPAP (breathing) machine, 165

CT scans, 132

cultural issues, 26–27

cyclic antidepressants: chronic pain and, 169; dosages of, 182; generic and brand names of, 174; quick reference to, 192; side effects of, 175

cyclothymia, 98–99

cytochrome P450 system, 277, 287

D

delusional disorder, 129

Dement, William, 162

dementia praecox, 129

dendrites, 29

dendritic spines, 29

dependent patients, 24

depression: antidepressant toxicity vs., 307; bipolar disorder and, 84–85, 95; books for patients about, 321; causes of, 78, 85–88; childhood and adolescent, 259–263; facts about, 77; grief and, 76; Parkinsonian side effects vs., 306; Prozac controversy and, 9–10; treatment-resistant, 186–187, 191

depressive disorders, 75–91; atypical depressions, 80, 83; biological depressions, 77, 79–80; bipolar disorder and, 265; childhood and adolescent, 259–263; clinical depressions, 76; diagnosis of, 75–76, 259–260; discontinuing treatment for, 249; educating patients about, 187, 189; electroconvulsive therapy for, 187, 190; etiology of, 85–88; facts about, 77; major unipolar depressions, 76–81; medications for, 80–81, 88–89, 173–189, 192–196, 260–263; minor depressions, 82–83; monoamine hypothesis of, 86–88; over-the-counter products for, 189, 238; patients medicated for, 25; phases of treatment for, 184–185; physiological consequences of, 88; postpartum depression, 84; premenstrual dysphoric disorder, 84; psychotherapy for, 89, 187; psychotic depressions, 81; quick reference to, 91; reactive depressions, 77; reactive-biological depressions, 80; recurrent and highly recurrent, 82; resistant to treatment, 186–187, 191; seasonal affective disorder, 83–84; symptoms of, 77, 79–80, 82, 91, 260; treatments for, 88–89, 173–196, 260–263. See also antidepressant medications

dermatological effects, 201, 204, 205

despair, 75, 80

desvenlafaxine, 176

dextroamphetamine, 179, 256

diabetes, 228–229

diagnosis: of ADHD, 254–255; of anxiety disorders, 105–108, 267–268; of Axis I and II disorders, 63–66, 67; of bipolar disorders, 93–95, 263–265; of borderline personality disorders, 145–147; of depressive disorders, 75–76, 259–260; of obsessive-compulsive disorder, 121–122; of physical illness, 68–73; of post-traumatic stress disorder, 139–140; of psychotic disorders, 127–131; of schizophrenia, 130–131; of substance abuse, 67–68, 151–153

Diagnostic and Statistical Manual of Mental Disorders (DSM-IV), 4; Axis I and II disorders, 63–66, 67

diazepam, 219

differential diagnosis, 64. See also diagnosis

diphenhydramine, 217

discontinuance syndrome, 51

discontinuation process, 239–241, 245, 248, 249

disorganized schizophrenia, 130

dissociation, 144

distribution of medications, 47–48, 276

disulfiram, 154

divalproex, 199, 203–205, 210, 301

DNA molecules, 35–36

dopamine: depressive disorders and, 86; lithium and, 202–203; second-generation antipsychotics and, 227; stimulant abuse and, 155–156

dopamine model of schizophrenia, 132–133, 223

dopamine receptors, 54

dosages: of antianxiety medications, 216; of anticonvulsants, 205; of antidepressants, 181, 182; of antipsychotics, 225; of bipolar medications, 199, 205; for children and adolescents, 253; errors in designating, 318; for geriatric patients, 285; of lithium, 199; need for adjusting, 244; noncompliance by missing, 57–58; of OTC products, 238

double depression, 82, 83

down-regulation, 34

drugs: anxiety caused by, 114; broad definition of, 45; childhood addiction to, 253–254; depression caused by, 78, 79, 86; interactions between, 51–52, 277–279, 289–303; mania caused by, 97; recreational use of, 67–68; safety issues related to, 317–319; sleep disorders caused by, 164; trade vs. generic names of, 313–315; withdrawal symptoms from, 218–219. See also medications; substance abuse

D-serine, 33

duloxetine, 169, 176, 180

dysregulation, 16, 101

dysthymia, 82

dystonic symptoms, 224, 306–307

E

eating disorders, 160–161

educating patients. See patient education

egodystonic symptoms, 64

egosystonic symptoms, 64

ejaculatory anhedonia, 186

elderly patients, 283–286

electroconvulsive treatment (ECT), 5, 6, 81, 187, 190

emotional brain, 38

emotional control, 141
enantiomers, 33
endocrine effects, 200
endogenomorphic depressions, 80
endogenous mental illness, 17
endoplasmic reticulum, 36
endorphins, 32, 161
enkephalins, 32
Ensam patch, 179
environmental factors, 18
enzyme induction, 278
enzyme inhibition, 52, 278
equilibrium, 276
escitalopram, 175, 180
estazolam, 215
eszopiclone, 166, 215
ethchlorvynol, 213
ethnic factors, 26, 287
etiology, 63–73; of anxiety disorders,
    108–116; of bipolar disorders, 100–103;
    of borderline personality disorders,
    147–148; of depressive disorders, 85–88; of
    obsessive-compulsive disorder, 122–124;
    of post-traumatic stress disorder, 140–
    142; of psychotic disorders, 132–134; of
    schizophrenia, 132–134
excretion of medications, 49–50
extrapyramidal symptoms (EPS), 224, 226,
    227

F

fasting, 160
fears, specific. *See* phobias
fetal development, 281–282
fight-or-flight response, 40–41, 109–110
financial concerns, 58
first messenger molecules, 30
first-generation antipsychotics (FGA), 224,
    225, 226–227, 232, 298
first-pass effect, 275
5-HT receptors, 54, 56
flashbacks, 141–142, 157
fluoxetine, 175, 180; controversy about, 9–10;
    intrusive symptoms and, 141
fluvoxamine, 175
folic acid, 238
Food and Drug Administration (FDA), 197,
    253
Frances, Allan, 145
Frank, Jerome, 23
Freud, Sigmund, 5, 75, 108
frontal cortex, 123
functional psychosis, 127

G

gabapentin, 117, 206, 265
gamma aminobutyric acid (GABA), 33, 110,
    214
gastrointestinal effects, 200, 204, 205
gene expression, 35–36
gene products, 36
generalized anxiety disorder (GAD), 107;
    biological factors in, 112; childhood onset
    of, 267; treatments for, 116–117, 269
generic names of medications, 313–315
genetic factors: alcoholism and, 153–154;
    bipolar disorder and, 102–103; clinical
    and practical implications of, 287–288;
    depression and, 86; drug metabolism and,
    286–287; membrane transporters and, 287;
    mental illness and, 7; psychopathology
    and, 43; schizophrenia and, 132
genital anesthesia, 186
geriatric patients, 283–286
ginkgo biloba, 238
glucocorticoid receptors (GRs), 41
glutamate, 33, 134, 142
glutethimide, 213
glycine, 33
goiter, 200
G-protein mediated second messenger
    system, 34, 35
grand mal seizures, 190, 226
grief, 75–76
guanfacine, 257, 258

H

Halcion, 218
half-life of medications, 49
hallucinogens, 157, 158
hand tremors, 200
hematological effects, 201, 204
hepatitis, 226, 227
herbal remedies, 235–238; antidepressant,
    189; documented benefits of, 238;
    guidelines for therapists, 237; need for
    research on, 237; problems with, 236; side
    effects of, 236, 238
heroin, 156
heterocyclic antidepressants, 174, 240
high-intensity light therapy, 83–84
hippocampus, 41
Hippocrates, 16
history: of biological psychiatry, 4–13; of
    patient medication use, 285
homeostasis, 34
Horowitz, Mardi, 137

human genome, 36
Human Genome Project, 286, 287
human relationship, 273
Hume, David, 237
hydroxyzine, 217
hyperactivity, 255
hyperarousal, 141
hypercortisolemia, 87, 88
hypersomnia, 85
hypertensive reaction, 177, 179
hyperthermia, 226
hypnotics, 166–167, 213, 215, 221, 240
hypomania, 84, 93–94
hypothalamic-pituitary-adrenal (HPA) axis, 41, 102, 112
hypothalamic-pituitary-thyroid (HPT) axis, 41
hypothalamus, 37–38, 40–41
hypothyroidism, 200
hysteroid-dysphoric borderline personality, 146, 148, 149

I

idiosyncratic effects, 51
illness. *See* medical disorders
iloperidone, 228
I'm Dancing as Fast as I Can (Gordon), 218
imipramine, 5, 173
impulse-control disorders (ICDs), 122
inattention, 255
indigenous cultures, 27
information processing, 40
information sheets. *See* patient information sheets
informed consent, 252
inhalants, 157
inhibited temperament, 267
inorgasmia, 186
insomnia: anxiety-related, 117; causes of, 163–164; treatments for, 166–167, 213. *See also* sleep disorders
Institute of Safe Medication Practices (ISMP), 317
insulin shock, 5
integrative approaches, 4
interactions, drug, 51–52, 277–279, 289–303; antipsychotics, 298–299; benzodiazepines, 303; bipolar medications, 300–301; buproprion, 295; lithium, 301; mirtazapine, 297; monoamine oxidase inhibitors, 296; mood stabilizers, 300–301; psychostimulants, 302; selective serotonin reuptake inhibitors, 291–292; serotonin

and norepinephrine reuptake inhibitors, 293–294; tricyclic antidepressants, 290
intercellular communication, 30
interpersonal psychotherapy, 12
intoxication, 152
intrusive symptoms, 141–142
ion-channel mediated process, 34
ionic actions, 34
iproniazid, 6, 173
isocarboxazid, 196

J

Joint Commission, 317

K

kava kava, 238
kidney function, 49, 201
kindling, 19, 101, 142
Klein, Donald, 146
Klerman, G. L., 10
Kraepelin, Emil, 4, 5, 100
Kramer, Peter, 66

L

lactation issues, 282–283
lamotrigine, 203–204, 205, 210, 301
Latino patients, 26
L-dopa, 155
learned helplessness, 18, 85
learning disorders, 159
levetiracetam, 206
Librium, 7
ligands, 30, 53
light therapy, 83–84
limbic system: anxiety disorders and, 110, 112; depressive disorders and, 86; functions of, 38, 40
Lindeman, Eric, 137
lipid metabolism, 228, 229
lipophilic drugs, 53
lisdexamphetamine, 256
Listening to Prozac (Kramer), 66
lithium, 199–203; aggressive behavior and, 169; bipolar disorders and, 100, 265, 266; blood level monitoring of, 202; child and adolescent use of, 265, 266; cultural context for using, 26; discontinuation problems, 239, 241; dosage guidelines for, 199; drug interactions with, 301; history of psychiatric use of, 199; mechanism of action for, 202–203; patient information sheet on, 331–333; pregnancy/lactation issues for, 202, 282–283; quick reference to,

211; schizophrenia and, 135; side effects of, 200–202, 203, 247, 266; signs of toxicity or overdose, 248; treatment guidelines for, 199

lithium carbonate, 7

liver function, 204, 213, 236

locus coeruleus (LC), 110, 111, 116

lorazepam, 115, 119, 213

LSD (lysergic acid diethylamide), 157

lurasidone, 228

M

maintenance treatment phase, 185

major unipolar depressions, 76–81; atypical depressions, 80; biological depressions, 77, 79–80; bipolar disorder and, 265; childhood signs and symptoms of, 260; discontinuing treatment for, 249; efficacy of medications for, 80; phases of treatment for, 184–185; reactive depressions, 77; reactive-biological depressions, 80; recurrent and highly recurrent, 82; resistant to treatment, 186–187

malaria therapy, 5

managed care, 11–12

mania: childhood-onset, 263; depression and, 84; diagnosis of, 93–94; drugs causative of, 97; medical conditions associated with, 95; medications for, 197, 265; stages of acute, 94; treatments for, 197, 265

manic-depressive illness. *See* bipolar disorders

MAOIs. *See* monoamine oxidase inhibitors

meclobemide, 179

medical disorders, 68–73; anxiety associated with, 108, 113–114, 118; checklists for diagnosing, 72, 73; cognitive functioning and, 70–71; depression caused by, 78, 79, 86; mania and, 95; neurochemistry and, 71–72; onset of new conditions and, 245; physical symptoms indicative of, 73; psychiatric disorders due to, 68–73; psychotic disorders caused by, 127–128; sleep disorders caused by, 164; unexplained relapse and, 244

medications: absorption of, 46–47, 275–276; antianxiety, 213–221, 267–268; antidepressant, 88–90, 173–196, 260–263; antipsychotic, 223–233, 270; arguments in favor of, 8–9; biotransformation of, 48–49, 277; bipolar, 103, 197–211; bodily distribution of, 47–48, 276; books for patients about, 321–322; cellular-level effects of, 53; child and adolescent use

of, 251–271; combinations of, 206–207; discontinuation of, 239–241, 245, 248, 249; dosage adjustments to, 244; educating patients about, 187, 189, 207–208, 220, 231, 319; effects of, 51; excretion of, 49–50; failure to respond to, 243–244; geriatric patients and, 283–286; interactions between, 51–52, 277–279, 289–303; managed care and, 11–12; meanings attributed to, 21–25; media attention on, 8–10; noncompliance issues, 11, 57–60; patient information sheets, 323–338; pregnancy/lactation issues, 281–283; psychotherapy vs., 8–10; receptor actions and, 53–56; safety issues related to, 317–319; side effects of, 51, 57, 58–59, 185–186, 245, 246–247; signs of toxicity or overdose, 248; sleep, 166–167; special populations and, 281–288; therapeutic index for, 279; trade vs. generic names of, 313–315; withdrawal symptoms from, 218–219, 245. *See also* drugs; treatments

melatonin, 238

membrane transporters, 287–288

memory impairments, 58, 59

mental status exam, 309–312

Mental Status Examination in Neurology, The (Strub and Black), 309

meprobamate, 7, 213

mescaline, 157

messenger molecules, 32–33, 35, 36

messenger RNA (mRNA), 36

metabolic disorders, 17, 88

metabolic drug interactions, 51–52, 277–279, 289–303

metabolism of medications, 48–49, 277; genetic variations in, 286–287; in young clients, 253

metabolites, 48, 277

metabotropic actions, 34–35

methadone, 156

methylphenidate: ADHD and, 8–9, 256; controversy about, 8–9; depression and, 179

methyprylon, 213

Michaels, Robert, 66

microdosing, 58

minor depressions, 76, 82–83

minor side effects, 245, 246–247

mirtazapine, 176, 177, 180, 195, 297

mixed episodes, 95–96

mixed function oxidase (MFO) system, 277

monoamine hypothesis of depression, 86–88

monoamine oxidase (MAO), 87, 173

monoamine oxidase inhibitors (MAOIs), 173, 177, 179, 180; anxiety disorders and, 113, 118, 119; development of, 173; discontinuation symptoms, 240; dosages of, 182; drug interactions with, 296; seasonal affective disorder and, 83; self-injurious behavior and, 162; side effects of, 177, 179, 246

Mood Disorder Questionnaire, 85

mood disorders. *See* depressive disorders

mood stabilizers. *See* bipolar medications

morality issues, 22

morphine, 156

"Mourning and Melancholia" (Freud), 75

MRI scans, 132

N

naltrexone, 154, 160

names of medications: common errors related to, 317; trade vs. generic, 313–315

narcissistic patients, 25

National Patient Safety Goal, 317

nefazodone, 177, 180

Nemeroff, Charles, 140

nerve cells, 29–30

nervous system: autonomic, 41–42; conduction and transmission, 30–31; divisions of, 40; effects of receptor binding, 32; intercellular communication, 30; nerve cells, 29–30; neuronal malfunction, 35–36; parasympathetic, 41–42; peripheral, 41–42; receptors, 33–35; sympathetic, 41–42

neuroanatomy, 36–37

neurobiological impairment, 252

neurobiology, 29–43; ADHD and, 255; brain structures and, 37–42; cellular nervous system and, 29–36; neuroanatomy and, 36–37; psychopathology and, 43

neurochemistry, 7, 71–72

neurocognitive mental status exam, 309–312

neuroendocrine pathways, 41, 110

neuroimaging techniques, 11–12, 18–19, 36

neuroleptic malignant syndrome (NMS), 226

neuroleptics, 223

neurologic side effects, 200, 204, 205

neuromodulators, 32

neuromuscular symptoms, 200

neurons, 29–30; malfunction of, 35–36; structure of, 30

neurophysiological models of schizophrenia, 134

neuroprotective substances, 203, 252

neurotic anxiety, 108, 115, 118

neurotransmitters, 29–30; effects on receptors, 32; neuronal malfunction and, 35–36; typology of, 32–33

neurovegetative symptoms, 80

nicotine, 157

NIMH website, 263

nitric oxide, 33

N-methyl-D-aspartate (NMDA) receptor, 134

nonadherence/noncompliance, 11, 57–60, 244

noradrenergic hypothesis, 115

norepinephrine, 42; depressive disorders and, 86; lithium and, 202–203

norepinephrine reuptake inhibitors (NRIs), 173, 177; dosages of, 182; side effects of, 176, 177

NREM sleep, 163

O

obesity, 167–168

object relations theory, 85

obsessive-compulsive disorder (OCD), 106, 121–125; behavioral techniques for, 124; books for patients about, 322; childhood and adolescent, 267; diagnosis of, 121–122; discontinuing treatment for, 249; etiology of, 122–124; facts about, 122; medications for, 123, 124–125, 268; patients medicated for, 24; psychotherapy and, 124; quick reference to, 125; Tourette syndrome and, 159; treatments for, 124–125, 268

obsessive-compulsive personality disorder (OCP), 122

olanzapine, 228, 229

omega-3 fatty acids, 189, 238

opiates, 156–157, 158

organic psychosis, 127

organs: effects of nervous system activity on, 42; fetal development of, 282

orlistat, 168

overdose, 248

over-the-counter (OTC) products, 235–238; antidepressants, 189; documented benefits of, 238; guidelines for therapists, 237; herbal remedies, 189, 235–238; need for research on, 237; problems with, 236; side effects of, 236, 238

oxazepam, 213

oxcarbazepine, 206

oxytocin, 270

P

pain, chronic, 169

paliperidone, 228

panic attacks: anxiety symptoms vs., 105–106; medications for, 119; stress-induced, 112

panic disorder, 108; adolescent onset of, 268; biological factors in, 115–116; discontinuing treatment for, 249; separation anxiety and, 112; treatments for, 118–119

paranoid patients, 24

paranoid schizophrenia, 130

parasympathetic nervous system, 41–42

Parkinsonian side effects, 224, 306

paroxetine, 175, 180

pathophysiology, 64

patient compliance, 11, 57–60, 231, 244

patient education, 319, 321–322; on antianxiety medications, 220; on antidepressant medications, 187, 189; on antipsychotic medications, 231; on bipolar medications, 207–208

patient information sheets, 323–338; on antianxiety medications, 326–327; on anticonvulsant mood stabilizers, 328–330; on antidepressants, 323–325; on antipsychotics, 336–338; on lithium, 331–333; on psychostimulants, 334–335

Paxil, 175, 261

periodic limb movements in sleep (PLMS), 165–166

peripheral nervous system, 41–42

personality traits: biochemical disorders and, 66, 67; psychological disorders and, 63–66

PET scans, 11, 18–19, 132

pharmacodynamics, 46

pharmacogenetics, 286–288; clinical and practical implications of, 287–288; drug metabolism and, 286–287; membrane transporters and, 287

pharmacokinetics, 45–52, 275–279; absorption, 46–47, 275–276; biotransformation, 48–49, 277; distribution, 47–48, 276; drug interactions, 51–52, 277–279, 289–303; ethnic variables, 26, 287; excretion, 49–50; medication effects, 51; metabolism, 48–49, 277, 286–287; therapeutic index, 279

pharmacological effect, 51

pharmacology, 45–56; age-specific, 285; cellular-level effects and, 53; pharmacokinetic factors and, 45–52; receptor actions and, 53–56

phencyclidine (PCP): abuse of, 152, 157; model of schizophrenia, 134

phenelzine, 179, 196

phenothiazines, 223

phentermine, 167

phobias, 107, 113; childhood onset of, 268; treatments for, 117–118, 269

physical illness. See medical disorders

polydipsia, 26

polyuria, 26

postpartum depression, 84

postsynaptic neuron, 30–31

post-traumatic stress disorder (PTSD), 106, 137–144; childhood onset of, 267–268; diagnosis of, 139–140; discontinuing treatment for, 249; etiology of, 140–142; facts about, 140; medications for, 141, 142, 143–144, 269; psychotherapy for, 142–143; quick reference to, 144; stress response syndrome and, 137–138; symptoms of, 139; treatments for, 142–144, 269

potentially serious side effects, 245, 246–247

pragmatic practitioners, 10

pregabalin, 206

pregnancy issues, 202, 281–283

premenstrual dysphoric disorder (PMDD), 84

presynaptic neuron, 30

primary psychoses, 129

progressive neurobiological impairment, 252

propoxyphene, 156

propranolol, 117, 135, 217

protein binding, 276

protein signaling network theory, 102

Prozac, 9–10, 175, 180

psilocybin, 157

psychiatric disorders: alcohol abuse and, 154; anxiety symptoms due to, 108, 114, 118; biological factors in, 43; differentiating drug side effects from, 305–307; medical disorders as cause of, 68–73; sleep disorders and, 163–164; unexplained relapse of, 244

psychiatry: contemporary changes in, 3–4; history of biological psychiatry, 4–13

psychodynamic models, 85

psychological factors: biology and, 16–20, 43; nonadherence based on, 58–60; pharmacologic treatment and, 21–25; stressful life events, 43, 140–142

psychological masquerade, 68–69

psycho-neuro-immunology, 18

psychopathology, 39, 43

psychopharmacology: child and adolescent, 251–271; cultural context of, 26–27; history of, 4–13; managed care dilemma and, 11–12; new discoveries in, 273; psychodynamics of, 21–25; reasons for learning about, 13–14 psychosomatic medicine, 17

psychostimulants. *See* stimulants

psychosurgery, 5–6

psychotherapy: anxiety disorders and, 116, 117, 118, 119; arguments in favor of, 9; bipolar disorders and, 103, 208; book for patients about, 322; brain functioning and, 18–19; depressive disorders and, 89, 187; human relationship in, 273; managed care and, 11–12; medication vs., 8–10; obsessive-compulsive disorder and, 124; post-traumatic stress disorder and, 142–143; schizophrenia and, 231

psychotic depressions, 81

psychotic disorders, 127–136; anticholinergic effects vs., 306; book for patients about, 322; childhood onset of, 269–270; diagnosis of, 127–131; discontinuing treatment for, 249; educating patients about, 231; etiology of, 132–134; facts about, 128; length of treatment for, 230–231; medical conditions as cause of, 127–128; medications for, 135–136, 223–233, 270; primary psychoses, 129; psychotherapy for, 231; quick reference to, 136; schizophrenia, 129–131, 230, 231; symptoms of, 129, 130, 131; treatments for, 135–136, 223–233, 270. *See also* antipsychotic medications

psychotropic medications: interactions between, 289–303; managed care and, 11–12; new discoveries in, 273; noncompliance issues with, 57–60; OCD treatment with, 124; prescribers of, 13; side effects of, 246–247. *See also* medications

PTSD. *See* post-traumatic stress disorder

published resources, 321–322

Q

quazepam, 215

quetiapine, 228, 229, 265

Quinlan, Karen Ann, 220

R

ramelteon, 166

rapid cycling bipolar disorder, 100

rapid neuroleptization, 230

reactive-biological depressions, 80

reactive depressions, 77

reactive dysphoria, 75

reboxetine, 177

receptors: binding of neurotransmitters to, 32; drug effects and, 53–56; impact of stress on, 34; intracellular actions and, 33–35; side effects and, 53–56; specific actions of, 55, 56

regulated systems, 34

relapse: common reasons for, 244; schizophrenia and, 231

REM sleep, 163, 215

Remeron, 186, 195, 297

renal disease, 201

repetition compulsion, 141

residual ADHD, 161

resistance, 25

restless legs syndrome (RLS), 165–166

reuptake transporter pump, 32

risks of medication use: children and adolescents and, 253–254; genetic factors and, 286–288; geriatric patients and, 283–286; pregnancy/lactation and, 281–283

risperidone, 228, 229

Ritalin, 8–9, 179, 256

RNA molecules, 36

S

sadness, 75, 80

Saint-John's-wort, 189, 236, 238

SAM-e, 189, 238

schizoaffective disorder, 129

schizophrenia, 129–131; diagnosis of, 130–131; discontinuing treatment for, 249; dopamine model of, 132–133, 223; educating patients about, 231; etiology of, 132–134; length of treatment for, 230–231; medications for, 135–136, 223–233; neurophysiological models of, 134; phencyclidine model of, 134; psychotherapy and, 231; quick reference to, 136; relapse and, 231; symptoms of, 130, 131; treatments for, 135–136, 223–233; types of, 130

schizophreniform disorder, 129

schizotypal borderline personality, 147, 148, 149

seasonal affective disorder (SAD), 83–84

second messenger systems, 34, 35–36

secondary gain, 59

second-generation antipsychotics (SGA), 206, 225, 227–229, 233, 299

sedation side effects, 224, 226, 227

sedatives, 213, 221, 223

seizures, 190, 226

selective serotonin reuptake inhibitors (SSRIs), 173, 175–176; aggressive behavior and, 169; anxiety disorders and, 112, 117, 118, 268, 269; child and adolescent use of, 261, 268, 269; chronic pain and, 169;

discontinuation symptoms, 240; dosages of, 182; drug interactions with, 291–292; eating disorders and, 160; obsessive-compulsive disorder and, 123, 268; premenstrual dysphoric disorder and, 84; quick reference to, 193; seasonal affective disorder and, 83; self-injurious behavior and, 162; side effects of, 175, 176, 181, 246

selegiline, 179, 196

self-mutilation, 141, 161–162

separation anxiety, 112, 113, 267, 269

serotonin: anxiety disorders and, 111; depressive disorders and, 86; lithium and, 203; seasonal affective disorder and, 83; second-generation antipsychotics and, 227; self-mutilation and, 162

serotonin and norepinephrine reuptake inhibitors (SNRIs), 173, 176; discontinuation symptoms, 240; dosages of, 182; drug interactions with, 293–294; quick reference to, 194; side effects of, 176

serotonin receptors, 54, 56

sertraline, 175, 180

sexual dysfunction, 185–186

shared psychotic disorder, 129

Shea, Shawn, 57, 60

shell shock, 137

Sherrington, C. S., 7

sibutramine, 161, 168

side effects, 51; of antianxiety medications, 213; of anticonvulsants, 204–205, 247, 266; of antidepressants, 174–175, 176, 177, 179, 181, 183, 185–186; of antipsychotics, 224, 226–229; differentiating from psychiatric symptoms, 305–307; geriatric patients and, 284, 286; of lithium, 200–202, 203, 247, 266; management of, 227; noncompliance due to, 11, 57, 58–59, 60; of OTC products, 236, 238; reassessing medication based on, 227; receptor actions and, 53–56; sensitivity to, 58–59; severity classifications for, 245; of stimulants, 179, 257; summary table of, 246–247

signaling mechanisms, 34

single-compartment model, 276

sleep: deprivation symptoms, 162; preparing for, 164–165; stages of normal, 163

sleep apnea, 165

sleep disorders, 162–167; anxiety and, 117; causes of, 117, 163–164; depression and, 80, 85, 117; OTC products for, 238; patterns indicative of, 162–163; primary, 165–166; treatments for, 166–167

sleep hygiene, 164–165

sleep medications, 166–167

SNRIs. *See* serotonin and norepinephrine reuptake inhibitors

social anxiety disorder, 107, 267, 269

social phobias, 107; biological factors in, 113; childhood onset of, 267; treatments for, 117–118

socioeconomic status, 26

somatic therapies, 5–6

special populations, 281–288

SPECT scans, 11

SSRIs. *See* selective serotonin reuptake inhibitors

STAR-D program, 184

steady state, 49–50

STEP-BD study, 207

stigma, 59–60

stimulants: abuse of, 155–156; ADHD treatment with, 256–257; child and adolescent use of, 253, 256–257; discontinuation of, 240; drug interactions with, 302; misdiagnosed use of, 258; patient information sheet on, 334–335; prescribing for depression, 179; quick reference on, 158; side effects of, 179, 257

stimulus-response specificity, 20–21

stress: acute reactions to, 137–138; anxiety associated with, 107, 117; biology altered by, 140–142; brain functioning and, 43; depression and, 86; impact on receptors, 34; psychopathology and, 43; relapse caused by, 244; sleep disorders and, 163. *See also* post-traumatic stress disorder

stress response syndrome, 137–138

Stress Response Syndromes (Horowitz), 137

substance abuse, 151–158; alcoholism and, 153–155; anxiety from, 108, 114, 118; benzodiazepines and, 218; child and adolescent, 253–254; diagnosis of, 67–68, 151–153; disorders mimicked by, 153; *DSM-IV-TR* definition of, 152; facts about, 152; fears and concerns about, 58, 60; hallucinogens and, 157; medications for, 154–157, 158; opiates and, 156–157; psychotic symptoms and, 128; quick reference on, 158; stimulants and, 155–156; symptoms of, 158; treatments for, 154–157, 158

substance P, 32

suicide: borderline personality patients and, 149; childhood antidepressant use and, 261–263; major depression and, 77; noncompliance based on fears of, 58; Prozac use and, 9–10

switching, 185
symbol errors, 318
sympathetic nervous system, 41–42
symptoms: of ADHD, 254–255; of anxiety disorders, 106; of benzodiazepine withdrawal, 218–219; of bipolar disorders, 94, 104, 263, 264; of borderline personality disorders, 146; of depressive disorders, 77, 79–80, 82, 91, 260; of post-traumatic stress disorder, 139; of psychotic disorders, 129, 130, 131; of schizophrenia, 130, 131; of substance abuse, 158
synapse, 7, 30, 31

T

tardive dyskinesia, 224, 231, 270, 306–307
target symptoms, 64
Taylor, Robert, 68
TCAs. *See* tricyclic antidepressants
temazepan, 213
teratogenesis, 202, 281, 282
terminal boutons, 29
Terr, Lenore, 140
therapeutic index, 279
therapeutic window, 199
Thorazine, 6, 223
thyroid function, 200
tiagabine, 206, 217
Tofranil, 6
tolerance, 152, 244
topiramate, 160, 205, 206
Tourette syndrome, 159
toxicity, 48, 64–65, 248
trade names of medications, 313–315
tranquilizers, 10
transcranial magnetic stimulation (TMS), 187
transfer RNA (tRNA), 36
transient psychosis, 138, 148, 157
transmission, 7, 31
tranylcypromine, 179, 196
trauma: acute reactions to, 137–138; biology altered by, 140–142. *See also* post-traumatic stress disorder
treatment-resistant depression (TRD), 186–187, 191
treatments: for ADHD, 256–259; for aggression, 168–169; for alcohol-related disorders, 154–155; for anxiety disorders, 116–119, 213–221, 268–269; for autism spectrum disorders, 270; for bipolar disorders, 103, 197–211; for borderline personality disorders, 148–149; for chronic pain, 169; for depressive disorders, 88–89, 173–196; for eating disorders, 160, 161; for obesity, 167–168; for obsessive-compulsive disorder, 124–125; for post-traumatic stress disorder, 142–144; for psychotic disorders, 135–136, 223–233, 270; for schizophrenia, 135–136; for self-injurious behavior, 162; for sleep disorders, 166–167; for substance abuse, 154–157, 158. *See also* medications
Treatments for Adolescents with Depression Study (TADS), 261
triazolam, 166
trichotillomania, 162
tricyclic antidepressants (TCAs), 174–175; child and adolescent use of, 260; dosages of, 182; drug interactions with, 290; side effects of, 174–175, 181, 246
troublesome side effects, 245, 246–247
tybamate, 213
tyramine, 178, 179

U

up-regulation, 34

V

vagal nerve stimulation (VNS), 187
Valium abuse, 218
van der Kolk, Bessel A., 140
vegetative symptoms, 80
venlafaxine, 169, 176, 180, 261
vesicles, 31
Viagra, 186
vilazodone, 177, 180

W

Ward, Nicholas, 82
weight gain, 186, 201, 226, 228
Wellbutrin, 160, 177, 180, 186, 195, 295
white blood cell (WBC) count, 204
Winter Blues (Rosenthal), 84
withdrawal symptoms, 152, 218–219, 240, 245

X

Xanax, 218

Y

yohimbine, 238

Z

zaleplon, 166, 215
ziprasidone, 228, 229
zolpidem, 166, 215

MORE BOOKS *from*
NEW HARBINGER PUBLICATIONS

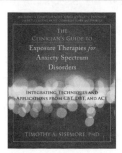

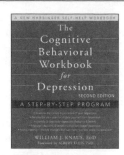

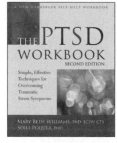

THE CLINICIAN'S GUIDE TO EXPOSURE THERAPIES FOR ANXIETY SPECTRUM DISORDERS

Integrating Techniques & Applications from CBT, DBT & ACT

US $49.95 / ISBN: 978-1608821525
Also available as an e-book at newharbinger.com

THE COGNITIVE BEHAVIORAL WORKBOOK FOR DEPRESSION, SECOND EDITION

A Step-by-Step Program

US $24.95 / ISBN: 978-1608823802
Also available as an e-book at newharbinger.com

THE PTSD WORKBOOK, SECOND EDITION

Simple, Effective Techniques for Overcoming Traumatic Stress Symptoms

US $22.95 / ISBN: 978-1608827039
Also available as an e-book at newharbinger.com

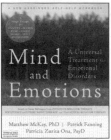

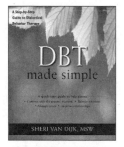

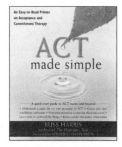

MIND & EMOTIONS

A Universal Treatment for Emotional Disorders

US $21.95 / ISBN: 978-1608820153
Also available as an e-book at newharbinger.com

DBT MADE SIMPLE

A Step-by-Step Guide to Dialectical Behavior Therapy

US $39.95 / ISBN: 978-1608821648
Also available as an e-book at newharbinger.com

ACT MADE SIMPLE

An Easy-To-Read Primer on Acceptance & Commitment Therapy

US $39.95 / ISBN: 978-1572247055
Also available as an e-book at newharbinger.com

new harbinger publications, inc.
1-800-748-6273 / newharbinger.com

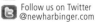 Like us on Facebook

 Follow us on Twitter
@newharbinger.com

(VISA, MC, AMEX / prices subject to change without notice)

Don't miss out on new books in the subjects that interest you.
Sign up for our **Book Alerts** at nhpubs.com/bookalerts

Sign up to receive QUICK TIPS for Therapists—
fast and free solutions to common client situations mental health professionals encounter.
Written by New Harbinger authors, some of the most prominent names in psychology today,
Quick Tips for Therapists are short, helpful emails that will help enhance your client sessions.

Sign up online at **nhpubs.com/quicktips**

Quick Reference to Psychotropic Medication®

To the best of our knowledge, recommended doses and side effects listed below are accurate. However, this is meant as a general reference only, and should not serve as a guideline for prescribing of medications. Physicians, please check the manufacturer's product information sheet or the *PDR* for any changes in dosage schedule or contraindications. (Brand names are registered trademarks.) Note: Doses are for adults. Elderly patients generally require lower doses.

ANTIDEPRESSANTS

Generic	Brand	Usual Daily Dosage Range	Sedation	ACH[1]	Selective Action on Neurotransmitters[2] NE	5-HT
imipramine	Tofranil	150–300 mg	++	++	++	+++
desipramine	Norpramin	150–300 mg	+	+	+++++	0
amitriptyline	Elavil	150–300 mg	++++	++++	+	++++
nortriptyline	Aventyl, Pamelor	75–125 mg	++	++	+++	++
protriptyline	Vivactil	15–40 mg	++	++	++++	+
trimipramine	Surmontil[3]	100–300 mg	++++	+++	++	++
doxepin	Sinequan, Adapin[3],	150–300 mg	++++	++	+++	++
	Silenor	3–6 mg				
maprotiline	Ludiomil	150–225 mg	++	++	+++++	0
amoxapine	Asendin	150–400 mg	++	+	++++	+
trazodone	Desyrel, Oleptro	150–400 mg	+++	0	0	+++++
fluoxetine	Prozac, Sarafem	20–80 mg	+	0	0	+++++
bupropion SR	Wellbutrin SR[4]	150–300 mg	+	0	++	0
sertraline	Zoloft	50–200 mg	+	0	0	+++++
paroxetine	Paxil, Pexeva	20–50 mg	+	+	+	+++++
venlafaxine XR	Effexor XR	75–350 mg	+	0	++	+++
fluvoxamine	Luvox	50–300 mg	+	+	0	+++++
mirtazapine	Remeron	15–45 mg	++	++	+++	+++
citalopram	Celexa	10–40 mg	+	0	0	+++++
escitalopram	Lexapro	5–20 mg	+	0	0	+++++
duloxetine	Cymbalta	40–60 mg	+	0	++++	++++
atomoxetine	Strattera	60–120 mg	+	+	+++++	0
vilazodone	Viibryd	10–40 mg	+	0	0	+++++
MAO INHIBITORS						
phenelzine	Nardil[5]	30–90 mg	+	0	+++	+++
tranylcypromine	Parnate[5]	20–60 mg	+	0	+++	+++
isocarboxazid	Marplan[5]	10–40 mg	+	0	+++	+++
Selegiline transdermal	Emsam[5]	6–12 mg	+	0	+++	+++

1 ACH: anticholinergic side effects.
2 NE: norepinephrine; 5-HT: serotonin.
3 Uncertain, but likely, effects.
4 Atypical antidepressant. Uncertain effects but likely to be a dopamine agonist, and indirect increase in norepinephrine.
5 MAO inhibitors operate via a different mechanism of action from other antidepressants, and increase NE, 5-HT, and dopamine.

ANTIOBSESSIONAL

Generic	Brand	Dose Range[1]	Sedation	ACH Effects
clomipramine	Anafranil	150–300 mg	++++	++++
fluoxetine	Prozac[1]	20–80 mg	+	0
sertraline	Zoloft[1]	50–200 mg	+	0
paroxetine	Paxil[1]	20–60 mg	+	+
fluvoxamine	Luvox	50–300 mg	+	+
citalopram	Celexa	10–40 mg	+	0
escitalopram	Lexapro[1]	5–30 mg	+	0

1 Often higher doses are required to control obsessive-compulsive symptoms than the doses generally used to treat depression.

BIPOLAR MEDICATIONS

Generic	Brand	Daily Dose Range	Serum[1] Level
lithium	Eskalith, Lithonate	600–2400	0.6–1.5
carbamazepine	Tegretol, Equetro	600–1600	4–10+
oxcarbazepine	Trileptal	1200–2400[2]	
divalproex	Depakote, Depakene	750–1500	50–100
lamotrigne	Lamictal	50–500	n/a
olanzapine	Fluoxetine	6/25–12/50 mg[3]	2
topiramate	Topamax	50–300	n/a

1 Lithium levels are expressed in mEq/l; carbamazepine and valproic acid levels are expressed in mcg/ml.
2 Not well established
3 Available in 6/25, 6/50, 12/25, and 12/50 mg formulations

PSYCHOSTIMULANTS

Generic	Brand	Daily Doses[1]
methylphenidate	Ritalin	5–50 mg
methylphenidate	Concerta[2]	18–54 mg
methylphenidate	Metadate	5–50 mg
methylphenidate	Methylin	10–60 mg
dexmethylphenidate	Focalin	5–40 mg
dextroamphetamine	Dexedrine	5–40 mg
lisdexamphetamine	Vyvanse	30–70 mg
d- and l-amphetamine	Adderall	5–40 mg
modafinil	Provigil	100–400 mg
armodafinil	Nuvigil	150–250 mg

1 Note: Adult doses.
2 Sustained release.

HYPNOTICS[1]

Generic	Brand	Daily Doses[1]
temazepam	Restoril	15–30 mg
triazolam	Halcion	0.25–0.5 mg
quazepam	Doral	7.5–15 mg
zolpidem	Ambien	5–10 mg
	Intermezzo	1.75 mg
zaleplon	Sonata	5–10 mg
eszopiclone	Lunesta	1–3 mg
ramelteon	Rozerem	4–16 mg
diphenhydramine	Benadryl	25–100 mg
doxepin	Silenor	3–6 mg

1 To treat initial insomnia